Adult Neurogenic Language Disorders: Assessment and Treatment

A Comprehensive Ethnobiological Approach

Second Edition

Adult Neurogenic Language Disorders: Assessment and Treatment

A Comprehensive Ethnobiological Approach

Second Edition

Joan C. Payne, PhD

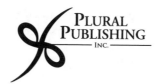

PLURAL
PUBLISHING
INC.

KH

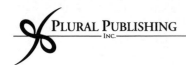

5521 Ruffin Road
San Diego, CA 92123

e-mail: info@pluralpublishing.com
Website: http://www.pluralpublishing.com

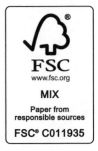

FSC
www.fsc.org
MIX
Paper from
responsible sources
FSC® C011935

Typeset in 10.5/13 Palatino by Flanagan's Publishing Services, Inc.
Printed in the United States of America by McNaughton & Gunn, Inc.

Library of Congress Cataloging-in-Publication Data

Payne, Joan C., author.
  Adult neurogenic language disorders : assessment and treatment : a comprehensive ethnobiological approach / Joan C. Payne. — Second edition.
      p. ; cm.
  Includes bibliographical references and index.
  ISBN 978-1-59756-503-5 (alk. paper) — ISBN 1-59756-503-2 (alk. paper)
  I. Title.
  [DNLM: 1. Language Disorders—ethnology—United States. 2. Healthcare Disparities—ethnology—United States. 3. Language Disorders—etiology—United States. WL 340.2]
  RC423
  616.85'5—dc23
                                                                    2013045700

11/17/16

Contents

COMPANION WEBSITE

Purchase of *Adult Neurogenic Language Disorders: Assessment and Treatment. A Comprehensive Ethnobiological Approach, Second Edition* comes with complimentary access to supplementary instructor materials on the companion website.

The companion website is located at:
http://www.pluralpublishing.com/publication/anld2e/

To access the materials, you must login with a passcode.

Instructor passcode: Please contact Plural Publishing at information@pluralpublishing.com in order to receive your code.

Introduction

In the first edition of *Adult Neurogenic Language Disorders: Assessment and Treatment. A Comprehensive Ethnobiological Approach* (1997), the first chapter emphasized understanding family dynamics across ethnic groups as these related to how aging adults are viewed and cared for within diverse families. From the literature, it was quite apparent that culture plays a significant role in familial responsibility for older adult care. Culture also determines how families cope and react to disabilities in older adult family members.

Because the literature also reported differences in health status for ethnic groups, the second chapter was devoted to explaining how chronic and disabling health conditions differ in prevalence and severity for some ethnic groups but not others. The third chapter sought to explain why some members of ethnic groups may be more comfortable with alternative medicine than with Western health care and what types of barriers prevent them from participating in primary and rehabilitative health services. Three additional chapters provided information on specific disabilities that impair language and cognition: dementia, traumatic brain injury, and cerebrovascular accidents. Within these chapters, issues on differences among ethnic groups for these disabilities were infused throughout to enable the clinician to understand how these disorders might differ between and within groups of diverse patients.

Other equally important issues have emerged during the 15 years between the first and now the most current edition. The second edition should be viewed as a further discussion of cultural diversity and its role in neurogenic communication disorders. The first two chapters of this book describe national legislative and demographic changes, the effects of health disparities, and the need for culturally competent speech-language pathology services for an increasingly multicultural, multilingual patient population.

It has not been the usual practice to begin a text on neurogenic language disorders with a discussion of health disparities; however, changing events that will impact the profession for decades call for attention to this area. Hence, Chapter 1 begins the inquiry into future demographic projections, specific health legislation, and pervasive health disparities, with emphasis on health conditions that cause disorders of language and cognition for persons who are at risk. The legislation for health care reform was enacted to eliminate barriers to health care experienced by many ethnic group members. Health disparities legislation created a national institute designed to conduct research on ways to bridge the gap between those who have enjoyed access to health care and those who have not. These developments, together with ongoing projections of major population changes over the next 40 years, strongly suggest that all health care providers, including the profession of speech-language pathology, invest in culturally competent service delivery to an increasingly multilingual and multicultural patient population. Recommendations for future research are included because an aggressive research agenda is needed to provide more evidence-based information to practitioners and students in training.

Hence, Chapter 1, on health disparities, lays the groundwork for the discussion on culturally competent service delivery in the following chapter. Chapter 2, written with Wilhelmina Wright-Harp, examines bias in assessment and treatment and provides recommendations for culturally competent care that are appropriate for clinicians and organizations that provide services to adults with neurogenic language impairments. Within this chapter are resources culled from related disciplines as well as from speech-language pathology.

Cultural competence is not a new issue for speech-language pathologists and audiologists. Several articles have appeared in print recently that address how clinicians should prepare for a multicultural population of patients in the health care setting (Chin, 2000), for adults with dysphagia (Riquelme, 2004), for adults with neurogenic language disorders (Payne, 2011), and for adults with hearing disorders (Scott & Jones, 2003; Wolf, 2004). These articles, taken together with policy statements on cultural competence from the American Speech-Language-Hearing Association (2004, 2005, 2011), are positive indicators that the profession has begun the process of structuring new paradigms for service delivery for an increasingly diverse population. It is in this spirit that Chapters 1 and 2 address critical issues in diversity for consideration by the academy, researchers, and practitioners in a text on four major neurogenic disorders: dementia, traumatic brain injury, aphasia, and right hemisphere disorders.

Chapter 3 reviews basic information on neural structures necessary for language and cognition and their functions within the central nervous system. This review is updated to include those structures identified in the literature as having specific roles in memory, attention, learning, and language. Current literature on the major disorders that impair language and cognition describe recent neuroimaging procedures that make earlier and more definitive diagnoses possible. Where changes in brain structure due to Alzheimer's disease could be seen only after a patient's death, newer neuroimaging techniques allow researchers to see changes in brain structure and function early in the progression of the disease. Additionally, advances in neuroimaging enable researchers to identify the interdependence of structures for language and confirm that structures like the cerebellum and the substantia innominata in the basal forebrain play more active roles in language, learning, and memory than previously thought.

Chapter 4 focuses on dementia and related disorders, including evaluation and treatment. The most recent classifications and descriptions of dementia are discussed in this chapter as well as current trends in assessment and treatment of language and cognitive disturbances.

Chapter 5, co-authored with colleagues Wilhelmina Wright-Harp and Alaina Davis, is devoted to understanding traumatic head injury, its effects, and patient management. In this chapter, head injury prevalence across the general population will be discussed in detail; however, attention is also given to topics that are being discussed widely in the mass media: head injuries from sports and missile blast combat injuries.

Chapter 6 details causes of aphasia with emphasis on cerebrovascular accidents and other sources of focal lesions, along with aphasia identification, classifications, assessment, and treatment. Consequences of right hemisphere lesions are also discussed in this chapter, as well as appropriate assessment and treatment strategies.

As the chapters unfold, it is clear that a more traditional view of the typical adult with neurogenic language disorders will need to be rethought as part of an ongoing research agenda. In some instances, some perspectives about patients with neurogenic disorders may need to be abandoned altogether if the profession is to be ready to document evidence-based assessment and intervention strategies that are appropriate for a diverse population.

In service delivery, speech-language pathologists will need to be aware of the resources and policy statements provided by the American Speech-Language-Hearing Association on cultural competence. These resources are invaluable to enable clinicians to be respectful of and sensitive to different worldviews, primary languages, ethnic group identification, socioeconomic status, cultural values, and family structures. Given the nation's long history of health disparities, speech-language pathologists will also need to be cognizant of possible differences in severity of language and cognitive disorders and other functional disabilities that may accompany a lifetime of poor or no health care, poverty, and discrimination.

To that end, this book seeks to describe neurogenic language disorders not just as a distinct set of disordered behaviors, but as disorders that affect patients and their families within the larger context of significant changes in the national landscape. Hence, the major purposes of the second edition are: (1) to provide clinicians with the most current information on assessment and management of language and cognitive communication disorders in adults; (2) to alert clinicians

about possibilities for variations in clinical presentations evidenced by diverse patient populations; (3) to offer alternative strategies for assessment and treatment for patients from diverse communities; and (4) to provide clinicians with the rationale and resources for culturally competent and appropriate assessment and treatment. Each chapter includes a list of study questions to provoke thinking about the topics. At the conclusion of the book, a glossary of terms is provided to further explain the nomenclature used throughout the text. Although the second edition was written for graduate students in training, it is hoped that practitioners in speech-language pathology will find this edition to be a useful reference for assessing and treating adults with neurogenic language disorders as well.

REFERENCES

American Speech-Language-Hearing Association. (2004). *Knowledge and skills needed by speech-language pathologists and audiologists to provide culturally and linguistically appropriate services.* Retrieved from http://www.asha.org/policy

American Speech-Language-Hearing Association. (2005). *Cultural competence* [Issues in Ethics]. Retrieved from http://www.asha.org/policy

American Speech-Language-Hearing Association. (2011). *Cultural competence in professional service delivery* [Position statement]. Retrieved from http://www.asha.org/policy

Chin, J. (2000). Cultural competence. Viewpoint. Culturally competent health care. *Public Health Reports, 115*(1), 25–34.

Payne, J. C. (2011, November 1). *Cultural competence in treatment of adults with cognitive and language disorders.* Retrieved from http://www.asha.org/Publications/leader/2011/111101/Cultural-Competence-in-Treatment-of-Adults-with-Cognitive-and-Language-Disorders.htm

Riquelme, L. F. (2004, April 13). Cultural competence in dysphagia. Retrieved from http://www.asha.org/Publications/leader/2004/040413/f040413b3.htm

Scott, D., & Jones, R. (2003). *Cultural competence in audiology*. Rockville, MD: American Speech-Language-Hearing Association.

Wolf, K. E. (2004, April 13). *Cultural competence in audiology*. Retrieved from http://www.asha.org/Publications/leader/2004/040413/f040413b2.htm

Acknowledgments

Most especially, I thank my loving and supportive husband, Robert.

A special thanks to the contributors: Wilhelmina Wright-Harp and Alaina Davis.

Thank you Ted, Traci, Christian, Zoe and Solomon, Marvin and Catey, and Maceo.

Thank you Johnetta, William, Erica, and Jadae.

To my graduate students:

"Which of these, then do you think proved to be a neighbor to the man who fell among robbers? He said, 'the one who showed him mercy.' And Jesus said to him, 'You go and do likewise'" (Parable of the Good Samaritan, Luke 10: 36–37).

Contributors

Alaina S. Davis, MS, CCC-SLP
Speech-Language Pathologist
Department of Communication Sciences and Disorders
Howard University
Washington, DC
Chapter 5

Joan C. Payne, PhD
Professor and Interim Chair
Department of Communication Sciences and Disorders
School of Communications
Howard University
Washington, DC

Wilhelmina Wright-Harp, PhD, MS, BS, CCC-SLP
Associate Dean and Associate Professor
School of Communications
Howard University
Washington, DC
Chapters 2 and 5

This work is dedicated to the memories of the late Dr. Joseph Arthur Payne, Jr. and the late Dr. Gretchen Bradley Payne. In the words of the great Negro spiritual, "I done done what you told me to do."

This book is also dedicated to the late Drs. Sadanand Singh, John Black, Ayub Khan Ommaya, Jesse Barber, and Bertha Minus, and to the late Roland Frederick Bradley.

SECTION I

Contemporary Issues in Neurogenic Communication Disorders

CHAPTER 1

Health Disparities: Implications for Neurogenic Communication Disorders

HEALTH DISPARITIES DEFINED

The National Institutes of Health (2004) defines health disparities as the difference in the incidence, prevalence, morbidity, mortality, and burden of diseases and other adverse health conditions that exist among specific population groups. A health disparity population is one in which there is a significant disparity in the overall rate of disease incidence, prevalence, morbidity, mortality, or survival rates in the population compared with the health status of the general population (United States Public Law 106–525, p. 2498).

Health disparities are a national health care crisis (DHHS [Department of Health and Human Services], Agency for Healthcare Research and Quality, 2007; Healthy People 2010, 2020) that requires changes in both national health care policy and service delivery (Healthy People; National Institutes of Health, 2002; DHHS, 2010, 2011a, 2011b, 2012). Millions of persons have been affected by disparities in health status and health care because of decades of racial and cultural inequities. Identifying, reducing, and eliminating health disparities have therefore become national research, service, and outreach priorities.

Despite public health information and improvements in the quality of health care, health disparities continue to exist because of a number of sociodemographic factors. Said another way, Caesar and Williams (2002) posit that health disparities are related to a long-standing national history of poverty, discrimination in access to health care, poor or nonexistent medical care early in life among the poor and ethnic subgroups, differences in collective wealth within neighborhoods in which affected populations live, and hazardous living and working situations. Within many low-income communities, the stressors of high unemployment, poverty, dangerous working environments, and substandard housing can be directly attributed to the health profiles of the residents. Hence, it may be inferred that differences in ethnicity, economic status, culture, and human ecology play major roles in patterns of disease and health.

Additionally, and most particularly concerning groups with health disparities, problems with quality of health care are decreasing while problems with access to health care are increasing (The Institute of Medicine, 2002). In 2005, Americans received about 34% of health care services they should have received. By 2009, this had fallen to 30% of services. In 2002, 24% of Americans encountered difficulties accessing health care. By 2009, this had increased to 26% of Americans (DHHS, 2012).

Lack of insurance, more than any other demographic or economic barrier, negatively affects the quality of health care received by ethnic populations. Persons from racial and ethnic minorities are significantly less likely than the rest of the population to have health insurance. These persons constitute about one-third of the U.S. population but make up more than half of the 50 million people who are uninsured (DHHS, 2011a).

RELEVANT LEGISLATION: IMPLICATIONS FOR NEUROGENIC LANGUAGE DISORDERS

Two significant laws have been enacted to address health disparities. To meet the challenge of decreasing health disparities, in 2000, United States Public Law 106-525, also known as the Minority Health and Health Disparities Research and Education Act, was signed into law. This law authorized the establishment of the National Center for Minority Health and Health Disparities, now the National Institute for Minority Health and Health Disparities. The institute's mission is that of providing a platform for generating new research and knowledge on the causes and interventions appropriate to eliminating health disparities.

The second law enacted is designed to reduce health disparities by making health care available and affordable to all citizens. Two important federal statutes were signed into law in 2010. On March 23, President Obama signed into law H.R. 3590, the Patient Protection and Affordable Care Act (PPACA). This act and the Health Care and Education Reconciliation Act of 2010 (H.R. 4872), which amended the PPACA, are designed to provide health insurance to millions of Americans who have been marginalized because of: (1) pre-existing conditions and/or (2) insufficient income to purchase health insurance. Many of the individuals who will benefit from health reform are poor and/or people of color.

This new legislation will not be fully implemented for adults until 2014. Rose (2013) observes:

> As healthcare reform gradually unfolds more people will soon have access to health insurance, and because those individuals who were disenfranchised were largely from minority groups with lower socioeconomic status, it is inevitable that cultural competency will be a necessary factor in terms of moving forward in serving all patients optimally. (p. 2)

The PPACA legislation includes rehabilitative and habilitative services as part of the basic benefit package that insurance companies must provide. By the year 2014, the legislation will roll out essential health benefits to provide health care for the 24 million Americans who are currently uninsured. The addition of these individuals who may be able to access covered services, including speech-language pathology and audiology services, will greatly increase the number of people who can be served.

In response to this changing clinical environment, a working committee of the American Speech-Language-Hearing Association (2012, hereafter ASHA), called the ASHA Changing Health Care Landscape Summit, developed the statement that speech-language pathologists should:

> expand the clinical paradigm beyond traditional [Communication Sciences and Disorders] services to include patient–provider communication strategies, services to communication-vulnerable (not necessarily disordered) populations participating in health care services, and providing consultation regarding altering and enabling the communication environment in care venues such as ICUs and stroke units. (p. 7)

This is a crucial time for speech-language pathologists to become familiar with both health disparities and health care reform because, over the next three to five decades, several factors will converge to change the clinical profiles of adults with neurogenic language disorders in important ways. Major demographic changes in the country will usher in an era of unparalleled population growth of older nonwhite ethnic groups, who, because of health disparities, may be living with major, chronic diseases that impair language and cognition. Furthermore, as of 2014 under the PPACA, "states must cover all persons under the age of

65 with incomes of less than 133% of the Federal poverty level using expansion of the Medicaid program," which includes 16 million recipients (Havens, 2012, p. 3), many of whom may need speech-language pathology services.

Finally, special populations of aging adults, some of whom have been significantly underrepresented in the health care system, may now be eligible to receive speech-language pathology services. Among the underrepresented are those living with AIDS, returning veterans with multisystem and missile blast head injuries, incarcerated men and women, and the homeless. It is anticipated that most speech-language pathologists will accept the increased scrutiny and challenges associated with health care reform and will work closely with others to achieve desired health care outcomes (Cornett, 2010).

DEMOGRAPHIC PROJECTIONS: THE CHANGING CLINICAL LANDSCAPE

For the purpose of uniformity, designations of ethnic groups will follow those of the U.S. Census. According to population projections in the United States, African Americans (non- Hispanic), Asian American/Pacific Islanders, Hispanics (all ethnic groups), and American Indian/Alaska Natives will grow in population at a more rapid rate than that of non-Hispanic whites over the next 50 years. The percentage of African Americans and races from countries other than Europe is expected to increase from 10.2% in 1990 to 15.3% in 2020 and to 21.3% by 2050 (Vincent & Velkoff, 2010).

Older adult population numbers will vary with age over time. Non-Hispanic whites are becoming an older aging group than those of non-European ethnic origins. The impending demographic changes in the United States, brought about largely by immigration, will change the country's population characteristics over the next several decades in a dramatic way. According to the U.S. Bureau of the Census (Vincent & Velkoff, 2010), non-Hispanic whites accounted for 49.6% of all births in the 12-month period that ended in July 2011. In that same period, ethnic minorities, including Hispanics, African Americans, Asians, and those of mixed race, reached 50.4%, representing a majority for the first time in this country's history, while the population of non-Hispanic whites of European ancestry stagnated. It is projected that by 2040, the largest populations in the nation will be persons of color. This means that by the middle of the 21st century, over half of the United States will be African, Hispanic, Asian, and Native Americans, making the current terminology of majority and minority meaningless. Although non-Hispanic white Americans as a group will remain in the majority, racially ethnic groups will become an ever larger and important force in the aging of America (Vincent &Velkoff, 2010).

U.S. Census projections also point to a significant increase in the number of older ethnic adults, those 65 years and older and the oldest old, that is, those 85 years and older. By 2060, the U.S. population will be considerably older and more racially and ethnically diverse. For the first time, the older population is projected to outnumber those who are under 18 years of age. Populations of persons aged 65 and older are expected to more than double between 2012 and 2060, from 43.1 million to 92.0 million and will represent just over one in five U.S. residents by the end of the period, up from one in seven currently. The increase in the number of the oldest

old will be even more dramatic—those 85 and older are projected to more than triple, from 5.9 million to 18.2 million, reaching 4.3% of the total population. Of those age 65 and older in 2060, 56.0% are expected to be non-Hispanic white, with 21.2% Hispanic and 12.5% non-Hispanic persons of African descent making up the majority of persons of color (U.S. Bureau of the Census, 2012).

The American Speech-Language-Hearing Association (2005, 2011a) has already begun to address health disparities, demographic projections and cultural competence in position papers that relate to ethical considerations in the treatment of diverse populations. Most of the chronic diseases and conditions that can compromise language and cognition occur most frequently in mature or older adults, such as stroke and dementia. Many of the persons who are aging now have also been victims of health disparities. Given the national population projections, it seems reasonable to assume that the numbers of culturally and ethnically diverse aging adults with language and cognitive disorders secondary to neurological damage will continue to increase rapidly as well. And these previously underserved adults will now have more of the means to access speech-language pathology assessment and treatment.

PROFESSIONAL AND RESEARCH ISSUES

Currently, there is a dearth of information about cultural, ethnic, and linguistic diversity available to practitioners who provide services to older persons with neurogenic language disorders. According to Horton-Ikard, Munoz, Thomas-Tate, and Keller-Bell (2009), there are too few resources or too little evidence with which to educate current and future practitioners about cultural diversity and cultural competence. There are only a small percentage of academicians who specialize in multicultural research and teaching, and there are a limited number of instructors who include multicultural competence in their area of specialty.

This lack of information and resources affects a significant number of professionals in speech-language pathology. Currently, more than one-third of certified speech-language pathologists work in health care settings, including hospitals, speech and hearing clinics, home health agencies, skilled nursing facilities, and other, similar settings. The largest number, 24,080, practice in hospitals and skilled nursing facilities, where they are most likely to work with older persons with neurogenic language disorders (ASHA, 2011b; 2011c; 2011d). To further illustrate the point, in a 2011 ASHA membership survey of 1,431 respondents, 4.9% felt that they were "not at all qualified to address cultural and linguistic influences on service delivery and outcomes." Among respondents working in health care settings, 4% of 175 respondents working in hospitals, 9.6% of 136 respondents working in residential health care settings, and 6.7% of 268 persons working in nonresidential health care settings indicated that they did not feel at all qualified. Members working in college or university settings fared better. Although no respondents felt that they were not qualified at all, only 13.9% of 115 respondents rated themselves as "very qualified" to address cultural and linguistic influences on service delivery and outcomes. While the number of respondents is only a small representative sample of the ASHA membership, their answers may be very reflective of the level

of comfort held by a much larger number of professionals who work with patients with neurogenic language disorders or who educate future clinicians who will work with this population (ASHA, 2011c).

A rigorous national research agenda on culturally and ethnically diverse adults with neurogenic language disorders should lead the way to raising awareness in speech-language pathology about service delivery that meets the needs of all persons regardless of their cultural, ethnic, or linguistic backgrounds. The dilemma is that despite significant national health issues and trends, researchers in speech-language pathology have been less aggressive than those in other health disciplines about investigating the relationship of disease prevalence, population projections, and the possible impact of legislation on health disparities and health care reform to adult neurogenic language disorders.

In an editorial comment, Hammer (2012) remarked that few studies have been submitted to the *Journal of Speech-Language Pathology* that address the cultural, racial/ethnic, and socioeconomic diversity that exists within the adult population. Indeed, Ellis (2009) notes that there is a dearth of information on cultural, ethnic, and language differences among adults with neurogenic language disorders and that information about "communication outcomes is needed, which will in turn enhance clinical service provision for all clients regardless of race/ethnicity" (p. 311). Furthermore, Graham (2003) also observes that there is a need for new research and research training initiatives that will help to create interventions and treatments that are appropriate for all populations. Certainly, without systematic investigations about which assessment and therapy approaches represent best practices for diverse adults with neurogenic disorders, there will continue to be little in the way of information about evidence-based assessment and intervention strategies for this clinical population.

The paucity of available research also translates into how well clinicians are being prepared for the inevitable changes in the clinical landscape. Presently, there is little consensus in the professional literature for how the academy should integrate, or integrally infuse, multicultural information in speech-language pathology curricula in a way that sensitizes future clinicians about culturally and ethnically diverse adult clients (Stockman, Boult, & Robinson, 2004). Of particular concern for speech-language pathologists who evaluate and treat adults with neurogenic language disorders are the following:

1. Several major diseases and conditions that compromise language and cognition, including stroke, dementia, and traumatic brain injuries, have not decreased in scope, severity, or prevalence for persons of color according to results of large-scale study data.

2. The prevalence of these diseases and conditions is significantly correlated with age, ethnicity, income, education, and geographic region.

3. Chronic diseases that pose significant stroke and dementia risks for persons in some ethnic groups are often poorly diagnosed and treated (suboptimal care) and portend a more grim prognosis because of a variety of social and economic barriers.

4. Research findings strongly suggest that adults who are poor and ethnic recover functional skills more slowly after catastrophic illness than their non-Hispanic white cohorts (Horner,

Matchar, Divine, & Feussner, 1991; Horner, Swanson, Bosworth, & Matchar, 2003).

Given these dynamics, speech-language pathologists should anticipate that their patients with neurogenic language disorders will be increasingly diverse in age, severity of functional limitations, previous health status, income, education, primary and secondary languages, and cultural/ethnic identities. Therefore, clinicians will need to assess and treat neurogenic language and cognitive disorders using culturally competent approaches to patient diagnoses and management (DHHS, Office of Minority Health, 2001, 2008; Payne, 2011). The following sections will address specific health disparities in diseases and conditions that can and do impair language and cognitive functioning in adults.

STROKE AND DISPARITIES IN STROKE RISK FACTORS

Cerebrovascular accidents (CVAs) are implicated in both aphasia and dementia. Although the mortality rate of persons who suffer CVAs has declined, significant numbers of persons survive with functional impairments, including language and cognitive disorders. Those who are identified as health disparity populations are most likely to have earlier and more severe CVAs because of chronic diseases like hypertension, heart disease, cavernous venous malformations (CVMs), and diabetes; lifestyle contributors such as obesity and alcoholism, which are acknowledged risk factors; and limited access to optimal health care.

Hypertension

Hypertension is a precursor to stroke and dementia. "High blood pressure" and "hypertension" are used interchangeably. *Hypertension* refers to systolic and diastolic blood pressure readings that are higher than normal, indicating that the body needs to work harder to circulate the blood. A positive relationship exists between diagnosed hypertension and age. Approximately 2.7% of persons 18 to 24 years old and 58.9% of persons 65 years and older report that they have received a hypertension diagnosis (Sung, Ostchega, & Louis, 2008).

There is variation in hypertension rates within ethnic groups. African Americans have the highest rates of hypertension, but Mexican Americans, American Indians/Alaska Natives, Filipino Americans, and Pacific Islanders also have a significant prevalence of hypertension. For many persons in these groups, there has been a history of discrimination, high unemployment, suboptimal health care, and substandard housing that may have contributed to the prevalence of hypertension in addition to lifestyle indicators.

Specific biopsychosocial determinants of hypertension may provide an understanding of racial disparities with respect to the prevalence of hypertension in nonwhite ethnic groups. It has been suggested that feelings of anger and frustration resulting from institutionalized racial discrimination are emotional causative pathways to the pathophysiology contributing to the health disparities experienced by African Americans and other persons of color (Carlson & Chamberlain, 2004). There may be associations among racism, stress exposure, and reactivity as well as associations with established hypertension-related risk factors, such as obesity, low levels of physical activity, and alcohol use. The effects appear to vary by level of racism. Racism may increase risks for hypertension, but these effects emerge more clearly at the level of institutional racism when compared with racism encountered at an individual level. However, all levels of racism may influence the prevalence of hypertension and raise the barriers to lifestyle change (Brundolo, Love, Pencille Schoenthaler, & Ogedegbe, 2011).

African Americans and Hypertension

African Americans are the most frequently studied ethnic group on measures of hypertension. Research findings verify that African Americans are most at risk, followed by Mexican Americans (Quiñones, Liang, & Ye, 2012). Biological substrates have been examined, including a possible effect of lower levels of specific enzymes that protect the cardiovascular system in African American adolescents (Federation of American Societies for Experimental Biology, 2010). Table 1–1 shows the prevalence of hypertension in African Americans over age 20 compared with non-Hispanic whites. Table 1–2 gives the percentage of African Americans in 2010 who had hypertension and were 18 years and older. Table 1–3 shows the disparity between African Americans and non-Hispanic whites in percentage of hypertension under control between 2005 and 2008.

As can be seen in these tables, African Americans have higher rates of hypertension compared with non-Hispanic whites. Moreover, fewer African Americans have their hypertension under control compared with non-Hispanic whites.

Table 1–1. Age-Adjusted Percentage of Persons 20 Years of Age and Over Who Have High Blood Pressure, 2007–2010. National Health and Nutrition Examination Survey

	Non-Hispanic Black	Non-Hispanic White	Non-Hispanic Black/ Non-Hispanic White Ratio
Men	40.5	31.1	1.3
Women	44.3	28.1	1.6

Source: CDC. (2012). Health United States, 2011, Table 70. http://www.cdc.gov/nchs/data/hus/hus11.pdf

Table 1–2. Age-Adjusted Percentage of Persons 18 Years of Age and Over Who Have High Blood Pressure, 2010. National Health Interview Survey (NHIS)

African Americans	Non-Hispanic White	African Americans/ Non-Hispanic White Ratio
34.1	23.9	1.4

Source: CDC. (2011). Summary Health Statistics for U.S. Adults: 2010. Table 2. http://www.cdc.gov/nchs/data/series/sr_10/sr10_252.pdf

Table 1–3. Percent of Adults Age 18 and Over With Hypertension Whose Blood Pressure Is Under Control, 2005–2008

Non-Hispanic Black	Non-Hispanic White	Non-Hispanic Black/ Non-Hispanic White Ratio
38.6	44.1	0.9

Source: T2_1_2_1: 2011 National Healthcare Quality and Disparities Reports. March 2012. Agency for Healthcare Research and Quality, Rockville, MD. http://www.ahrq.gov/research/findings/nhqrdr/nhqrdr11/2_heartdiseases/T2_1_2_1.h

Centers for Disease Control and Prevention, National Center for Health Statistics, National Health and Nutrition Examination Survey.

Hispanic Americans and Hypertension

Among Hispanic Americans, there appears to be a strong inverse relationship between socioeconomic status and hypertension. Mexican American males have the highest rates of hypertension of any Hispanic group. As seen in Table 1–4 and Table 1–5, however, as a group, Mexican Americans have lower percentages of hypertension compared with non-Hispanic whites.

Those Mexican American males with the lowest socioeconomic profiles have significantly worse cardiovascular disease profiles than those in higher socioeconomic status groups. Advanced age and increased acculturation, rather than socioeconomic status, are considered to be important factors associated with the

Table 1–4. Age-Adjusted Percentage of Persons 20 Years of Age and Over Who Have High Blood Pressure, 2007–2010

	Mexican American	Non-Hispanic White	Mexican/Non-Hispanic White Ratio
Men	28.6	31.1	0.9
Women	27.8	28.1	1.0

Source: CDC. (2012). Health United States, 2011, Table 70. http://www.cdc.gov/nchs/data/hus/hus11.pdf

Table 1–5. Age-Adjusted Percentage of Persons 18 Years of Age and Over Who Have High Blood Pressure, 2010. National Health Interview Survey (NHIS)

Hispanics	Non-Hispanic White	Hispanic /Non-Hispanic White Ratio
22.5	23.9	0.9

Source: CDC. (2011). Summary Health Statistics for U.S. Adults: 2010. Table 2. http://www.cdc.gov/nchs/data/series/sr_10/sr10_252.pdf

prevalence of hypertension in older Mexican Americans (De Arellano, 1994). However, Mexican American women are less likely than non-Hispanic white women to have high blood pressure (DHHS, Office of Minority Health, 2011).

American Indian/Alaska Natives and Hypertension

American Indian/Alaska Native adults are 1.3 times as likely as non-Hispanic white adults to develop hypertension. An estimated 2 million American Indians and Alaska Natives, while sharing certain genetic traits, belong to groups with distinct social, cultural, political, and biomedical attributes. They, like other ethnic groups, have a history of high poverty rates and unemployment, lower educational attainment, and increased susceptibility to certain diseases. Hypertension has been reported less frequently among Native Americans compared with other U.S. groups, but hypertension diagnoses are increasing. This change in hypertension rates is strongly associated with obesity and diabetes (Galloway, 2005; Rhoades, 1996). Table 1–6 illustrates the percentages of persons over age 18 who had high blood pressure among American Indian/Alaska Natives in 2010. Table 1–7 shows 2012 differences in percentages of American Indian/Alaska Natives with hypertension by gender.

Asian American/Pacific Islanders and Hypertension

In general, Asian Americans have lower rates of hypertension than non-Hispanic whites. Among Asian Americans, Pacific Islanders are more at risk for diseases associated with obesity, including hypertension, as seen in Table 1–8. Filipino Americans have the highest rates of

Table 1–6. Age-Adjusted Percentage of Persons 18 Years of Age and Over Who Have High Blood Pressure, 2010. National Health Interview Survey (NHIS)

American Indian/ Alaska Native	Non-Hispanic White	American Indian/AlaskaNative/ Non-Hispanic White Ratio
30.0	23.9	1.3

Source: CDC. (2011). Summary Health Statistics for U.S. Adults: 2010. Table 2. http://www.cdc.gov/nchs/data/series/sr_10/sr10_252.pdf

Table 1–7. Age-Adjusted Percentages of Persons 18 Years of Age and Over Who Have High Blood Pressure by Gender, 2012. National Health Interview Survey

	American Indian/Alaska Native	Non-Hispanic White	American Indian/ Alaska Native/ Non-Hispanic White Ratio
Men and women	34.5	25.7	1.3
Men	38.7	26.7	1.4
Women	30.2	24.7	1.2

Source: CDC. (2010). Health Characteristics of the American Indian and Alaska Native Adult Population: United States, 2004-2008. Table 4. http://www.cdc.gov/nchs/data/nhsr/nhsr020.pdf

Table 1–8. Age-Adjusted Percentage of Persons 18 Years of Age and Over Who Have High Blood Pressure, 2010

Asians	Non-Hispanic White	Asian/Non-Hispanic White Ratio
20.5	23.9	0.9

Source: CDC. (2011). Summary Health Statistics for U.S. Adults: 2010. Table 2. http://www.cdc.gov/nchs/data/series/sr_10/sr10_252.pdf

hypertension among Asian groups. Fewer Filipino women have their blood pressure under control, which is the reverse of many of the gender trends (Centers for Disease Control and Prevention [hereafter CDC], 2008, 2011). Table 1–9 shows percentages of Native Hawaiian/Pacific Islanders with hypertension compared with non-Hispanic whites. As can be seen, Native Hawaiian/Pacific Islanders have significantly higher hypertension prevalence.

Obesity

Obesity has been increasing across all U.S. groups since 1980 and places an individual at greater risk for hypertension and diabetes. *Overweight* and *obesity* refer to weight that is considered unhealthy for a given height. Body mass index (BMI) indicates the amount of body fat. The higher the BMI, the more likely it is that the adult is at risk for chronic diseases and condi-

Table 1–9. Age-Adjusted Percentage of Persons 18 Years of Age and Over Who Have High Blood Pressure, 2010. National Health Interview Survey

Native Hawaiian/ Pacific Islander	Non-Hispanic White	Native Hawaiian/Pacific Islander/ Non-Hispanic White Ratio
40.8	23.9	1.7

Source: Summary Health Statistics for U.S. Adults: 2010. Table 2 http://www.cdc.gov/nchs/data/series/sr_10/sr10_252.pdf

tions. An adult who has a BMI between 25 and 29.9 is considered overweight. An adult who has a BMI of 30 or higher is considered obese (CDC, 2012a).

Concomitant diagnoses of diabetes and hypertension significantly increase the risk for stroke. Ethnic disparities for obesity are seen at higher prevalence rates among African American women, Hispanic Americans (especially Mexican Americans and Puerto Ricans), American Indians/Alaska Natives, Pacific Islanders, and Native Hawaiians compared with non-Hispanic whites (Smith et al., 2005). The risks from obesity are such that these ethnic groups are more likely than non-Hispanic whites to suffer from CVAs or strokes at an earlier age and are less likely to recover fully from strokes (Payne & Stroman, 2004).

Obesity is a significant risk factor for stroke because of the relationship to coronary artery disease. Ischemic (clot-caused) stroke and coronary artery disease share many of the same disease processes and risk factors. A meta-analysis of 25 prospective cohort studies with 2.3 million participants demonstrates a direct, graded association between excess weight and stroke risk. Overweight increased the risk for ischemic stroke by 22%, and obesity increased it by 64%. There was no significant relationship between overweight or obesity and hemorrhagic (bleeding-caused) stroke, however. A repeat analysis that statistically accounted for blood pressure, cholesterol, and diabetes weakened the associations, suggesting that these factors mediate the effect of obesity on stroke (Strazzullo et al., 2010). High cholesterol, age at diagnosis, poor disease management, language barriers, limited access to health services, lack of health insurance, tobacco use, and limited physical activity are other risk factors that can also worsen the outcome and prognoses for recovery (Payne, 1997).

Diabetes

According to the American Diabetes Association (2013), type 2 diabetes affects adults and is the most common diabetic form. In type 2 diabetes, either the body does not produce enough insulin or the cells ignore the insulin. Insulin is necessary for the body to be able to use glucose for energy. When food is eaten, the body breaks down all of the sugars and starches into glucose, which is the basic fuel for the cells in the body. Insulin takes the sugar from the blood into the cells. Cells use the hormone insulin, made in the pancreas, to help process blood glucose into energy.

People develop type 2 diabetes because the cells in the muscles, liver, and fat do not use insulin properly. Eventually, the pancreas cannot make enough insulin for the body's needs. As a result, the amount of glucose in the blood increases while the cells are starved of energy. Over the years, high blood glucose damages nerves and blood vessels, leading to complications such as heart disease and stroke (American Diabetes Association, 2013).

Significant sociodemographic disparities in prevalence and incidence of diagnosed diabetes exist in the United States among adults. Racial/ethnic disparities in prevalence and incidence of diagnosed diabetes had not decreased as of 2008, and socioeconomic disparities have worsened with the downturn of the U.S. economy (CDC, 2011). The prevalence of diabetes in African Americans is nearly 70% higher than in non-Hispanic whites. American Indians, Hispanics, African Americans, and some Asian Americans, Native Hawaiians, and Pacific Islanders, including Japanese Americans and Samoans, are at particularly high risk for developing type 2 diabetes (National Institutes of Health, 2004).

Cavernous Malformations

An additional risk factor for stroke in Hispanic Americans are cavernous malformations (CMs), which are found more in this population than in any other ethnic group. Cerebral CM is a vascular disease of the brain that causes headaches, epilepsy, seizures, and cerebral hemorrhage (Gault, Sain, Hu, & Awad, 2006; Gunel et al., 1996). Vascular lesions may remain clinically silent or lead to a number of neurological symptoms, including focal neurological deficits (Marchuk et al., 1995).

Affected persons in this population may have inherited the same mutation from a common ancestor (Gunel et al., 1996). More recently, researchers have determined that the gene mutation for CMs can occur as sporadic or autosomal-dominant inherited conditions. Approximately 50% of Hispanic patients with cerebral CMs have the familial form, compared with 10% to 20% of non-Hispanic white patients. There is no difference in the pathological findings or presentation in the sporadic and familial forms. To date, familial CMs have been attributed to mutations at three different gene loci (CCM1 on 7q21.2, CCM2 on 7p15-p13, and CCM3 on 3q25.2-q27) (Dashti, Hoffer, Hu, & Selman, 2006). Familial cases with CCM1 mutations may have less severe clinical manifestations than other familial cases (Gault et al., 2006).

Heart Disease

"Native American" refers to a person having origins in any of the original peoples of North, Central, and South America and who maintains a tribal affiliation or community attachment. Native Americans include both American Indian and Alaska Natives. Native Americans have among the highest rates of risk factors for cardiovascular disease compared with other racial/ethnic groups, and the highest prevalence of stroke in non-institutionalized adults (Barnes, Adams, & Powell-Griner, 2010; Rosamond et al., 2008).

Despite recent large-scale efforts to eliminate health disparities in ethnic and minority populations, the impact among American Indian and Alaska Natives to date has been relatively limited. Indeed, over the past several decades the incidence and prevalence of cardiovascular risk factors have risen significantly, including the development of an epidemic of diabetes.

Evidence suggests that these higher rates of cardiovascular risk factors, including tobacco abuse, diabetes, high blood pressure, and elevated cholesterol levels, may be placing an inordinate burden of cardiovascular disease on the American Indian and Alaska Native populations (American Heart Association, 2007).

The rates of heart disease and stroke among American Indians and Alaska Natives are now higher than in the general U.S. population as well as in U.S. non-Hispanic whites. Recent evaluations suggest that these rates are also higher than among other ethnic or racial populations in the United States (Galloway, 2005). The limited data available on American Indians/Alaska Natives show that these groups frequently contend with issues that prevent them from receiving quality medical care, including cultural barriers, geographic isolation, inadequate sewage disposal, and low income (DHHS, 2011).

Stroke Prevalence

Health disparities among ethnic groups in stroke incidence and prevalence are well documented (Hayes, Greenlund, Denny, Kennan, & Croft, 2005; Keppel, Pearcy, & Wagener, 2001; Kessela et al., 2004; Trimble & Morgenstern, 2008). Although the mortality rate from stroke has declined nationally, research findings suggest that, with the exception of some Asian American groups like the Pacific Islanders, African Americans, Hispanic Americans, and American Indians/Alaska Natives are the highest risk populations for strokes compared with non-Hispanic whites (Thom et al., 2006).

Three trends are consistently reported about disparities among and within ethnic groups. These issues are summarized as:

1. differences in racial predisposition for types of strokes;
2. variations in the severity of stroke-related disabilities across ethnic groups; and
3. correlations among ethnicity, stroke, and disabilities.

Differences in Racial Predisposition for Types of Stroke

Earlier studies note that compared with Hispanic Americans, non-Hispanic whites are more likely to have ischemic heart disease, transient ischemic attacks, and ischemic causes of potential cardiogenic emboli. In addition, cardiac disease, including atrial fibrillation, myocardial infarction, angina, and congestive heart failure, was found to be less prevalent in both African Americans and Hispanics compared with non-Hispanic whites (Bruno & Qualls, 1994; Sacco, Kargman, & Zamanillo, 1995). Non-Hispanic whites may have a higher prevalence of hyperlipidemia, myocardial infarction, and stroke at an older age than other racial/ethnic groups, and cardioembolic stroke, including atrial fibrillation, is more prevalent compared with many minority groups.

By contrast, in a study of 792 cohorts over an 8-year period in four U.S. communities, after accounting for established baseline risk factors, African Americans, particularly males, had a 38% greater risk of incident ischemic stroke compared with non-Hispanic whites. Of the 267 incident definite or probable strokes, 83% ($n = 221$) were categorized as ischemic strokes, 10% ($n = 27$) were intracerebral hemorrhages, and 7% ($n = 19$) were subarachnoid hemorrhages. The age-adjusted incidence rate (per 1,000 person-years) of total strokes was highest among African American men (4.44), followed by African American women (3.10), non-Hispanic white men (1.78), and non-Hispanic white women (1.24) (Rosamond et al., 1999).

Results from the Northern Manhattan Stroke Study conducted over a period of 3 years show that African Americans and Hispanics also have a higher incidence rate of stroke than non-Hispanic whites. Stroke incidence increased with age and was greater in men than in women. The average annual age-adjusted stroke incidence rate at age ≥20 years, per 100,000 population, was 223 for African Americans, 196 for Hispanics, and 93 for non-Hispanic whites. African Americans had a 2.4-fold and Hispanics a 2-fold increase in stroke incidence compared with non-Hispanic whites. Cerebral infarct accounted for 77% of all strokes, intracerebral hemorrhage for 17%, and subarachnoid hemorrhage for 6% (Sacco et al., 1998).

Native Americans/Alaska Natives have a higher incidence of stroke compared with non-Hispanic whites or African Americans. The case-fatality rate for first stroke is also higher in American Indians than in the U.S. non-Hispanic white or African American population in the same age range, and American Indian/Alaska Native adults are 60% more likely to have a stroke than their non-Hispanic adult cohorts. In a study of over 4,549 American Indian participants aged 45 to 74 years at enrollment in the Strong Heart Study, through December 2004, 306 (6.8%) of 4,507 participants without prior stroke suffered a first stroke at a mean age of 66.5 years. Nonhemorrhagic cerebral infarction occurred in 86% of participants with incident strokes; 14% had hemorrhagic stroke (Zhang et al., 2008). American Indian/Alaska Native women have twice the rate of stroke as non-Hispanic white women. American Indian/Alaska Native adults are more likely to be obese and have high blood pressure compared with non-Hispanic white adults (American Heart Association, 2007).

There is also evidence of increased prevalence of stroke among Mexican Americans compared with non-Hispanic whites. Data indicate an incidence of 168/10,000 in Mexican Americans and 136/10,000 in non-Hispanic whites for first-time strokes in the same time period (Morgenstern et al., 2004). In addition, Mexican Americans have an increased incidence of intracerebral hemorrhage and subarachnoid hemorrhage compared with non-Hispanic whites and have an increased incidence of ischemic stroke and transient ischemic attack at younger ages.

Asians, specifically Chinese and Japanese, have high stroke incidence rates (He, Klang, Wu, & Whelton, 1995). Stroke incidence and mortality rates in Japan were very high for most of this century and exceeded those for heart disease. As in the United States, stroke death rates in Japan have fallen dramatically since World War II. In recent years stroke incidence rates in Japanese men in Hawaii were similar to those of white Americans and between the rates of Japanese men in Japan and in California (Sacco et al., 1997). However, within the group of Asian Americans, Pacific Islanders/Native Hawaiians in general have developed several of the high-risk factors that can lead to heart attacks and stroke, such as higher rates of obesity, hypertension, and cigarette smoking. Cerebrovascular disease can be more prevalent in some U.S. island territories. For example, the death rate from stroke is three times higher in American Samoa compared with the U.S. national non-Hispanic white population (CDC, 2011).

Differences in type of stroke have been investigated in earlier studies. African Americans, Asians, and Hispanics have more involvement of the intracerebral arteries than do non-Hispanic whites (Caplan, 1994; Caplan, Gorelick, & Hier, 1986; Feldman et al., 1990; Horner, Matchar, Divine, & Feussner 1991). This difference is important in determining the severity of strokes, as mortality and severe functional disabilities are more likely seen in hemorrhagic strokes than in ischemic infarcts (Gresham et al., 1995).

Further evidence for the influence of racial differences in differential diagnoses is explained by Gresham and his associates (1995), who note that if a patient were a menstruating woman or of African or Asian descent, the lesion would most likely be at an intracerebral arterial site. It is not clear why Africans and Asians have more intracranial hemorrhages except to note that high blood pressure, a major factor in intracranial hemorrhage, has been correlated with living in areas of high social stress (Schafer, Bruun, & Richter, 1973a, 1973b). Genetics do not appear to be solely responsible for the prevalence of hypertension incidence among African Americans, given the variations in hypertension incidence among blacks in Africa, the Caribbean, and the United States (Bernard, 1993).

Feldman and his associates (1990) also found that the distribution of cerebrovascular lesions was affected by race in that African Americans, Japanese, and Chinese have more intracranial occlusive cerebrovascular disease, while non-Hispanic whites have more extracranial disease. The distribution of lesions in Chinese adults is not explained by differences in incidence of transient ischemia, hypertension, diabetes, hypercholesterolemia, or ischemic heart disease between the groups. Ethnic group identification appears to be the only factor that correlates with disease distribution.

Geographical Disparities: The Stroke Belt

Disparities for stroke and related disorders have been identified for geographical region in the United States. These regional influences coexist not only for stroke mortality and morbidity, but for obesity and lower socioeconomic income for African Americans as well. Ten states (Alabama, Arkansas, Georgia, Kentucky, Louisiana, Mississippi, North Carolina, South Carolina, Tennessee, and Virginia) are categorized as southeastern by the CDC (2005; Liao, Greenlund, Croft, Keenan, & Giles, 2009), as seen in Figure 1–1. Higher stroke mortality in the United States has long been evidenced among African Americans and other residents of southeastern states. A greater proportion of African Americans live in the southeastern states that make up the so-called stroke belt than elsewhere in the country; however, variations in socioeconomic characteristics and risk factors have also been associated with disparities in stroke, and these variations have been associated with region and race.

The findings by the CDC and others indicate a higher prevalence of stroke in 10 southeastern states than in 13 non-southeastern states sampled and the District of Columbia. African Americans who live in the southeastern states have the highest prevalence of strokes. The greater proportion of African Americans in the Southeast accounts for some of the higher prevalence in this group of states. Differences in educational level and prevalence

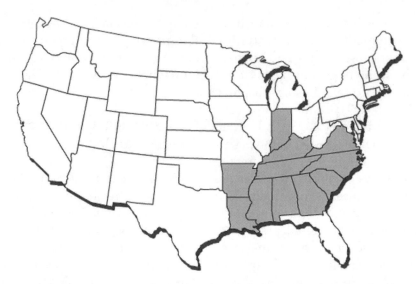

Figure 1–1. State map of the United States showing the Stroke Belt, a region with higher stroke incidences (National Heart, Lung and Blood Institute, part of the United States Department of Health and Human Services / Wikimedia Commons / Public Domain).

of risk factors such as diabetes and high blood pressure accounted for approximately half of the difference in stroke prevalence between southeasterners and nonsoutheasterners and approximately three-fourths of the difference in prevalence between blacks and whites (Richardson, Liao, & Tucker, 2005).

Variations in the Severity of Stroke-Related Disabilities Across Ethnic Groups

Data from the Framingham Disability Study (Pinsky et al., 1985) suggest that a number of factors predict stroke-related disability, such as long-term or current hypertension, increased BMI, and diabetes mellitus. Using these parameters, the Charleston Heart Study (Kell et al., 1989) evaluated African American males and females over the age of 60 and found

that disability was predicted by elevated systolic blood pressure, high serum cholesterol, and obesity for women and by systolic hypertension for men. Incidence of disability was greatest among African American females, followed by non-Hispanic white females, African American males, and non-Hispanic white males.

There is consensus that African Americans and Hispanic Americans return to function more slowly than non-Hispanic whites. This may be due to the more severe first-time stokes noted in this population (Miles & Bernard, 1992). In addition, Hispanic and African American stroke patients are twice as likely as non-Hispanic whites to experience a recurrent stroke within 2 years of their first stroke (Scheinart et al., 1998).

Motor impairments, for example, from ischemic strokes, were found to be greater in African Americans than in their non-Hispanic white cohorts (Horner et al.,

1991). In a related study Berges, Kuo, Ottenbacher, Seale, and Ostir (2012) investigated functional independence measure (FIM) scores in 900 adults over age 55 after stroke. At the 3-month follow-up, both Hispanic and African American patients had lower FIM scores compared with non-Hispanic whites. Their findings indicated that racial/ethnic group, age, length of stay, and medical comorbidities were significant predictors of total FIM ratings over four time points after stroke. Others (Hinojosa, Rittman, Hinojosa, & Rodriguez, 2009) observed a relationship among functional recovery of motor skills, amount of caregiver support, and personal resources of the patient in persons from Puerto Rico and African Americans.

DEMENTIA

Today, 1 in 10 people 65 and older, or approximately 5 million adults, has Alzheimer's disease (AD), yet only half of these adults have actually been diagnosed with the disease. It is estimated that by 2050, as many as 16 million persons will have AD. Dementia affects all ethnic groups; however, stroke risk factors and prevalence determine the types of dementia diagnosed in persons of specific ethnic groups.

Although ethnic group identity as an independent variable does not appear to be predictive of cognitive decline, it does appear that cortical infarcts and multiple infarcts in multiple sites are associated with increased odds of dementia. Cortical, multiple, or large infarcts may be associated with lower global cognitive function (Aggarwal et al., 2012).

Even allowing for discrepancies in methodologies and possible test bias, the most frequent findings are that African Americans and Hispanics have a higher prevalence and incidence of dementia and AD than non-Hispanic whites. Native Americans appear to have lower rates of AD in comparison with non-Hispanic whites. Asian Americans had rates of dementia comparable to non-Hispanic whites; however, whether there is the same proportion of AD compared with vascular dementia among Asian Americans and Asian immigrants remains uncertain (Gurland et al., 1999).

Despite some evidence of racial differences in the influence of genetic risk factors for AD and other dementias, genetic factors do not appear to account for these large prevalence differences across racial groups. Instead, health conditions that increase one's risk for AD and other dementias, such as high blood pressure and diabetes, are more prevalent in African American and Hispanic communities. Lower levels of education and other socioeconomic characteristics in these communities may also increase risk.

High blood pressure, more common among African Americans and a risk factor for stroke, can lead to a greater risk for developing AD. African Americans may have a higher rate of vascular (stroke-related) dementia, and the number of African Americans entering the age of AD risk (age 65 or older) is expected to more than double to 6.9 million by 2030 (Lloyd-Jones et al., 2010).

The presence of an apolipoprotein E (ApoE)-epsilon 4 allele is a determinant of AD in non-Hispanic whites, but African Americans and Hispanics have an increased frequency regardless of their ApoE genotype. This finding strongly suggests that other genes or risk factors may contribute to the increased risk for AD in African Americans and Hispanics (Tang et al., 1998). Hispanics also have higher rates of vascular disease and may be at greater risk for developing AD compared with non-Hispanic whites. According to a growing body of evidence, risk factors for vascular disease—including diabetes, high blood pressure, and high cholesterol—may be risk factors for AD and stroke-related dementia (Tatemichi et al., 1992).

Alzheimer's disease and other dementias have been studied extensively in older non-Hispanic whites, African Americans, and Hispanics. Gurland and his associates (1999) found that most people in the United States living with AD and other dementias are non-Hispanic whites. However, older African Americans and Hispanics are proportionately more likely than older whites to have AD and other dementias. Data indicate that in the United States, older African Americans are probably about two and a half times as likely to have AD and other dementias as older non-Hispanic whites (Demirovic et al., 2003), and Hispanics are approximately one and a half to two times as likely to have AD and other dementias as older non-Hispanic whites (Tang et al., 2001).

Manley and Mayeux (2004) found that disparities in significant risk factors, many of which are seen as contributors to stroke or as stroke risk factors, are also risk factors for dementia and may explain in part the differences among ethnic groups for AD and vascular dementia. These are described as:

1. disparities among African Americans, Hispanics, and Pacific Islanders in the prevalence of stroke and the possibility that silent infarcts decrease cognitive reserve and the brain's ability to compensate for AD pathology (cognitive reserve, or a buffer of extra neu-rological networks developed from stimulating experiences, is less well researched, but years of education or occupational attainment may increase one's ability to delay severe disability from cognitive decline);

2. disparities in hypertension prevalence that places African Americans at higher risk for neurovascular pathology often found among people diagnosed with AD, such as cerebral amyloid angiopathy, white-matter lesions, and vascular endothelial damage;

3. disparities in diabetes prevalence for African Americans and Hispanics, which may mean that the greater possibility of a stroke or a small-vessel disease heightens the risk of AD and dementia diagnoses;

4. disparities in myocardial infarction and coronary artery disease in African Americans and Hispanics, which have been associated with higher rates of dementia and presence of diffuse plaques in the brain. In a recent large-scale study by Luchsinger, Tang, Stern, Shea, and Mayeux (2001), one-third of the risk for stroke-associated dementia found for African Americans and Hispanics was attributable to diabetes compared with 17% among non-Hispanic whites;

5. disparities in head injury prevalence, a reported risk factor for AD in which an insult to the brain leads to increased production of β-amyloid containing diffuse plaques an increased risk for traumatic brain injury has been reported among ethnic minority populations (Bruns & Hauser, 2003) in that African Americans are more likely to have a history of head injury and worse functional outcomes (Kraus & McArthur, 1996; Staudenmayer, Diaz-Arrastia, de Oliveira,

Gentilello, & Shafi, 2007) than African Americans with vascular dementia (Gorelick et al., 1994); and

6. disparities in possible protective factors for nonwhite women, such as estrogen replacement therapy, anti-inflammatory drugs, and a diet rich in antioxidants (Payne, 1997).

The influence of ethnic and sociocultural dynamics on dementia help-seeking behaviors is less well understood. There is consensus that missed diagnoses are more common for ethnic adults than for non-Hispanic whites and that early signs and symptoms of declining mental status may evoke little concern for the person or the family, or may be viewed as the stigma of mental illness. Terms such as "worration" "spells," "nerves," "going off," and "not right in the head" may be used to explain the early stages of dementia (Advisory Panel on Alzheimer's's Disease, 1993; Ethnic Elders Care, 2012) and may help to explain why ethnically diverse adults and their families do not seek health care services until the middle or advanced stages of dementia.

This disparity is of increasing concern because the proportion of older Americans who are African American and Hispanic is projected to grow in coming years. If the current racial and ethnic disparities in diagnostic rates continue, the proportion of individuals with undiagnosed or late-stage diagnosis of dementia will increase.

HIV/AIDS

The CDC (2012a) estimated that about 56,000 people in the United States contracted the human immunodeficiency virus (HIV) in 2006. There are two types of HIV, HIV-1 and HIV-2. In the United States, unless otherwise noted, the term "HIV" primarily refers to HIV-1. Both types of HIV damage a person's body by destroying specific blood cells, called CD4+ T cells, which are crucial to helping the body fight diseases, but HIV-1 is considered to be the more virulent. Acquired immune deficiency syndrome, or AIDS, is the most severe manifestation of HIV. AIDS is the late stage of HIV infection, when a person's immune system is severely damaged and has difficulty fighting diseases and certain cancers (CDC, 2012b).

AIDS has been implicated in both dementia and strokes (Bedos et al., 1995; Cole et al., 2004; Gordon & Thompson, 1995). Once a disease that affected primarily gay white men, AIDS prevalence has risen significantly in heterosexual adult women and men. Approximately 1.1 million adults and adolescents are living with HIV infection in the United States, with 48,200 to 64,500 persons newly infected each year (CDC, 2011). The non-Hispanic gay white male population continues to comprise a substantial proportion of persons newly infected with HIV, but the proportion of HIV infections among racial/ethnic minorities and women has increased substantially.

In particular, African American men and women are estimated to have an HIV incidence rate 7 times that of non-Hispanic whites (CDC, 2005; CDC, 2011). In 2002, the AIDS diagnosis rate among African Americans was almost 11 times the rate among non-Hispanic whites. African American women had a 23 times greater diagnosis rate than non-Hispanic white women. African American men had almost a 9 times greater rate of AIDS diagnosis than non-Hispanic white men. In addition, the AIDS incidence per 100,000 population among Hispanics in 2000 was

22.5, more than 3 times the rate for non-Hispanic whites (National Institutes of Health, 2004). In 2010, African Americans accounted for 44% of the new HIV infections, followed by non-Hispanic whites (31%) and Hispanics/Latinos (21%) (CDC, 2012c). Additional estimates of AIDS prevalence come from the DHHS Office of Minority Health (2012):

◆ African American males have 7.6 times the AIDS rate as white males.
◆ African American women have almost 20 times the HIV rate as non-Hispanic white women.
◆ American Indian/Alaska Native women have 3 times the AIDS rate as non-Hispanic white women.
◆ Hispanic females have 4 times the AIDS rate as non-Hispanic white females.
◆ Native Hawaiian/Pacific Islanders are 2.2 times as likely to be diagnosed with AIDS as the non-Hispanic white population.

AIDS has become increasingly an area of concern for mature adults. HIV surveillance data show that 11% of all new HIV cases are being diagnosed in adults aged 50 and older (Wooten-Bielsky, 1999). Older adults are now contracting HIV from intravenous drug use as well as sexual contact (CDC, 2012d). Statistics also show that new AIDS cases rose faster in the over-40 population than in people aged 39 and under (CDC, 2011).

Impaired cognition and stroke are two of the major symptoms linked to AIDS diagnoses. Cognitive impairment occurs in 55% to 65% of people with AIDS affecting activities of daily living as well as concentration, memory, think-ing, language, emotional expression, social behavior, and the ability to focus on specific stimuli (Ziefert, Leary, & Boccellari, 1995). Cole and his associates (2004) observed that AIDS is highly correlated with both ischemic and intracerebral hemorrhagic strokes.

Disparities associated with HIV/AIDS among African Americans extend to access to HIV care and quality of care. African Americans with HIV are more likely to experience a 3-month delay in HIV diagnosis and access to HIV care than non-Hispanic whites. These disparities in access to HIV screening and care are attributed to social determinants and gaps in the health system. Disparities related to access to HIV screening and care are attributed to social stigma, health behaviors, higher levels of environmental stress, depression, and unemployment within the African American community. For African Americans, gaps in the health system also contribute to the disparities associated with HIV/AIDS due to lack of insurance, low income, lack of awareness of the Ryan White program, language and cultural barriers that impede access to prevention programs, and reduced geographic access to HIV care programs (CDC, 2005).

CHRONIC ALCOHOL ABUSE

Chronic alcohol abuse, defined as more than three or four drinks per day (depending on gender), is associated with permanent damage to the cerebrovascular system, organic brain syndrome, increased cardiovascular risks, and cognitive and memory impairment.

Results from an early study conducted in North Carolina suggest that the older alcoholic may be nonwhite, separated or divorced, with less than a high school education, lives with someone other than family, and demonstrates moderate to severe cognitive deficits. Feelings of loneliness and depression were directly related to increased drinking in older men and women (Blazer, George, Woodbury, Manton, & Jordan, 1984).

Nakamura and his colleagues (1990) studied the responses on alcohol consumption of Anglo-American, African American, and Mexican American non-institutionalized residents in San Diego, California. Respondents between the ages of 55 and 64 represented the largest proportion of the study sample. The results suggest that male, unmarried, early-onset drinkers are most likely to be severe abusers of alcohol in later life.

In urban areas in the United States, all ethnic minority groups experience a higher density of alcohol outlets compared with non-Hispanic whites (Romley, Cohen, Ringel, & Sturm, 2007). Recent data from the National Institute on Alcohol Abuse and Alcoholism (2006) show that current drinking is most prevalent among non-Hispanic white and Hispanic men and lowest for Asian American women. Alcohol use in adults age 18 or older is most prevalent for non-Hispanic whites (59.8%), lowest for Asian Americans (38.0%), and similar for Native Americans (i.e., American Indians and Alaska Natives; 47.8%), Hispanics (46.3%), and African Americans (43.8%). Native Americans have the highest prevalence (12.1%) of heavy drinking (i.e., five or more drinks on the same occasion for five or more of the past 30 days), followed by non-Hispanic whites (8.3%) and Hispanics (6.1%). A larger percentage of Native Americans (29.6%) also are binge drinkers, with somewhat lower percentages for non-Hispanic whites (25.9%), Hispanics (25.6%), and African Americans (21.4%).

Relative to other ethnic groups, the proportion of Asian Americans (2.7%) and blacks (4.7%) who are heavy drinkers and Asian Americans (13.3%) who are binge drinkers is low.

Among Hispanics, higher acculturation is associated with a greater risk for alcohol abuse (Caetano, Ramisetty-Mikler, & Rodriguez, 2009). In addition, social disadvantage, as defined by racial/ethnic stigma, may contribute to ethnic disparities in alcohol problems for Hispanics and African Americans (Mulia, Ye, Greenfield, & Zemore, 2009).

Chae and others (2008) found a greater risk for alcohol dependence for Asian American individuals who report experiences of unfair treatment and for individuals who indicate low ethnic identification but who experience racial/ethnic discrimination. Native Americans of both genders have the highest prevalence of weekly heavy drinking, whereas Hispanic men have the highest prevalence of daily heavy drinking.

Race and ethnicity are other factors to consider related to alcohol abuse in older adults. Native Americans, Asian, Hispanic, and African Americans have been reported to consume higher amounts of alcohol, placing these diverse populations at greater risk for a head injury and other acute and chronic disorders. Moreover, the level of bodily and head injury severity has been shown to be greater for certain racial ethnic groups including Asian, Hispanics, and African Americans (Sorani, Lee, Kim, Meeker, & Manley, 2009). These researchers also confirmed a higher mortality rate among African Americans and that Hispanics seemed to function slightly better than all other racial/ethnic groups at discharge (Sorani et al., 2009).

Both drinking and the development of alcohol-related problems are complex events with multiple causes. Ethnic groups in the United States, therefore, have to contend with a host of factors with the potential to have adverse effects on these behaviors. Immigrant groups must go through a process of acculturation to U.S. society that can lead to increased personal stress and tension within families. Together with African Americans and Native Americans, these groups also can face socioeconomic disadvantage and potential racial/ethnic discrimination. These two latter factors in turn often are associated with, for example, poor job opportunities, residential segregation, life in unsafe neighborhoods, overexposure to alcohol advertising, police profiling and brutality, and lack of access to adequate health care (Chartier & Caetano, 2010). According to the *2010 National Survey on Drug Use and Health* (Substance Abuse

and Mental Health Services Administration, 2011):

◆ Non-Hispanic whites in 2010 were more likely than other racial/ethnic groups to report current use of alcohol (56.7%) (Figure 1–2). The rates were 45.2% for persons reporting two or more races, 42.8% for blacks, 41.8% for Hispanics, 38.4% for Asians, and 36.6% for American Indians or Alaska Natives.

◆ The rates of alcohol dependence or abuse for the racial/ethnic groups in 2010 were similar to the rates in 2002 and 2009, except that among African Americans, aged 12 or older, the rate of alcohol dependence or abuse in 2010 (5.7%) was lower than

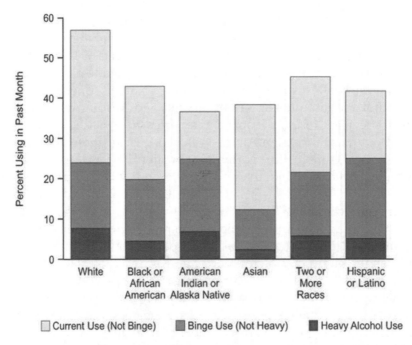

Figure 1–2. Current, binge, and heavy alcohol use among persons aged 12 or older, by race/ethnicity: 2010 (Substance Abuse and Mental Health Services Administration, 2011).

that in 2009 (7.0%) and in 2002 (7.1%).

◆ Moreover, among persons aged 18 or older who reported two or more races, the rate of substance dependence or abuse in 2010 (9.6%) was lower than that in 2009 (14.4%). See Figure 1–1 for alcohol use among persons 12 and older by race and ethnicity.

◆ The rate of binge alcohol use was lowest among Asians (12.4%). Rates for other racial/ethnic groups were 19.8% for blacks, 21.5% for persons reporting two or more races, 24.0% for whites, 24.7% for American Indians or Alaska Natives, and 25.1% for Hispanics. See Figure 1–2 for binge drinking and heavy alcohol use by race/ethnicity.

DRUG USE

An estimated 22.6 million Americans aged 12 or older were illicit drug users in 2010, meaning they had used an illicit drug during the month prior to the survey interview. This estimate represents 8.9% of the population aged 12 or older. Illicit drugs include marijuana/hashish, cocaine (including crack), heroin, hallucinogens, inhalants, or prescription-type psychotherapeutics used nonmedically. The most commonly used drug was marijuana (Substance Abuse and Mental Health Services Administration , 2011). See Figure 1–3 for prevalence of drug use by type.

Another drug, not mentioned above, that has serious negative consequences for long-term abusers, is methamphetamine. Twenty-one areas in the United

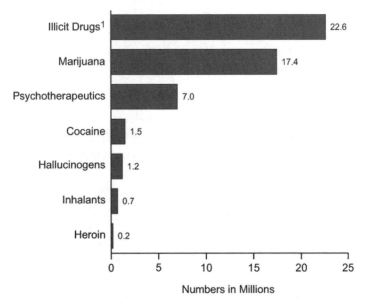

Figure 1–3. Drug abuse by drug type. Illicit drugs include marijuana/hashish, cocaine (including crack), heroin, hallucinogens, inhalants, or prescription-type psychotherapeutics used non-medically (Substance Abuse and Mental Health Services Administration, 2011).

States have been identified as areas of concern. Methamphetamine continues to be a problem in the West, with indicators persisting at high levels in Honolulu, San Diego, Seattle, San Francisco, and Los Angeles; and it continues to spread to other areas of the country, including both rural and urban sections of the South and Midwest. In fact, methamphetamine was reported to be the fastest growing problem in metropolitan Atlanta. According to the National Institute on Drug Abuse (2006), long-term methamphetamine users experience addiction, characterized by compulsive drug seeking and use. Addiction leads to functional and molecular changes in the brain. Abusers exhibit symptoms that can include anxiety, confusion, mood disturbances, and insomnia. They also can display a number of psychotic features, including paranoia, visual and auditory hallucinations, and delusions (for example, the sensation of insects creeping under the skin). Psychotic symptoms can sometimes last for months or years after methamphetamine abuse has ceased, and stress has been shown to precipitate spontaneous recurrence of methamphetamine psychosis in formerly psychotic methamphetamine abusers.

Chronic methamphetamine abuse also significantly changes the brain. Specifically, there are alterations in the activity of the dopamine system that are associated with reduced motor speed and impaired verbal learning. Recent studies on chronic methamphetamine abuse have also revealed severe structural and functional changes in areas of the brain associated with emotion and memory, which may account for many of the emotional and cognitive problems observed in chronic methamphetamine abusers. Although some of the effects of methamphetamine abuse appear to be somewhat reversible, some of the changes caused by this drug are extremely long lasting. Moreover, the increased risk for stroke from the abuse of methamphetamine can lead to irreversible damage to the brain.

Drug use has been associated with cerebrovascular accidents (Reeves, McMillan & Fitzgerald, 1995), seizure and movement disorders (Sloan et al., 1998), and cognitive decline (Enewoldson, 2004). The main illicit drugs associated with stroke are cocaine, amphetamines, Ecstasy, heroin/opiates, phencyclidine (PCP), lysergic acid diethylamide (LSD), and cannabis/marijuana (Esse, Fossati-Ballani, Traylor, & Martin-Schild, 2011). Most strokes tend to occur within an hour of use, especially for crack and intravenous cocaine, and most of the others within 3 hours. The surge in blood pressure is thought to blame for acute rupture. Resulting hemorrhages may be intracerebral (basal ganglia, thalamic, lobar, or brainstem), intraventricular, or subarachnoid. They may occur especially in individuals with pre-existing vascular malformations such as aneurysms and arteriovenous malformations (accounting for up to 50% of intracranial hemorrhage with cocaine). Any level of the nervous system may be affected, from the cortex to the neuromuscular junction (Enewoldson, 2004). Many drug users are polydrug users, and their drug use exposes them to neurological complications from HIV/AIDS, traumatic head injuries, and other medical problems.

Drug use varies by ethnic identity and age. In 2010, adults aged 26 or older were less likely to be current users of illicit drugs than youths aged 12 to 17 or young adults aged 18 to 25 (6.6 vs. 10.1 and 21.5%, respectively). As a group, African Americans reported more drug use, followed by non-Hispanic whites, Hispanics, Native Americans/Alaska Natives, and Asian Americans (Substance Abuse and Mental Health Services Administration, 2011). See Figure 1–4 for drug use by ethnicity and Figure 1–5 for drug use by age.

Issues with treatment for drug use include lack of health insurance, lack of transportation to treatment facilities, and an unreadiness to begin treatment. In addition, persons from ethnic groups report institutional barriers to treatment, such as inadequate referrals for treatment (Substance Abuse and Mental Health Services Administration, 2011).

For those aged 50 to 54, the rate increased from 3.4% in 2002 to 7.2% in 2010. Among those aged 55 to 59, current

illicit drug use increased from 1.9% in 2002 to 4.1% in 2010. These patterns and trends partially reflect the aging in these age groups of members of the baby boom cohort, whose rates of illicit drug use have been higher than those of older cohorts.

A major change in drug use is noted for adolescents. The annual *National Survey on Drug Use and Health* (Substance Abuse and Mental Health Services Administration, 2011) reported that 39% of non-Hispanic white teens between the ages of 12 and 17 admitted to using substances in the past year, compared with just 32% of African Americans and 24% of

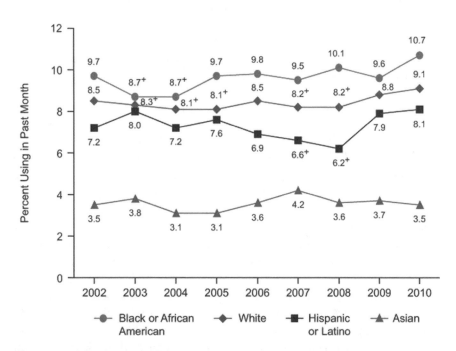

Figure 1–4. Past month illicit drug use among persons aged 12 or older, by race/ethnicity: 2002-2010. Sample sizes for American Indians or Alaska Natives and for persons of two or more races were too small for reliable trend presentation for these groups. Due to low precision, estimates for Native Hawaiians or Other Pacific Islanders are not shown. There were no statistically significant differences in the rate of current illicit drug use between 2009 and 2010 or between 2002 and 2010 for any of the racial/ethnic groups. However, there were significant increases in the rate for whites and Hispanics between 2008 and 2010. (Substance Abuse and Mental Health Services Administration, 2011)

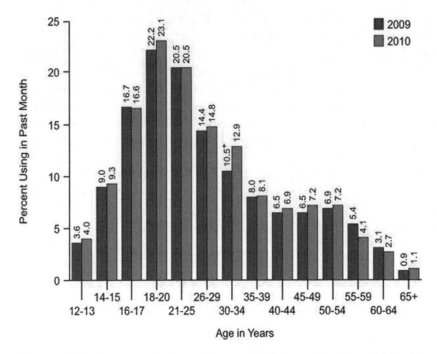

Figure 1–5. Drug use by age. *Source:* Substance Abuse and Mental Health Services Administration, 2011.

Asian Americans. This finding suggests that African American and Asian teenagers are less likely to use illegal drugs compared with their non-Hispanic white age cohorts. Hence, there may be a decrease in drug-related neurologic consequences among some ethnic adults over time. The downward trajectory in drug use among ethnic teens is encouraging because if the trend continues, there will be some ethnic adults who, in future, may not have drug-related health problems in general and neurologic complications from drug use in particular.

TRAUMATIC BRAIN INJURY

Traumatic brain injury (TBI) is an insult to the brain that is caused by an external force. Within the general popula-

tion, vehicular accidents, falls, and sport injuries are the most common sources of TBI. Interpersonal violence and industrial accidents and falls, however, may be far greater risk factors in TBIs for the most vulnerable persons in our society: those who live in low-income, high-crime communities, those who are homeless, and those who are incarcerated in the nation's prison system (Rosenthal & Ricker, 2000). Recent data from the CDC (2008) on the average number of hospitalizations by race indicate that African Americans have the highest incidence of TBI (74.1 per 100,000) compared with other racial/ethnic groups studied, including non-Hispanic whites (71.3 per 100,000) and American Indian/Alaska Native/Asian or Pacific Islanders, collectively (50.1 per 1000,000). Among this African American population, the highest incidence of TBI occurred in older adults (ages 65–74) at a rate of 96.5 per 100.000 (CDC, 2011).

Firearms (34.8%), motor-vehicle (31.4%), and fall-related TBIs (16.7%) were the leading causes of TBI-related death among individuals from nonwhite racial/ethnic groups. As a result, epidemiological studies have shown that members of minority racial/ethnic groups are at disproportionate risk of TBI (Bazarian, Pope, McClung, Cheng, & Flesher, 2003). Moreover, race- and ethnicity-based disparities in health care for persons with TBIs are well documented (Gary, Arango-Lasprilla, & Stevens, 2009; Shafi et al., 2007). These disparities have resulted in poorer outcomes following rehabilitation among at-risk racial/ethnic groups (O'Neill-Pirozzi et al., 2010; Strangeman et al., 2008).

Assaults are the second leading cause of head trauma (16%) in the general population (Barber & Webster, 1974; Desai et al, 1983; McCrary, 1992; Naugle, 1990). Head-injured patients in low-income communities are more likely to be older, have repeated head injuries, make low wages, or be unemployed. Nonwhite adults across the age spectrum in urban settings reveal a pattern of head injury that is unlike that of whites in terms of the frequencies of assault-related TBIs (McCrary, 1992).

In 2000, the nonfatal hospitalization rate for TBIs were 74 per 100,000 persons for African Americans, 76.3/100,000 for American Indian/Alaska Natives, and 62.9/100,000 for Anglo-Americans (Fau, Xu, Wald, & Coronado, 2010). The elevated rates are attributable in part to increased exposure to firearms and violence. It is likely that a combination of race and income places many persons at greatest risk because of hazardous or unsafe working conditions, assaults with firearms, and exposure to older, substandard housing and vehicles. Other causes of TBIs in multicultural populations are military injuries, homelessness, and incarceration.

Veterans With Traumatic Brain Injuries

The U.S. military is a multicultural organization with all races and ethnicities represented in all four branches of service. However, racial and ethnic disparities have been identified in veterans with head injuries (Egede, Dismukes, & Echols, 2012). From April 2007 through fiscal year 2009, 66,023 veterans were identified as possibly having a TBI through outpatient screening of individuals presenting to the VA for health care following deployment in Operation Enduring Freedom or Operation Iraqi Freedom. Of those identified through screening, 24,559 were confirmed to have sustained a TBI. Thirty-three percent of all patients with combat-related injuries and 60% of the patients with blast-related injuries seen at Walter Reed Army Medical Center had sustained a TBI (Okie, 2005). Additionally, a recent study of the Navy-Marine Corps Combat Trauma Registry revealed that battle-injured personnel were more likely than those injured outside of battle to have multiple TBIs (Galarneau, Woodruff, Dye, Mohrle, & Wade, 2008).

Many military personnel detailed to wars in Iraq (Operation Iraqi Freedom) and Afghanistan (Operation Enduring Freedom) in particular have been subjected to multi-blast missile injuries. Wallace (2006) defines blast injury as injury from barotraumas (increase or decrease of normal atmospheric pressure) due to detonated devices or weapons, such as rocket-propelled grenades, improvised explosive devices, projectiles, and land mines. Injuries can also come from the impact of blast-energized debris (penetrating and nonpenetrating), such as bomb fragments and related structural collapse, or from an individual's bodily displacement caused by the blast wind (Mashima, 2010).

Homelessness and TBI

A relationship between homelessness and TBI has been identified. Homelessness affects people of all ages and ethnicities. According to the U.S. Department of Housing and Urban Development's Annual Homeless Assessment Report to Congress (2012), on a given night in January 2010, 407,966 individuals were homeless in shelters, transitional housing programs, or on the streets (this number does not include persons in family households) and 109,812 individuals were chronically homeless, a 1% decrease from the previous year. Over 50% of those persons were African American, Hispanic, and other single or multiple races. Among all sheltered individuals over the course of a year (October 2009–September 2010), 62% were male and 38% were female. Approximately 45.3% were under age 30; 54.7% were over age 31. While 41.6% were classified as white, non-Hispanic, 58.4% were African American, Hispanic, other races, and multiple races. An estimated 19% of the persons sheltered had hypertension. A significant finding is that homelessness also affects veterans living in poverty. Of those, About one in four Hispanic and African American veterans living in poverty became homeless (Current Statistics on the Prevalence and Characteristics of People Experiencing Homelessness in the United States, 2011).

Examining TBI as a causal effect in homelessness, Solliday-McRoy, Campbell, Melchert, Young, and Cisler (2004) conducted a study involving 90 homeless men. Eighty percent were found to have cognitive impairment. Another report on homelessness and TBI provides data on over 3,000 comprehensive psychiatric evaluations of persons experiencing homelessness. At least one-half of those evaluated reported histories of blows to the head sustained as the result of childhood physical abuse or motor vehicle crashes, falls, or sporting injuries (Highley, 2008). While not described in this report, it is likely that the homeless are also victims of interpersonal violence and TBI after becoming homeless.

Incarceration and TBI

There is also a correlation between incarceration and TBIs. African Americans and Hispanics are disproportionately represented in the prison system in the United States. At the end of 2005, there were 1,525,924 persons incarcerated in state and federal prisons; 40% of these inmates were African Americans, 35% were non-Hispanic whites, and 20% were Hispanics (Harrison & Beck, 2006). Hence, African Americans comprise about 12% of the U.S. population but two-fifths of the prison population.

The disparities are even more dramatic for males, and particularly for males in their twenties and thirties. In 2005, 8.1% of all African American males age 25 to 29 were in prison, compared with 2.6% of Hispanic males and 1.1% of white males. Although the absolute numbers are much smaller, the pattern for females is similar (Garland, Spohn, & Wodahl, 2008).

The CDC (2011) found that 25%–87% of inmates report having experienced a head injury or TBI compared with 8.5% in the general population. As noted in another study regarding the prevalence in correctional facilities, TBI can make adjustment to prison life difficult and can prevent offenders from successfully reentering communities upon release (Hagelson, 2010).

SUMMARY AND RECOMMENDATIONS

Health disparities are major concerns for all health practitioners and researchers and the focus of national attention. Ethnic minorities are disproportionately represented in prevalence data for hypertension, diabetes, stroke and stroke complications, AIDS, dementia, alcohol abuse, and TBIs. Ethnic minorities are also most likely to live and/or work in hazardous conditions, to become homeless, or to be incarcerated. Finally, health care in all dimensions has been uneven to persons who have health disparities. The National Healthcare Disparities Report (Agency for Healthcare Research and Quality, 2010, pp. 2 and 4) highlights specific key issues that require immediate attention from all health care professionals: (1) Health care and access are suboptimal especially for minority and low-income groups; (2) health disparities are not improving despite improvement in health care quality; and (3) certain services, geographic areas, and populations are in need of urgent attention.

The implications are clear: speech-language pathologists should anticipate that assessment and intervention will be administered to an increasingly diverse adult patient population with respect to age, income, education, primary and secondary diagnoses, previous health status, languages spoken in the home, and experiences with the health care system.

Of particular concern will be that patients may be more severely involved at younger ages, may present with a slower recovery rate from acute conditions or more severe chronic conditions, and may require a level of cultural competency necessary to provide sensitive and appropriate speech-language pathology services.

Although varying in magnitude by many clinical conditions and populations, disparities across many care environments are observed in almost all aspects of health care, such as quality of health care, access to care, and levels and types of care (Agency for Healthcare Research and Quality, 2004, 2007). The National Report on Healthcare Disparities (2010, p. 4) goes further to point out that disparities in quality of care are common. Several groups receive worse care than non-Hispanic whites, specifically adults over age 65, African Americans, Asians, American Indians and Alaska Natives, Hispanics, and the poor.

For many persons of color and particularly those who are low-income, participation in the speech-language therapy process may be challenging. Non-Hispanic whites are more likely to participate in all levels of evaluations and treatment, including preventive care, routine office visits, rehabilitation hospitals and clinics, and support organizations for patients and their families. They are also less likely to underutilize health services because of cost or because their health plans do not cover services.

Non-Hispanic whites and ethnic persons of color are most distinguished by their level of comfort with the health care system. Nonwhite ethnic individuals underutilize all types of health services and support groups in large cities. Financial issues are certainly prevalent in many communities of color, but elders of color often prefer informal, home, or community-based approaches to assessment and healing (Payne, 1997).

Barriers to use of health care services, including speech-language pathology, may be reflective of distrust of Western health care, perceptions of institutional racism, language and literacy differences, cultural variation in health beliefs, and physical barriers, including financial constraints and service accessibility. According to the National Report on Healthcare Disparities (Agency for Healthcare Research and Quality, 2010), these barriers still pervade the American health care system.

In light of the impact of a changing demography over the next 30 years, new legislation to reform the American health care system that will provide greater access for the underserved to primary and rehabilitative care, the aging of Americans, and the persistence of health disparities for diseases and conditions that impair language and cognition in adults, the following recommendations seem appropriate:

1. Greater emphasis needs to be placed in the academy on multicultural infusion in all speech-language pathology curricula, including case studies and instruction in effective interpersonal communication in the clinical setting.
2. Research is needed to measure whether those affected by health disparities are being adequately served by speech-language pathologists, and if not, what workforce priorities should be in place over the next 20 to 50 years to meet their needs.
3. Research is also needed to examine the appropriateness of standardized tests and measurements in the areas of syntax and morphology for

an increasingly diverse adult patient population.
4. Research is needed to develop innovative ways to assess and treat a diverse adult patient, such as revising existing tests, including translations of existing tests in more than one language, developing new protocols for informal assessments, and establishing new norms based upon accurate and changing percentages of ethnic older adults in field test data.
5. Finally, research is needed to investigate the efficacy of treatment procedures, including augmentative alternative communication, for an increasingly diverse adult patient population.

STUDY QUESTIONS

1. What law, enacted in 2010, will allow greater access to health care for adults who have been uninsured or underinsured?

2. Which Institute at the National Institutes of Health is dedicated to generating new knowledge about health disparities?

3. What are the population projections for older U.S. citizens by the year 2050? What is meant by the statement that the "terms majority and minority will be meaningless"?

4. What is the definition of a health disparity population?

5. What factors have caused health disparities among some groups in this country?

6. What are the issues for incorporating multicultural education into

speech-language pathology curricula presently?

7. Why should speech-language pathologists understand health disparities, health reform, and the changing demography in the United States?

8. Why should culturally competent services be increasingly mportant for speech-language pathologists in the next 10 to 40 years?

9. Which ethnic groups are most at risk for hypertension and diabetes?

10. Which ethnic groups have the highest prevalence of stroke?

11. How are hypertension and stroke implicated in dementia?

12. Who is most likely to have a cavernous venous malformation (CVM)? What are the consequences of CVM?

13. In what ways are non-Hispanic whites and other ethnic groups different in the types of stroke and cardiovascular disease?

14. Which ethnic group has the highest prevalence of alcoholism?

15. How has the prevalence of AIDS changed in this country? Which groups are now at risk?

16. How does AIDS affect neurologic status?

17. What are the prevalence data on Alzheimer's disease for ethnic older persons?

18. What are the major causes of traumatic brain injury (TBI) among ethnic older persons?

19. Who is likely to be homeless? How is TBI implicated in homelessness?

20. What is a missile blast injury? How is this injury related to returning veterans?

21. Which ethnic groups are most likely to be incarcerated? How is TBI a factor in incarceration?

22. What issues in health care still pervade the health care system for ethnic adults?

23. How are the issues in health disparities relevant for speech-language pathologists?

24. What are some of the research issues that still need to be addressed if speech-language pathologists are to provide optimal care for a diverse patient population with neurogenic language disorders?

25. Is there a dearth of information in the journals for the profession about health disparities? Why?

26. What are some of the barriers to the use of health care services?

27. How is drug use related to stroke?

28. What are some other health-related problems that drug users might have?

29. Why has drug use among mature adults increased?

30. Which ethnic adolescents are less likely to use drugs?

31. What are reported barriers to drug and alcohol treatment for persons from ethnic communities?

REFERENCES

Advisory Panel on Alzheimer's Disease. (1993). *Fourth report of the advisory panel on Alzheimer's disease.* 1992 (NIH Pub, No. 93-3520). Washington, DC: U.S. Government Printing Office.

Agency for Healthcare Research and Quality. (2004). *National Healthcare Disparities Report: Summary.* Rockville, MD: Author. Retrieved from http://www.ahrq.gov/qual/nhdr03/nhdrsum03.htm

Agency for Healthcare Research and Quality. (2007). *Key themes and highlights from the National Healthcare Disparities Report.* Rockville, MD: Author.

Agency for Healthcare Research and Quality. (2010). *National Healthcare Disparities Report.* Retrieved from http://www.ahrq.gov/research/findings/nhqrdr/nhdr10/pdf/nhdr10.pdf

Aggarwal, N. T., Schneider, J. A., Wilson, R. S., Beck, T. L., Evans, D. A., & De Carli, C. (2012). Characteristics of MR infarcts associated with dementia and cognitive function in the elderly. *Neuroepidemiology, 38,* 41–47.

American Diabetes Association. (2013). Facts about diabetes. Retrieved from http://www.diabetes.org/diabetes-basics/type-2/facts-about-type-2.html

American Heart Association. (2007). Heart disease and stroke statistics 2007 update. *Circulation, 115,* e69–e171. Retrieved from http://circ.ahajournals.org/gci/content/full/CIRCULATIONAHA.106.179918

American Speech-Language-Hearing Association. (2011a). *Cultural competence in professional service delivery* [Position statement]. Retrieved from http://www.asha.org/policy

American Speech-Language-Hearing Association. (2005). *Cultural competence* [Issues in Ethics]. Retrieved from http://www.asha.org/policy

American Speech-Language-Hearing Association. (2011b). *Current status of SLP employment in health care settings.* Retrieved from http://www.asha.org/careers/recruitment/healthcare/recruit_current

American Speech-Language-Hearing Association. (2011c). *2011 membership survey. CCC-SLP survey summary report: Number and type of responses.* Retrieved from http://www.asha.org

American Speech-Language-Hearing Association. (2011d). *SLP Health Care Survey Report: Workforce trends 2005–2011.* Retrieved from http://www.asha.org

American Speech-Language-Hearing Association. (2012). *ASHA Changing Health Care Landscape Summit (Executive summary).* Retrieved from http://www.asha.org/uploadedFiles/ASHA/Practice/Health-Care-Reform/Healthcare-Summit-Executive-Summary-2012.pdf#search=%22Changing%22

American Stroke Association. *Statistical Fact Sheets* (2011). Retrieved from http://www.strokeassociation.org.presenter.jhtml?identifier=2011

Annual Homeless Assessment Report to Congress. (2012). Retrieved from http://www.in.gov/ihcda/files/2010HomelessAssessmentReport.pdf

Barber, J. B., & Webster, J. C. (1974). Head injuries: Review of 150 cases. *Journal of the National Medical Association, 66,* 201–204.

Barnes, P. M., Adams, P. F., & Powell-Griner, E. (2010). *Health characteristics of the American Indian or Alaska Native adult population: United States, 2004–2008. Centers for Disease Control and Prevention.* Retrieved from http://www.cdc.gov/nchs/data/nhsr/nhsr020.pdf

Bazarian, J. J., Pope, C., McClung, J., Cheng, Y. T., & Flesher, W. (2003) Ethnic and racial disparities in emergency department care for mild traumatic brain injury. *Academic Emergency Medicine, 10,* 1209–1217.

Bedos, J-P., Chastang, C., Lucet, J-C., Kalo, T., Gachot, B., & Wolff, M. (1995). Early predictors of outcome for HIV patients with neurological failure. *Journal of the American Medical Association, 273,* 35–40.

Berges, I. M., Kuo, Y. F., Ottenbacher, K. J., Seale, G. S., & Ostir, G. V. (2012). Recovery of functional status after stroke in a tri-ethnic population. *PM&R: The Journal of Injury, Function and Rehabilitation, 4,* 290–295. doi:10.1016/j.pmrj.2012.01.010

Bernard, M. A. (1993). Health status of African American elderly. *Journal of the National Medical Association, 85,* 521–528.

Blazer, D., George, L., Woodbury, M., Manton, K., & Jordan K. (1984). The elderly alcoholic: A profile. In G. Maddox, L. Robbins, & N. Rosenberg (Eds.), *Nature and extent of alcohol problems among the elderly* (pp. 275–297). New York, NY: Springer.

Brondolo, E., Love, E. E., Pencille, M., Schoenthaler, A., & Ogedegbe, G. (2011). Racism and hypertension: a review of the empirical evidence and implications for clinical practice. *American Journal of Hypertension, 24,* 518–529.

Bruno, A., & Qualls, C. (1994). Clinical features of ischemic stroke in Hispanics and non-Hispanic whites in New Mexico: A study of

341 consecutive patients at two hospitals. *Ethnic Disorders, 4,* 77–81.

Bruns, J., & Hauser, W. A. (2003). The epidemiology of traumatic brain injury: A review. *Epilepsia, 44,* 2–10.

Caesar, L. G., & Williams, D. R. (2002, April 2). Socioculture and the delivery of health care: Who gets what and why. *The ASHA Leader.*

Caetano, R., Ramisetty-Mikler, S., & Rodriguez, L. A. (2009). The Hispanic Americans Baseline Alcohol Survey (HABLAS): The association between birthplace, acculturation and alcohol abuse and dependence across Hispanic national groups. *Drug and Alcohol Dependence 99,* 215–221.

Caplan, L. R. (1994). Neurologic management plan. In M. N. Ozer, R. S. Materson, & L. R. Caplan (Eds.), *Management of persons with stroke* (pp. 61–113). St. Louis, MO: Mosby.

Caplan, L. R., Gorelick, P. B., & Hier. D. B. (1986). Race, sex, and occlusive vascular disease: A review. *Stroke, 14,* 530.

Carlson, E. D., & Chamberlain, R. M. (2004). The black-white perception gap and health disparities research. *Public Health Nursing, 21,* 372–379.

Centers for Disease Control and Prevention. (2007). *HIV/AIDS Surveillance Report, 2005.* Vol. 17. Revised. Atlanta, GA: U.S. Department of Health and Human Services, CDC; pp. 1–54.

Centers for Disease Control and Prevention. (2008). *Health, United States, 2008.* Hyattsville, MD: National Center for Health Statistics.

Centers for Disease Control and Prevention. (2011). *Summary Health Statistics for U.S. Adults: 2010. Table 2.* Retrieved from http://www.cdc.gov/nchs/data/series/sr_10/sr10_252.pdf

Centers for Disease Control and Prevention. (2012a). *Defining overweight and obesity.* Retrieved from http://www.cdc.gov/obesity/adult/defining.html

Centers for Disease Control and Prevention. (2012b). Estimated HIV incidence in the United States, 2007–2010. *HIV surveillance supplemental report, 17* (No. 4). Retrieved from http://www.cdc.gov/hiv/topics/surveillance/resources/reports/#supplemental

Centers for Disease Control and Prevention. (2012c). *Basic information about HIV and AIDS.* Retrieved from http://www.cdc.gov/hiv/topics/basic/index.htm

Chae, D. H., Takeuchi, D. T., Barbeau, E. M., Bennett, G. G., Lindsey, J. C., Stoddard, A. M., &

Krieger, N. (2008). Alcohol disorders among Asian Americans: Associations with unfair treatment, racial/ethnic discrimination, and ethnic identification (the national Latino and Asian Americans study, 2002–2003). *Journal of Epidemiology and Community Health 62,* 973–979.

Chartier, K., & Caetano, R. (2010). Ethnicity and health disparities in alcohol research. *Alcohol Research and Health, 33,* 152–160.

Cole, J. W., Pinto, A. N., Hebel, J. R., Buchholz, D. W., Earley, C. J., Johnson, C. J., . . . Kittner, S. J. (2004). Acquired immunodeficiency syndrome and the risk of stroke. *Stroke, 35,* 51–56.

Cornett, B. S. (2010, August 3). *Health care reform and speech-language pathology practice.* Retrieved from http://www.asha.org/Publications/leader/2010/100803/Health-Care-Reform-SLP.htm

Current statistics on the prevalence and characteristics of people experiencing homelessness in the United States, 2011. Retrieved from http://homeless.samhsa.gov/ResourceFiles/hrc_factsheet.pdf

Dashti, S. R., Hoffer, A., Hu, Y. C., & Selman, W. R. (2006). Molecular genetics of familial cerebral cavernous malformations. *Neurosurgical Focus, 15,* e2.

De Arellano, A. R. (1994). The elderly. In C. W. Molina & M. Aguirre-Molina (Eds.), *Latino health in the U.S.: A growing challenge* (pp. 189–206). Washington, DC: American Public Health Association.

Demirovic, J., Prineas, R., Loewenstein, D., Bean, J., Duara, R., Sevush, S., & Szapocznik, J. (2003). Prevalence of dementia in three ethnic groups: The South Florida program on aging and health. *Annals of Epidemiology, 13,* 472–478.

Department of Health and Human Services, Office of Minority Health. (2001, March). *National standards for culturally and linguistically appropriate services in health care, executive summary.* Washington, DC: U.S. Government Printing Office.

Department of Health and Human Services, Agency for Healthcare Research and Quality. (2007). *Key themes and highlights from the national healthcare disparities report.* Rockville, MD: Author.

Department of Health and Human Services, Office of Minority Health. (2008). *Cultural competence.* Retrieved June 8, 2010, from http://www.minorityhealth.hhs.gov

Department of Health and Human Services, Office of Minority Health (2011a). *National partnership for action*: *HHS action plan to reduce racial and ethnic health disparities*. Retrieved from http://minorityhealth.hhs.gov/npa

Department of Health and Human Services, Office of Minority Health. (2011b). *The national stakeholder strategy for achieving health equity*. Retrieved from http://minorityhealth.hhs.gov/npa

Department of Health and Human Services. (2011, April). *HHS action plan to reduce racial and ethnic disparities: A nation free of disparities in health and health care*. Washington, DC: Author.

Department of Health and Human Services, Agency for Healthcare Research and Quality. (2012). *National healthcare disparities report*. Retrieved from http://www.ahrq.gov/research/findings/nhqrdr/nhdr12/nhdr12_prov.pdf

Department of Health and Human Services, Office of Minority Health. (2012). *HIV/AIDS data and statistics*. Retrieved from http://www.minorityhealth.hhs.gov

Desai, B. T., Whitman, S., Coonley-Hoganson, R., Coleman, T. E., Gabriel, G., & Dell, J. (1983). Urban head injury: A clinical series. *Journal of the National Medical Association, 75*, 875–881.

Egede, L. E., Dismuke, C., & Echols, C. (2012).. Racial/ethnic disparities in mortality risk among US veterans with traumatic brain injury. *American Journal of Public Health, 102* (Suppl. 2), S266–S271.

Ellis, C. (2009). Does race/ethnicity really matter in adult neurogenics? *American Journal of Speech-Language Pathology, 18*, 310–314.

Enevoldson, T. P. (2004). Recreational drugs and their neurological consequences. *Neurology, Neurosurgery, and Psychiatry, 75*, iii9–iii15. doi:10.1136/jnnp.2004.045732

Esse, K., Fossati-Bellani, M., Traylor, A., & Martin-Schild, S. (2011). Epidemic of illicit drug use, mechanisms of action/addiction and stroke as a health hazard. *Brain and Behavior, 1*, 44–54. doi:10.1002/brb3.7

Ethnic Elders Care. (2012). *African Americans and dementia*. Retrieved from http://www.ethnicelderscare.net/ethnicity&dementiaA.htm

Fau, M., Xu, L., Wald, M. M., & Coronado, V. G. (2010). *Traumatic brain injury in the United States: Emergency department visits, hospitalizations and deaths 2002–2006*. Atlanta, GA: Centers for Disease Control and Prevention, National Center for Injury Prevention and Control.

Federation of American Societies for Experimental Biology. (2010, April 26). Predicting risk for high blood pressure: Factors of hormone metabolism that may make African-Americans more susceptible. *Science Daily*. Retrieved from http://www.sciencedaily.com/releases/2010/04/100426113102.htm

Feldman, E., Daneault, J., Kwan, E., Ho, K. J., Pessin, M. S., Lagenberg, P., & Caplan, L. R. (1990). Chinese-white differences in the distribution of occlusive cerebrovascular disease, *Neurology, 40*, 1541–1545.

Galarneau, M. R., Woodruff, S. I., Dye, J. L., Mohrle, C. R., & Wade, A. L. (2008). Traumatic brain injury during Operation Iraqi Freedom: Findings from the United States Navy-Marine Corps Combat Trauma Registry. *Journal of Neurosurgery, 108*, 950–957.

Galloway, J. M. (2005). Cardiovascular health among American Indians and Alaska Natives: Successes, challenges, and potentials. *American Journal of Preventive Medicine, 29*, 11–17.

Garland, B. E., Spohn, C., & Wodahl, E. J. (2008, Fall). Racial disproportionality in the American prison population: Using the Blumstein method to address the critical race and justice issue of the 21st century. *Justice Policy Journal, 5*, 4–5.

Gary, K. W., Arango-Lasprilla, J. C., & Stevens, L. F. (2009). Do racial/ethnic differences exist in post-injury outcomes after TBI? A comprehensive review of the literature. *Brain Injury, 10*, 775–789.

Gault, J., Sain, S., Hu, L. J., & Awad, I. A. (2006) Spectrum of genotype and clinical manifestations in cerebral cavernous malformations. *Neurosurgery, 67*, 1890–1892.

Gordon, S. M., & Thompson, S. (1995). The changing epidemiology of human immunodeficiency infection in older persons. *Journal of the American Geriatric Society, 43*, 7–9.

Gorelick, P. B., Freels, S., Harris, Y., Dollear, T., Billingsley, M., & Brown, N. (1994). Epidemiology of vascular and Alzheimer's dementia among African Americans in Chicago, IL: Baseline frequency and comparison of risk factors. *Neurology, 44*, 1391–1396.

Graham, K. J. (2003, March 4). *Focus on minority health*. Retrieved from http://www.asha.org/Publications/leader/2003/030304/030304h.htm

Gresham, C. E., Duncan, P. W., Stason, W. B., Adams, J. H. P., Adelman, A. M., Alexander, D. N., . . . Trombly, C. A. (1995). *Post-stroke rehabilitation: Clinical practice guidelines*. No. 16. Public Health Service Agency for Health Care Policy and Research (AHCPR Publication No. 95-0662). Rockville, MD: U.S. Department of Health and Human Services.

Gunel, M., Awad, I. A., Finberg, K., Anson, J. A., Steinberg, G. K., Batjer, H. H., . . . Lifton, R. P. (1996). A founder mutation as a cause of cerebral cavernous malformation in Hispanic Americans. *New England Journal of Medicine, 334*, 946–951.

Gurland, B., Wilder, D., Lantigua, R., Stern, Y., Chen, J., Killeffer, E. H., & Mayeux, R. (1999). Rates of dementia in three ethno racial groups. *International Journal of Geriatric Psychiatry, 14*, 481–493.

Hagelson, S. R. (2010). Identifying brain injury in state juvenile justice, corrections and homeless populations: Challenges and promising practices. *Brain Injury Professional, 7*, 18–21.

Hammer, C. S. (2012). Do demographic and cultural differences exist in adulthood? *American Journal of Speech-Language Pathology, 21*, 181–182.

Harrison, P. M., & Beck, A. J. (2006). *Prisoners in 2005*. Washington, DC: U.S. Department of Justice.

Havens, L. A. (2012, July 31). The health care ruling and you. *The ASHA Leader, 17*, 1–3.

Hayes, D. K., Greenlund, K. J., Denny, C. H., Keenan, N. L., & Croft J. B. (2005). Racial/ethnic and socioeconomic disparities in multiple risk factors for heart disease and stroke United States, 2003. *Morbidity and Mortality Weekly Report, 54*, 113–116.

He, J., Klang, M. J., Wu, Z., & Whelton, P. K. (1995). Stroke in the People's Republic of China, I: Geographic variations in incidence and risk factors. *Stroke, 26*, 2222–2227.

Healthy People 2010. (2000). *Understanding and improving health* (2nd ed.). Washington, DC: U.S. Department of Health and Human Services.

Healthy People 2020. (2010, July 26). *An opportunity to address the societal determinants of health in the United States*. Secretary's Advisory Committee on Health Promotion and Disease Prevention Objectives for 2020. Retrieved from http://www.healthypeople.gov/2010/hp2020/advisory/SocietalDeterminantsHealth.htm.

Highley J. L. (2008). *Traumatic brain injury among homeless persons: Etiology, prevalence and severity*. Nashville, TN: Health Care for the Homeless Clinicians' Network, National Health Care for the Homeless Council.

Hinojosa, M. S., Rittman, M., Hinojosa, R., & Rodriguez, W. (2009). Racial/ethnic variation in recovery of motor function in stroke survivors: Role of informal caregivers. *Journal of Rehabilitation Research and Development, 46*, 223–232.

Horner, R. C., Matchar, D. B., Divine, G. W., & Feussner, J. R. (1991). Racial variations in ischemic stroke-related physical and functional impairments. *Stroke, 22*, 1497–1501.

Horner, R. D., Swanson, J. W., Bosworth, H. B., & Matchar, D. B. (2003). Effects of race and poverty on the process and outcome of inpatient rehabilitation services among stroke patients. *Stroke, 34*, 1027–1031.

Horton-Ikard, R., Munoz, M. L., Thomas-Tate, S., & Keller-Bell, Y. (2009). Establishing a pedagogical framework for the multicultural course in communication sciences and disorders. *American Journal of Speech-Language Pathology, 18*, 182–196.

Kell, J. E., Gazes, P. C., Sutherland, S. E., Rust, P. F., Branch, L. G., & Tyroler, H. A. (1989). Predictors of physical disability in elderly black and whites of the Charleston heart study. *Journal of Clinical Epidemiology, 42*, 621–629.

Keppel, K., Pearcy, J., & Wagener, D. (2001). Trends in racial and ethnic-specific rates for the health status indicators: United States, 1990-98. *Statistical Notes, 23*, 1–16.

Kissela, B., Schneider, A., Kleindorfer, D., Khoury, J., Miller R., Alwell K., . . . Broderick, J. (2004). Stroke in a biracial population: The excess burden of stroke among blacks. *Stroke, 35*, 426–431.

Kraus, J. F., & McArthur, D. L. (1996). Epidemiologic aspects of brain injury. *Neurology Clinic, 14*, 435–450.

Liao, Y., Greenlund, K. J., Croft, J. B., Keenan, N. L., & Giles, W. H. (2009). Factors explaining excess stroke prevalence in the US stroke belt. *Stroke, 40*, 3336–3341. doi:10.1161/STROKEAHA.109.561688

Lloyd-Jones, D., Adams, R. J., Brown, T., Carnethon, M., Dai, S., De Simone, G., & Wylie-Rosett, J. (2010). Heart disease and stroke statistics 2010 update. *Circulation, 121*, e46–e215.

Luchsinger, J. A., Tang, M. X., Stern, Y., Shea, S., & Mayeux, R. (2001). Diabetes mellitus and risk of Alzheimer's disease and dementia with stroke in a multiethnic cohort. *American Journal of Epidemiology, 154,* 635–641.

Manley, J., & Mayeux, R. (2004). Ethnic differences in dementia and Alzheimer's disease. National Research Council (US) Panel on Race, Ethnicity, and Health in Later Life. In N. B. Anderson, R. A. Bulatao, & B. Cohen (Eds.), *Critical perspectives on racial and ethnic differences in health in late life.* Washington, DC: National Academies Press. Retrieved from http://www.ncbi.nlm.nih.gov/books/NBK25532

Marchuk, D. A., Gallione, C. J., Morrison, L. A., Clericuzio, C. L., Hart, B. L., Kosofsky, B. E., . . . Prenger, V. L. (1995). A locus for cerebral cavernous malformations maps to chromosome 7q in two families. *Genomics, 20,* 311–314.

Mashima, P. A. (2010, November 2). *Using telehealth to treat combat-related traumatic brain injury.* Retrieved from http://www.asha.org/Publications/leader/2010/101102/Using-Telehealth-to-Treat-Combat-Related-Traumatic-Brain-Injury.htm

McCrary, M. (1992). Urban, multicultural trauma patients. *ASHA, 34,* 37–40.

Miles, T. P., & Bernard, M. A. (1992). Morbidity, disability, and health status of black American elderly: A new look at the oldest old. *Journal of the American Geriatric Society, 40,* 1047–1054.

Morgenstern, L. B., Smith, M. A., Lisabeth, L. D., Risser, J. M. H., Uchino, K., Garcia, N., . . . Moye, L. A. (2004). Excess stroke in Mexican Americans compared with non-Hispanic whites. *American Journal of Epidemiology, 160,* 376–383.

Mulia, N., Ye, Y., Greenfield, T. K., & Zemore, S. E. (2009). Disparities in alcohol-related problems among white, black, and Hispanic Americans. *Alcoholism: Clinical and Experimental Research, 33,* 654–662.

Nakamura, C. M., Molgaard, C. A., Stanford, E. P., Peddecord, K. M., Morton, D. J., Lockery, S. A., . . . Gardner, S. A. (1990). A discriminant analysis of severe alcohol consumption among older persons. *Alcohol & Alcoholism, 25,* 75–80.

National Institute on Alcohol Abuse and Alcoholism. (2006). *Alcohol use and alcohol use disorders in the United States: Main findings from the 2001–2002 National Epidemiologic Survey on Alcohol and Related Conditions (NESARC).*

Vol. 8. Bethesda, MD: National Institutes of Health.

National Institute on Drug Abuse. (2006). *Methamphetamines: Abuse and addiction.* Retrieved from http://www.drugabuse.gov/publications/research-reports/methamphetamine-abuse-addiction/what-scope-methamphetamine-abuse-in-united-states

National Institutes of Health. (2002). National Center on Minority Health and Health Disparities. *Strategic research plan and budget to reduce and ultimately eliminate health disparities,Volume I, Fiscal Years 2002–2006.* Bethesda, MD: Author.

National Institutes of Health. (2004). *Strategic plan fiscal years 2004-2008.* U.S. Department Of Health and Human Services NIH Health Disparities. Vol. I. Bethesda, MD: Author.

Naugle, R. I. (1990). Epidemiology of traumatic brain injury in adults. In E. D. Bigler (Ed.), *Traumatic brain injury: Mechanisms of damage, assessment, intervention, and outcome* (pp. 69–106). Austin, TX: Pro-Ed.

Okie, S. (2005). Traumatic brain injury in the war zone. *New England Journal of Medicine, 352,* 2043–2047.

O'Neil-Pirozzi, T. M., Strangman, G. E., Goldstein, R., Katz, D. I., Savage, C. R., Kelkar, K., . . . Glenn, M. B. (2010). A controlled treatment study of internal memory strategies (I-MEMS) following traumatic brain injury. *Journal of Head Trauma Rehabilitation, 25,* 43–51.

Payne, J. C. (1997). *Adult neurogenic language disorders: Assessment and treatment. An ethnobiological approach.* San Diego, CA: Singular.

Payne, J. C. (2011, November 1). *Cultural competence in treatment of adults with cognitive and language disorders.* Retrieved from http://www.asha.org/Publications/leader/2011/111101/Cultural-Competence-in-Treatment-of-Adults-with-Cognitive-and-Language-Disorders.htm

Payne, J. C., & Stroman, C. (2004). Communication disorders in African Americans. In I. Livingstone (Ed.), *Handbook of black American health: Policies and issues behind disparities in health.* Westport, CT: Greenwood Press.

Pinsky, J. L., Branch, L. G., Jette, A. M., Haynes, S. G., Feinleib, M., Coroni-Huntley, J. C., & Bailey, K. R. (1985). Framingham disability study: Relationship of cardiovascular risk factors among persons free of diagnosed cerebrovascular disease. *American Journal of Epidemiology, 122,* 644–656.

Quiñones, A. R., Liang, J., & Ye, W. (2012). Racial and ethnic differences in hypertension risk: New diagnoses after age 50. *Ethnicity & Disease, 22,* 175–180.

Reeves, R. R., McWilliams, M. E., & Fitz-Gerald, M. (1995). Cocaine-induced ischemic, cerebral infarction mistaken for a psychiatric syndrome. *Southern Medical Journal, 88,* 352–354.

Rhoades, E. R. (1996). American Indians and Alaska Natives—overview of the population. *Public Health Reports, 111*(Suppl. 1), 49–50.

Richardson, A., Liao, Y., & Tucker, P. (2005). *Regional and racial differences in prevalence of stroke—23 states and District of Columbia, 2003.* Centers for Disease Control and Prevention. Washington, DC: U.S. Government Printing Office.

Romley, J. A., Cohen, D., Ringel, J., & Sturm, R. (2007). Alcohol and environmental justice: The density of liquor stores and bars in urban neighborhoods in the United States. *Journal of Studies on Alcohol & Drugs, 68,* 48–55.

Rosamond, W., Flega, K., Furie, K., Go, A., Greenlund, K., Haase N., . . . Hong, Y. (2008). American Heart Association Statistics Committee and Stroke Statistics Subcommittee. Heart disease and stroke statistics–2008 update. Report from the American Heart Association Statistics Committee and Stroke Statistics Subcommittee. *Circulation, 117,* e25–e146. doi:10.1161/

Rosamond, W. D., Folsom, A. R., Chambless, L. E., Wang, C-H., McGovern, P. G., Howard, G., . . . Shahar, E. (1999). Stroke incidence and survival among middle-aged adults. Nine-year follow-up of the Atherosclerosis Risk in Communities (ARIC) cohort. *Stroke, 30,* 736–743.

Rose, P. R. (2013). *Cultural competency for the health professional.* Burlington, MA: Jones & Barlett.

Rosenthal, M., & Ricker, J. H. (2000). Traumatic brain injury. In R. Frank & T. Elliott (Eds.), *Handbook of rehabilitation psychology* (pp. 49–74). Washington, DC: American Psychological Association.

Sacco, R. L., Benjamin, E. J., Broderick, J. P., Dyken, M., Easton, J. D., Feinberg, W. M., . . . Wolf, P. A. (1997). Risk factors. *Stroke, 28,* 1507–1517.

Sacco, R. L., Boden-Albala, B., Gan, R., Chen, X., Kargman, D. E., Shea, S., . . . Hauser, W. A. (1998). Stroke incidence among white, black, and Hispanic residents of an urban community. *American Journal of Epidemiology, 147,* 259–268.

Sacco, R. L., Kargman, D. E., & Zamanillo, M. C. (1995). Race-ethnic differences in stroke risk factors among hospitalized patients with cerebral infarction: The Northern Manhattan stroke study. *Neurology, 45,* 659–663.

Schafer, S. Q., Bruun, B., & Richter, R. W. (1973a). The contribution of nonaneurysmal intracranial hemorrhage to stroke in New York City blacks. *Stroke, 4,* 928–932.

Schafer, S. Q., Bruun, B., & Richter, R. W. (1973b). Epidemiology of in-hospital death among black stroke patients. *Stroke, 4,* 923–927.

Scheinart, K. F., Tuhrim, S., Horowitz, D. R., Weinberger, J., Goldman, M., & Godbold, J. H. (1998). Stroke recurrence is more frequent in blacks and hispanics. *Neuroepidemiology, 17,* 188–198.

Shafi, S., de la Plata, C. M., Diaz-Arrastia, R., Bransky, A., Frankel, H., Elliott, A. C., . . . Gentilello, L. M. (2007). Ethnic disparities exist in trauma care. *Journal of Trauma Injury Infection & Critical Care, 63,* 1138–1142.

Sloan, M. A., Kittner, S. J., Feeser, B. R., Gardner, J., Epstein, A., Wozsniak, M. A. . . . Buchholz, D. (1998). Illicit drug–associated ischemic stroke in the Baltimore-Washington Young Stroke Study. *Neurology, 50,* 1688–1693.

Smith, S. C., Clark, L. T., Cooper, R. S., Daniels, S. R., Kumanyika, S. K., Ofili, E., . . . Tiukinhoy, S. D. (2005). Discovering the full spectrum of cardiovascular disease. Minority health summit 2003: Report of the obesity, metabolic syndrome, and hypertension writing group. *ASHA Conference Proceedings Circulation, 111,* e134–e139.

Solliday-McRoy, C., Campbell, T. C., Melchert, T. P., Young, T. J., & Cisler, R. A. (2004). Neuropsychological functioning of homeless men. *Journal of Nervous and Mental Disease, 192,* 471–478.

Sorani, M. D., Lee, M., Kim, H., Meeker, M., & Manley, G. T. (2009). Race/ethnicity and outcome after traumatic brain injury at a single, diverse center. *Journal of Trauma, 67,* 75–80.

Staudenmayer, K. L., Diaz-Arrastia, R., de Oliveira, A., Gentilello, L. M., & Shafi, S. (2007). Ethnic disparities in long-term functional outcomes after traumatic brain injury. *Journal of Trauma, 63,* 1364–1369.

Stockman, I., Boult, J., & Robinson, G. (2004, July) *Multicultural issues in academic and clinical education.* Retrieved from http://www.asha.org/Publications/leader/2004/040720/f040720b.htm

Strangeman, G. E., O'Neil-Pirozzi, T. M., Goldstein, R., Kelkar, K., Burke, D., Katz, D. I., . . . Glenn, M. B. (2008). Prediction of memory rehabilitation outcomes in traumatic brain injury by using functional magnetic resonance imaging. *Archives of Physical Medicine and Rehabilitation, 89*, 974–981.

Strazzullo, P., D'Elia, L., Cairella, G., Garbagnati, F., Cappuccio, F. P., & Scalfi, L. (2010). Excess body weight and incidence of stroke: meta-analysis of prospective studies with 2 million participants. *Stroke, 41*, e418–426.

Substance Abuse and Mental Health Services Administration. (2011). *Results from the 2010 National Survey on Drug Use and Health: Summary of national findings.* NSDUH Series H-41, HHS Publication No. (SMA) 11-4658. Rockville, MD: Author.

Sung, S. Y., Ostchega, Y., & Louis, T. (2008). *Recent trends in the prevalence of high blood pressure and its treatment and control, 1999–2008.* NCHS Data Brief No. 48, October 2010.

Tang, M. X, Cross, P., Andrews, H., Jacobs, D. M., Small, S., Bell, K., . . . Mayeux R. (2001). Incidence of AD in African-Americans, Caribbean Hispanics, and Caucasians in northern Manhattan, *Neurology, 56*, 49–56.

Tang, M. X., Stern, Y., Bell, M. K., Gurland, B., Lantiqua, R., Andrews, H., . . . Mayeux, R. (1998). The APOE-epsilon4 allele and the risk of Alzheimer's disease among African Americans, whites, and Hispanics. *Journal of the American Medical Association, 279*, 751–755.

Tatemichi, T. K., Desmond, D. W., Mayeux, R., Paik, M., Stern, Y., Sano, M., & Hauser, W. A. (1992). Dementia after stroke: Baseline frequency, risks, and clinical features in a hospitalized cohort. *Neurology, 6*, 1185–1193.

The Institute of Medicine. *Disparities in health care: Methods for studying the effects of race, ethnicity, and ses on access, use, and quality of health care, 2002.* Retrieved from http://www.iom.edu/~/media/Files/Activity%20Files/Quality/NHDRGuidance/DisparitiesGornick.pdf

Thom, T., Haase, N., Rosamond, W., Howard, H. J., Rumsfeld, J., Manolio, T., . . . Wolf, P. (2006). Heart disease and stroke statistics—2006 update: A report from the American Heart Association Statistics Committee and Stroke Statistics Subcommittee. *Circulation, 113*, e85–e151.

Trimble, B., & Morgenstern, L. B. (2008). Stroke in minorities. *Neurology Clinic, 26*, 1177–1190.

U.S. Bureau of the Census. (2012). U.S. Census Bureau projections show a slower growing, older, more diverse nation a half century from now. *United States Public Law 106-525* (p. 2498). Retrieved from https://www.census.gov/newsroom/releases/archives/population/cb12-243.html.

Vincent, G. K., & Velkoff, V. A. (2010). The next four decades, the older population in the United States: 2010 to 2050. *Current Population Reports, 25-1138.* Washington, DC: U.S. Census Bureau.

Wallace, G. L. (2006, July 11). *Blast injury basics: A primer for the medical speech-language pathologist.* Retrieved from http://www.asha.org/Publications/leader/2006/060711/f060711a4.htm

Wooten-Bielsky, K. (1999). HIV & AIDS in older adults. *Geriatric Nursing, 20*, 268–272.

Zhang, Y., Galloway, J. M., Welty, T. K., Wiebers D. O., Whisnant, J. P., Devereux, R. B., . . . Lee, E. T. (2008). Incidence and risk factors for stroke in American Indians: The Strong Heart Study. *Circulation, 118*, 1577–1584.

Ziefert, P., Leary, M., & Boccellari, A. (1995). *AIDS and the impact of cognitive impairment.* University of California, San Francisco AIDS Health Project.

CHAPTER 2

Delivering Culturally Competent Services to Adults With Neurogenic Cognitive-Language Disorders

Joan C. Payne with Wilhelmina Wright-Harp

Referencing Chapter 1, changing demographics signal national changes in the coming decades. This means that all health professionals, including speech-language pathologists, will be called upon to provide services to an expanding diverse adult patient population. Recent health care legislation assures access to many persons who have suffered health disparities, who are poor and previously uninsured, and who, because of a history of limited access to preventive health care, may have chronic diseases and conditions that will, in all likelihood, result in impaired cognition and language. It is therefore incumbent upon professionals in speech-language pathology to be aware of the coming changes in caseload diversity and to be well prepared to deliver culturally competent assessment and treatment to diverse adults with neurogenic communication disorders. As one writer noted, "the notion of cultural competence as a best practice is not just 'something nice to do'" (Riquelme, 2004).

A definition of cultural and linguistic competence for health professionals, such as speech-language pathologists and audiologists, according to the Office of Minority Health (2013) at the National Institutes of Health, is:

a set of congruent behaviors, attitudes, and policies that come together in a system, agency, or among professionals that enables effective work in cross-cultural situations. "Culture" refers to integrated patterns of human behavior that include the language, thoughts, communications, actions, customs, beliefs, values, and institutions of racial, ethnic, religious, or social groups. "Competence" implies having the capacity to function effectively as an individual and an organization within the context of the cultural beliefs, behaviors, and needs presented by consumers and their communities.

This means that not only individual professionals must become culturally competent service providers, but the organizations in which they work must make every effort to eliminate institutional barriers and provide an environment for services that are sensitive and respectful. The importance of culturally competent health services in eliminating health disparities and fostering health and wellness is described by the Office of Minority Health (2013) thusly:

> Cultural competency is one of the main ingredients in closing the disparities gap in health care. It's the way patients and doctors can come together and talk about health concerns without cultural differences hindering the conversation, but enhancing it. Quite simply, health care services that are respectful of and responsive to the health beliefs, practices and cultural and linguistic needs of diverse patients can help bring about positive health outcomes.

Specifically for the professions of speech-language pathology and audiology, the American Speech-Language-Hearing Association (ASHA) (2005)

issued a policy statement based upon the Code of Ethics for certified professionals:

> The Code of Ethics requires the provision of competent services to all populations and recognition of the cultural/linguistic or life experiences of both professionals and those they serve. Everyone has a culture. Therefore, cultural competence is as important to successful provision of services as are scientific, technical, and clinical knowledge and skills. Caution must be taken not to attribute stereotypical characteristics to individuals. Rather, an attempt should be made to gain a better understanding of one's own culture, as well as the culture of those one serves. All professionals must continually improve their level of competence for providing services to all populations. Members and certificate holders should explore resources available from ASHA and other sources.

More recently, ASHA (2011) issued a policy statement that defines professional competence as inclusive of cultural competence:

> It is the position of the American Speech-Language-Hearing Association . . . that professional competence in providing speech-language-hearing and related services requires cultural competence. Cultural competence is a dynamic and complex process requiring ongoing self-assessment and continuous expansion of cultural knowledge. Cultural competence involves understanding the unique combination of cultural variables that the professional and patient/client bring to interactions. These variables include, for example, age, ability, ethnicity, experience, gender, gender identity, linguistic background, national origin,

race, religion, sexual orientation, and socioeconomic status.

Cultural competence includes the following:

◆ valuing diversity: awareness and acceptance of differences
◆ conducting cultural self-assessment
◆ being conscious of the dynamics inherent when cultures interact
◆ having institutional cultural knowledge: integration of cultural knowledge within individuals and systems
◆ adapting to diversity and the cultural contexts of the communities served.

Historically, speech-language pathologists have been trained to assess and treat adult patients from the perspective of a Western specialist culture. The specialist is acculturated to be individualistic, secular, egalitarian, independent, innovative, time conscious, and future oriented. Many cultures outside of the Western specialist culture are best described as generalist cultures in which emphasis is placed on holism, spirituality, interdependence, acceptance of authority and tradition, orientation to the present, fluidity of time and orientation to the community. Generalists want to find someone with whom they can establish and maintain a trusting, personalized relationship. They are far more likely to be concerned about immediate health needs, are far less time conscious, and are more likely to seek health care when it is needed. The frustrations and lack of acceptance between the specialist health care provider and the culturally and ethnically diverse generalist patient occur when the provider does not understand the patient's system of values,

norms, and beliefs (Damon-Rodriguez, Wallace, & Kingston, 1994).

This incongruence is at the heart of the dilemma facing the profession. Mahendra and her colleagues on the ASHA Multicultural Issues Board (2004) identified eight key parameters of culture, which are: (1) the extent to which an individual or group is considered to be the key unit of society, (2) views of time and space, (3) language and communication styles, (4) roles, (5) importance of work, (6) class and status, (7) rituals and superstitions, and (8) beliefs and values. In the view of the authors, cultural competence "requires a commitment to life-long learning and enhancement of our knowledge, skills, and attitudes" (American Speech-Hearing-Language Association, 2004, p. 4).

WHERE WE ARE NOW IN PROFESSIONAL CULTURAL COMPETENCE

In the professional literature, professionals who treat and conduct research on adults with neurogenic cognitive and language disorders have already begun conversations about culture and cultural competency (Blackstone, Ruschke, Wilson-Stronks, & Lee, 2012; Centeno, 2005; Cheng, 2005; Ellis, Payne, Harris, & Fleming, 2013; Goldberg, 2007; Harris, Fleming, & Harris, 2012; Huer & Wyatt, 1999; Mahendra et al., 2005; Mashima, 2012; Moxley, Mahendra, & Vega-Barachowitz, 2004; Payne, 2011; Riquelme, 2006, 2013; Salas-Provance, 2012; Threats, 2005; Tomoeda & Bayles, 2002; Ulatowska et al., 2001; Williams & Harvey, 2013; Wolf, 2004; Wright-Harp, Mayo, Martinez, Payne, & Lemmon, 2012). In these conversations, two major themes emerge: eliminating bias in assessment, treatment, and counseling; and preparing the workplace to serve persons of diverse ethnicities and languages.

At the heart of the discussion about eliminating bias is how professionals can render fair and objective assessment and, from that assessment, appropriate and meaningful intervention. Effective and evidence-based practice in the assessment and treatment of culturally and linguistically diverse populations requires that the speech-language pathologist know about the pathophysiology of language and cognitive impairments as well as cultural and linguistic differences that affect communication. It is also essential to understand the culture and environment(s) in which the individual functions daily (American Speech-Hearing-Language Association, 2010; American Speech-Hearing-Language Association, 2011). The speech-language pathologist and the client/patient each bring their own backgrounds that will influence the therapy process (Ruoff, 2002). The success or failure of the process is dependent largely upon the clinician's ability to approach each client as being unique rather than using a "one size fits all" approach in service delivery, particularly in assessment of ethnically and culturally diverse individuals (Wright-Harp et al., 2012).

Eliminating Bias in Assessment and Treatment

Evaluating adults from various ethnic and cultural groups is challenging, particularly since the goal is to identify areas to target in rehabilitation. Many assessments have a sociocultural bias. Wyatt (1998) identified four sources of bias in normed tests that can lead to an inaccurate diagnosis. These are:

1. Linguistic bias, that is, assessment probes and desirable answers that are not in the familiar or customary language of the respondent.
2. Value bias, or questions that elicit different responses from the patient based upon his or her own interpretative frame of reference.
3. Situational bias or a mismatch in communication styles and expectations.
4. Format bias—for example, testing procedures that are unfamiliar or uncomfortable for the patient.

These sources of bias and the underrepresentation of individuals from racial/ethnic groups in test normative data hinder the clinician's ability to make objective and valid diagnoses of cognitive and communication disorders for individuals from diverse cultural and linguistic populations. Paul-Brown and Ricker (2003) comment that:

Accurate assessment of speech, language and cognitive functions on standardized norm-referenced measures may be difficult for culturally and linguistically diverse populations, or with populations who may not have the same level of requisite skills or experiences to perform adequately on tests. Furthermore, unless the clinician maintains an open, objective approach to assessment, there can be a "clash" between clinicians' values and those of the patient and/or family (e.g. not everyone thinks reading is important; not everyone values competitive employment). This is another important reason to focus on the assessment of the patient determined by individualized goals and the culture and context in which that person functions. (p. 52)

Assessment must be undertaken with consideration for each patient's educational background, culture, language, and experiences. Members of nonwhite ethnic groups may be penalized for use of linguistic features and/or cognitive styles influenced by features of their dialect, language, or cultural background. Although some assessments are in other languages, they may not represent the various dialects of those languages and may not have been translated by speakers who are native to the languages. Two assessments, the *Boston Naming Test* (BNT; Kaplan, Goodglass, & Weintraub, 1983; Nicholas, Brookshire, MacLennan, Schumacher, & Porrazzo, 1988) and the *Ross Information Processing Assessment–2* (RIPA-2; Ross-Swain, 1996), have reported ethnic biases. Pedraza, Graff-Radford, and Lucas (2009) investigated performance on the BNT by older African Americans and non-Hispanic whites and found that six items ("dominoes," "escalator," "muzzle," "latch," "tripod," and "palette") were identified to represent the strongest evidence for race/ethnicity-based differential item functioning. Similar findings were noted by Kennepohl, Shore, Nabors, and Hanks (2004), who observed that differences in cultural experience may be important factors in the neuropsychological assessment, including the BNT, of African Americans following traumatic brain injury. Other findings strongly suggest that the BNT needs modification to be effective for persons who speak English but live in other countries (Barker-Collo, 2001). Also, Davis and Wright-Harp (2012a, 2012b) and Wright-Harp (2006) report that the RIPA-2 lacked the sensitivity to carefully evaluate African Americans with traumatic brain injury.

Investigators and practitioners must be aware that the published norms for tests administered in English are not necessarily valid when the tests are administered in another language. Furthermore, they should not assume that test norms can be applied to distinct populations simply because they share a language. For example, there is evidence that several instruments developed in Spanish-speaking countries may not be functionally or linguistically equivalent when used among Spanish speakers in the United States (Manley & Mayeux, 2004). When test items have not been designed to account for responses that reflect different language, dialect, and/or cognitive styles of a particular racial/ethnic population, misdiagnosis may result. To limit the potential for misdiagnosis, the clinician must be knowledgeable of the rules of the individual's dialect or language (Wright-Harp, 2005, 2006).

As a first step for speech-language pathologists, it is necessary to evaluate standardized tests and to either avoid using those that have been identified as being culturally, educationally, or linguistically biased (Davis & Wright-Harp, 2012; Wright, 2006) or prepare to supplement the results with other, less biased measures (Ulatowska et al., 2001). When standardized tests are not appropriate for a given patient, the use of informal assessment and dynamic assessment procedures can be used successfully (Davis, Lucker, Wright-Harp, & Payne, 2011; Wright-Harp et al., 2012). Researchers reporting from South Africa, for example, describe how much better their patients responded when they modified the "Cookie Theft Picture" and the BNT to minimize Western cultural, language, and education bias in neurocognitive screening in South Africa (Mosdell, Balchin, & Ameen, 2010).

Other measures, including behavioral and pragmatic observations in natural contexts as well as spontaneous and structured language sampling, provide valuable information that standardized tests alone may not. Gathering information from a variety of sources helps minimize the risk of misdiagnosis. Possible sources of information include the family, caregivers, members of the community, other members of the interdisciplinary team, and if possible, the patient. Sampling communication in a variety of contexts gives the clinician a more accurate profile of an individual's functional communication ability and aids in determining the potential effectiveness of intervention and compensatory strategies (Brown & Wright-Harp, 2011; Grice & Wright-Harp 2004a, 2004b; Ulatowska et al., 2001). When evaluating bilingual and monolingual speakers whose dominant language is not English, interpreters, not family members, may be necessary to ensure accurate assessment of the individuals' cognitive and language skills.

Once assessment is completed, planning intervention should be undertaken with the same degree of sensitivity as the selection of appropriate assessments. Therapy should be client-centered in the context of understanding what the communicative environment of the client demands. This can be accomplished only when the clinician understands and respects the perspective of the patient and the patient's support networks. Ruoff (2002) recommends that the plan of therapy should be culturally sensitive and should include functionally relevant materials and accommodations that are considerate of the patient's worldview (for example, allowing extra time when using a translator). The clinician must also appreciate and understand linguistic differences and the patient's cultural views on disability and physical/psychological change (Wilson, 2002).

Eliminating Bias in Counseling

Effective and compassionate counseling for patients and their families from culturally and ethnically diverse backgrounds requires that the clinician should appreciate how difficult it may be for some persons to share their innermost feelings with others outside of their sphere of comfort, and then take steps to minimize this difficulty. Salas-Provance (2012) recommends that counselors greet their patients and families in their own language and bring special skills to the counseling session. These are: (1) being comfortable with issues of race, culture, and class; (2) creating an environment where the client is comfortable and can talk freely; and (3) building a trusting relationship. Both Salas-Provance (2012) and Payne (1997) advise that a warm but formal approach is preferred. The clinician should address patients by formal titles (Dr., Mr., Ms., or Mrs.).

There are demonstrated cultural and ethnic differences in how families function when the patient has sustained a major neurologic episode. Harris and her colleagues (2012) noted that among African American families, feelings of embarrassment or stigma, distrust of mainstream institutions and agents, religiosity, lack of knowledge, and denial become barriers to acceptance of speech-language pathology services. Liu and associates (2005) observed that Asian immigrants do not encourage members to express problems to those outside the in-group. This is particularly true of mental and/or physical problems that could carry a stigma. Emphasis on shame and guilt are sometimes used to enforce norms in the family and prevent Asians from reporting their problems in public.

It is critical that clinicians understand how family perceptions about assessment and treatment influence the clinical process and their expectations for recovery (Wright-Harp et al., 2012). Perceptions and viewpoints regarding disability vary among racial/ethnic groups (O'Neil-Pirozzi et al., 2010). Views of disability appear to be influenced more by geographic, ethnic, and/or cultural factors than by race, and these factors are associated with particular beliefs, attitudes, and behaviors around a particular disability that may affect the likelihood of seeking services and participating in treatment. Disability is variously viewed as a tragedy, a disgrace, shameful, the result of sin, and a punishment from God. People with disabilities are repeatedly seen as objects of pity, which produces guilt feelings in their family members and associates. They are frequently viewed as a burden to others, to their family, to themselves, and to society and are continually perceived to be useless and to behave in inappropriate ways (Pfeiffer et al., 2003). In light of these perceptual and cultural differences, Asian, African American, Native American, and Hispanic populations each have distinct and varied views on disability (National Council on Disability, 2003; Parette & Huer, 2002; Payne, 1997).

Counseling patients and their families from Native American communities may be unsuccessful unless the clinician appreciates the differences in communicative style and acceptance of a natural order of things as fate. If the clinician uses a more direct communication style, the Native American listener may perceive the communication style as intrusive or rude (Westby & Vining, 2004). Hispanic and Arab Americans view counseling as a collective rather than a traditional individualist society view with an emphasis on accepting the disability rather than curing it (Salas-Provance, 2012). Given how important appropriate counseling is to assisting the entire family to cope

and accept a patient's disability, it may be necessary for the clinician to seek advice from others in the patient's community, including respected persons from religious and health care arenas who understand the culture.

RECOMMENDATIONS FOR CLINICIAN CULTURAL COMPETENCE

Because a substantial number of professionals work in health care settings where persons with neurogenic disorders are seen, many of the professional conversations about cultural competence cite The Joint Commission's (2010) report, *Advancing Effective Communication, Cultural Competence, and Patient- and Family-Centered Care: A Roadmap for Hospitals.* This is particularly important because most adults with neurogenic disorders are seen in hospitals or other health settings where over one-third of speech-language pathologists are delivering services. The American Speech-Language-Hearing Association (n.d.) reports that 38% of speech-language pathologists work in health care settings; 13% of these work in hospitals, and 9% work in skilled nursing facilities.

There remains a need to bridge the divide between speech-language pathologists who are specialists and culturally diverse persons with neurogenic disorders who are more likely to be generalists. Researchers agree that speech-language pathologists and audiologists are highly qualified and in the unique position to assume leadership in providing the highest quality of health-related services to patients regardless of their ethnic background, age, socioeconomic status, education, language, gender, sexual orientation, or country of birth. It is in this spirit that there are common threads in the recommendations offered in the conversations within and to the professions that encourage speech-language pathologists to:

I. **Provide health communication that is clear, easy to understand, in the patient's language, and reflective of the communication context of the patient.**
   a. Use illustrations that reflect ethnic diversity.
   b. Prepare text that is easy to read and in the patient's language.
   c. Provide verbal information through an interpreter.
   d. Tailor messages to the context of the patient, whether high-context (nonverbal communication and silence are valued) or low-context (spoken and written communication are valued).
   e. Avoid cultural faux pas: using the patient's first name, telling jokes, asking for personal information before trust has been established.

II. **Respect divergent views on health and wellness.**
   a. Ask the patient to describe his or her views on the illness or disability.
   b. Become informed about how health care decisions are made in the patient's community.
   c. Be aware of how differences in perceptions of disability and coping styles vary within cultures and are often tied to religion among some cultures.

III. **Respect differences in family structures.**
   a. Be mindful that there is no model of the perfect family

and that cultural norms often govern the hierarchy and membership status within families.
   b. Understand that in some cultures, families are largely patriarchal; in others, the eldest member speaks for the family; in still others, families are matriarchal or multigenerational; these arrangements work for the families involved.
   c. Appreciate that families may be racially mixed or have same-gender parents.

IV. **Respect diverse views on time and personal space.**
   a. Consider that time is relative and meaningful in different ways in different cultures.
   b. Respect that use of personal space is culture driven and that there are cultural variations in how personal and social spaces are defined.
   c. Understand that in some religions, personal space is delineated according to gender and/or marital status.

V. **Respect the important rituals (holidays, religious observances) of other groups.**
   a. Schedule appointments around important holidays and religious activities for patients.
   b. Become familiar with important rituals and their significance to patients.
   c. Honor requests for activities within therapy that symbolize important rituals to the patient and the patient's family.
   d. Understand the role of organized religion in the

lives of patients and their views on the power of prayer in healing.

VI. **Be flexible about assessment.**

a. Use more informal testing, such as proverbs and narratives, to tap into verbal and comprehension abilities in culturally diverse adults that may not be obvious in standardized testing.

b. Assess higher cognitive functioning and use of abstract language from cartoons and humorous stories from sources in other communities or countries and in the patient's preferred language.

c. Use indirect ways to assess, such as observations and family interviews.

d. Appreciate that culture drives communication styles and that differences in communication styles are not disordered.

VII. **Respect different views on health care.**

a. Know that cultures differ in the ways that illness is explained and in what is acceptable to hear about illness.

b. Be sensitive to the fact that technology-driven Western health care is not always preferable to alternative health care within a cultural community.

c. Be aware that distrust of Western health care is rooted in the national history of discrimination.

VIII. **Respect language differences.**

a. Provide a translator for patients whose primary language is not English.

b. Appreciate that one's language is a deeply personal aspect of culture.

IX. **Respect other views of work.**

a. Be knowledgeable that in some countries, work is defined differently than in the United States.

b. Understand that status in some communities may be defined by parameters other than work or by the type of work done.

X. **Respect the family's autonomy in decision making.**

a. With the permission of the patient, include all members of the extended family in conversations about the patient's progress.

b. Validate the opinions of the family.

c. Do not presume that the family has no knowledge of communication disorders; interview the family on this issue and build from there.

XI. **Respect cultural differences in emotional expression.**

a. Be aware that a smile does not necessarily mean agreement; it sometimes means confusion or respect.

b. Do not be offended by differences in how a patient can look the clinician in the eyes.

XII. **Become flexible about intervention.**

a. Use telehealth with persons who cannot come to therapy.

b. Select appropriate augmentative and alternative communication devices for a multilingual population.

c. Use stimuli that are functionally relevant for the patient.

d. Tailor therapy for the patient's needs.

XIII. Involve the family.

a. Involve the patient and the family in decision making for therapy goals.

b. Educate the family about the disorder that caused the communication impairment.

c. Provide support and information on resources in the family's preferred language.

Cultural competence for the professional means that the clinician endeavors to be culturally intelligent about patients who are culturally and ethnically diverse. The clinician, however, works within an employment setting, whether a hospital, clinic, or private practice. This setting establishes the tone and the agenda for cultural inclusion and sensitivity within the organization.

RECOMMENDATIONS FOR CULTURAL COMPETENCE WITHIN ORGANIZATIONS

Institutional policies determine whether the culture of the organization will be inclusive or exclusive. In 2000, the Office of Minority Health, in the Department of Health and Human Services (DHHS), published the first National Standards for Culturally and Linguistically Appropriate Services in Health Care (National CLAS Standards), which provided a framework for all health care organizations to best serve the nation's increasingly diverse communities. In the fall of 2010, the Office of Minority Health in DHHS launched the National CLAS Standards Enhancement Initiative in order to revise the standards to reflect the past decade's advance-

ments, expand their scope, and improve their clarity to ensure understanding and implementation. With the enhancement initiative, the National CLAS Standards will continue into the next decade as the cornerstone for advancing health equity through culturally and linguistically appropriate services. The 15 enhanced CLAS Standards are shown in Table 2–1.

The CLAS Standards mandate that organizations work in partnership with the communities of the persons they serve and engage in continuous dialogues. These dialogues are to ensure that persons with communication disorders from diverse populations are well served by these organization. For example, the Blueprint (Office of Minority Health, DHHS, n.d.) for the CLAS Standards for health communication materials recommend that organizations consult local librarians to build an appropriate collection of health materials and that organizations use focus groups made up of the target population to assess the diversity shown in graphics and to point out culturally offensive or embarrassing content.

Another recommendation from the Blueprint, to provide responsive and appropriate service delivery to a community, leads to the creation of an organizational culture that ensures accountability to the community. Members of the community become active participants in the health and health care process as well as in the design and improvement of services to meet their needs and desires.

Other recommendations from the Blueprint are to recruit and hire persons representative of and sensitive to the community who will be trained in culturally competent service delivery by the organization. The purpose of these recommendations is to create an environment in which culturally diverse individuals

Table 2–1. Enhanced CLAS Standards

Principal Standard	
1	Provide effective, equitable, understandable, and respectful quality care and services
Governance, Leadership, and Workforce	
2	Advance and sustain governance and leadership that promotes CLAS
3	Recruit, promote, and support a diverse governance, leadership, and workforce
4	Educate and train governance, leadership, and workforce in CLAS
Communication and Language Assistance	
5	Offer communication and language assistance
6	Inform individuals of the availability of language assistance
7	Ensure the competence of individuals providing language assistance
8	Provide easy-to-understand materials and signage
Engagement, Continuous Improvement, and Accountability	
9	Infuse CLAS goals, policies, and management accountability
10	Conduct organizational assessments
11	Collect and maintain demographic data
12	Conduct assessments of community health assets and needs
13	Partner with the community
14	Create conflict and grievance resolution processes
15	Communicate the organization's progress in implementing and sustaining CLAS

Note: The enhanced National CLAS Standards and *The Blueprint* are the culmination of the DHHS Office of Minority Health's 2010–2012 Enhancement Initiative.

Source: Office of Minority Health. (n.d.). *National Standards for Culturally and Linguistically Appropriate Services (CLAS) in Health and Health Care.* U.S. Department of Health and Human Services. Retrieved from https://www.thinkculturalhealth.hhs.gov/Content/clas.asp

feel welcomed and valued. This purpose applies to the staff and leadership of the organization and to the governance of the organization. It is necessary to ensure that diverse viewpoints and multicultural perspectives are well represented in the major decisions of the organization. This does not mean that the entire workforce has to look like the persons from the community, but it does mean that there should be some representation in the workforce from the cultural and ethnic groups represented in the patient population. It also means that persons hired by the organization must be open to and educated about diversity in order to engage in culturally appropriate assessment and treatment.

Finally, the organization has a responsibility to provide translators for patients who have difficulty with English. It also has an obligation to engage in ongoing collection and monitoring of demographic data about the service communities. In the first instance, patients who speak a language other than English are entitled to competent translators who can provide them with the means to achieve their goals in therapy. The organization, likewise, has a responsibility to identify population groups within the service area and to allocate organizational resources to patient needs, service planning, and quality of care.

RESOURCES FOR CULTURALLY COMPETENT SERVICE DELIVERY

The Office of Multicultural Affairs in ASHA has developed a series of tools that are helpful to clinicians who wish to self-appraise their cultural knowledge and become more culturally intelligent about a variety of topics related to cultural competence. These resources include the Cultural Competence Checklists (Personal Reflection, Policies and Procedures, Service Delivery), the Self-Assessment for Cultural Competence, and the Cultural Competence Awareness Tool, which is an interactive Web-based tool that allows the user to assess areas that need strengthening in cultural competence. These tools can be accessed at http://www.asha.org/practice/multicultural/self.htm. The National Black Association for Speech-Language-Hearing (NBASLH) is accessible at http://www.nbaslh.org. NBASLH publishes the e-journal *Echo*, which has articles on issues affecting African Americans. Readers can also access the Asian-Indian Caucus at http://www.asianindiancaucus.org; the Asian Pacific Islander Caucus at http://www.ashaapicaucus.org/; the Hispanic Caucus at http://

www.ashahispaniccaucus.com/; and the Native American Caucus at http://libarts.wsu.edu/speechhearing/overview/nap-caucus.asp

ASHA has published policy statements regarding services to culturally and ethnically diverse populations. The reader is referred to the following sites for ASHA position papers on best practices in service delivery to diverse persons:

◆ Clinical Management of Communicatively Handicapped Minority Language Populations, available at http://www.asha.org/docs/html/PS1985-00219.html

◆ Knowledge and Skills Needed to Provide Culturally and Linguistically Appropriate Services, available at http://www.asha.org/docs/html/KS2004-00215.html

◆ ASHA's Policies and Procedures Related to Working with Multicultural Populations, available at http://www.asha.org/practice/multicultural/issues/pp.htm

SUMMARY

In this chapter, policy statements on ethics and best practices from ASHA mandate that certified professionals in speech-language pathology and audiology engage in culturally competent service delivery. The parameters of this service delivery have been identified in the professional literature, in the report of the Joint Commission for hospitals, and by the Office of Minority Health of DHHS. Using current research and the national enhanced CLAS Standards, recommendations are given for individual practitioners and for organizations. The enhanced CLAS Standards are designed to help organizations to develop culturally competent health services to diverse adults. There are resources available through the Office of Multicultural Affairs of ASHA to assist clinicians in strengthening their cultural knowledge through a variety of online tools. Additional resources and their websites can be accessed to further develop an information base for cultural competence.

STUDY QUESTIONS

1. What are the CLAS Standards?

2. What are the issues of bias in assessment that can result in misdiagnoses?

3. How are professional ethics aligned with culturally competent service delivery?

4. In what ways can culturally competent service delivery decrease the effects of health disparities?

5. Contrast specialist and generalist perspectives on health care.

6. What are proxemics? How might proxemics differ between cultural groups?

7. What is at least one issue in counseling persons from diverse cultural and ethnic backgrounds?

8. How are views of disability different between cultural and ethnic groups?

9. Define linguistic and cultural competence generally.

10. What is ASHA's definition of cultural competence?

11. How does Wyatt (1998) describe the four sources of bias in normed tests?

12. What do researchers suggest as sources of bias in the *Boston Naming Test*?

13. What are possible strategies for informal assessment?

14. What are eight key parameters of culture, according to the ASHA Multicultural Board (2004)?

15. In what ways can clinicians demonstrate respect for language differences?

16. Why is it necessary to be flexible about time for some culturally diverse patients?

17. In what ways might family structures be different across cultural groups?

18. What tools are available through ASHA to assist clinicians in becoming culturally competent?

19. What is meant by, "one size fits all"? Why is this not an effective strategy for assessment or treatment?

20. What should clinicians consider when counseling patients from Native American communities?

21. Why is it important to use culturally relevant materials in therapy?

22. In what ways can clinicians show respect for rituals observed by culturally diverse patients?

23. How should the service delivery organization engage the community of the clients it serves?

24. What is meant by institutional racism and how does it affect service delivery?

25. Are all tests in Spanish appropriate for Spanish-speaking clients? Why or why not.

26. Why is it important to understand and respect divergent views on health care and health-seeking behaviors?

27. What should clinicians consider when counseling diverse families about the effects of disabilities?

28. What should clinicians consider when developing written information about communication disorders for clients and their families?

29. Is it always necessary to have persons representative of the cultural communities on staff in organizations that provide speech and language services? Why or why not?

30. How should clinicians interpret emotional expression from culturally diverse clients?

REFERENCES

American Speech-Language-Hearing Association. (n.d.). *Current status of SLP employment in health care settings.* Retrieved from http://www.asha.org/careers/recruitment/healthcare/HospitalConsiderations/

American Speech-Language-Hearing Association. (2004). *Knowledge and skills needed by speech-language pathologists and audiologists to provide culturally and linguistically appropriate services [Knowledge and skills].* Retrieved from http://www.asha.org/policy

American Speech-Language-Hearing Association. (2005). *Cultural competence* [Issues in ethics]. Retrieved from http://www.asha.org/policy

American Speech-Language-Hearing Association. (2010). *Cultural competence checklist: Personal reflection.* Retrieved from http://www.asha.org/uploadedFiles/practice/multicultural/personalreflections.pdf

American Speech-Language-Hearing Association. (2011). *Cultural competence in professional service delivery* [Position statement]. Retrieved from http://www.asha.org/policy

Barker-Collo, S. L. (2001). The 60-item Boston Naming Test: Cultural bias and possible adaptations for New Zealand. *Aphasiology, 15,* 85–92. doi:10.1080/02687040042000124

Blackstone, S. W., Ruschke, K., Wilson-Stronks, A., & Lee, C. (2012). Converging communication vulnerabilities in health care: An emerging role for speech-language pathologists and audiologists. *Perspectives on Communication Disorders and Sciences in Culturally and Linguistically Diverse Populations, 18,* 3–11.

Brown, J., & Wright-Harp, W. (2011). Cultural and generational factors influencing proverb recognition. *Contemporary Issues in Communication Sciences and Disorders (CICSD), 38,* 111–122.

Centeno, J. G. (2005). Working with bilingual individuals with aphasia: The case of a Spanish-English bilingual client. *Perspectives on Communication Disorders and Sciences in Culturally and Linguistically Diverse Populations, 12,* 2–7.

Cheng, L-R. L. (2005). Successful clinical management requires cultural intelligence. *Perspectives on Neurophysiology and Neurogenic Speech and Language Disorders, 15,* 16–19.

Damon-Rodriguez, J., Wallace, S., & Kingston, R. (1994). Service utilization and minority elderly. *Gerontology and Geriatrics Education, 15,* 45–63.

Davis, A., Lucker, J., Wright-Harp, W., & Payne, J. (2011, April). *Familiarity of figurative expressions from culturally-related music in African American adults.* Mini-seminar presented at the annual convention of the National Black Association for Speech-Language-Hearing (NBASLH), Washington, DC.

Davis, A. S., & Wright-Harp, W. (2012a, February). *Assessment and treatment in traumatic brain injury.* Poster session presented at the annual convention of the DC Speech and Hearing Association, Rockville, MD.

Davis, A. S., & Wright-Harp, W. (2012b, February). *A comparison of performance of African Americans and Caucasian Americans on the RIPA-2.* Poster session presented at the annual convention of the DC Speech and Hearing Association, Rockville, MD.

Ellis, C., Payne, J., Harris, J., & Fleming, V. (2013). *Issues in neurogenic communication disorders: Past, present and future.* Short course presented at the 2013 convention of the National Black Association for Speech-Language-Hearing, Washington, DC.

Goldberg, L. R. (2007). Service-learning as a tool to facilitate cultural competence. *Perspectives on Communication Disorders and Sciences in*

Culturally and Linguistically Diverse Populations, 14, 3–7.

Grice, A., & Wright-Harp, W. (2004a). The narrative performance of adolescents and emerging adults. NIDCD research symposium in aphasiology. Proceedings of the Clinical Aphasiology 34th Conference. *Aphasiology, 19*, 3–9.

Grice, A., & Wright-Harp, W. (2004b). *The use of narratives by African American adolescents with traumatic brain injury.* Paper presented at the annual convention of the American Speech-Language-Hearing Association, Philadelphia, PA.

Harris, J. L., Fleming, V. B., & Harris, C. L. (2012). A focus on health beliefs: What culturally competent clinicians need to know. *Perspectives on Communication Disorders and Sciences in Culturally and Linguistic Diverse Populations, 19*, 40–48.

Huer, M. B., & Wyatt, T. (1999). Cultural factors in the delivery of AAC to the African American community. *Perspectives on Communication Disorders and Sciences in Culturally and Linguistically Diverse Populations, 5*, 5–9.

Kaplan, E., Goodglass, H., & Weintraub, S. (1983). *The Boston Naming Test.* Philadelphia, PA: Febiger.

Kennepohl, S., Shore, D., Nabors, N., & Hanks, R. (2004). African American acculturation and neuropsychological test performance following traumatic brain injury. *Journal of the International Neuropsychological Society, 10*, 566–577.

Liu, D., Hinton, L., Tran, C., Hinton, D., & Barker, J. C. (2010). Re-examining the relationships among dementia, stigma, and aging in immigrant Chinese and Vietnamese family caregivers. *Journal of Cross-Cultural Gerontology, 23*, 283–299. doi:10.1007/s10823 008-9075-5

Mahendra, N., Ribera, J., Sevcik, R., Adler, R., Cheng, L-R. L., Davis-McFarland, D., . . . Villanueva, A. (2005). Why is yogurt good for you? Because it has live cultures. *Perspectives on Neurophysiology and Neurogenic Speech and Language Disorders, 15*, 3–7.

Mashima, P. A. (2012). Using technology to improve access to health care for culturally and linguistically diverse populations. *Perspectives on Communication Disorders and Sciences in Culturally and Linguistically Diverse Populations, 19*, 71–76.

Moxley, A., Mahendra, M., & Vega-Barachowitz, C. (2004, April 13). Cultural competence in health care. *The ASHA Leader*, 1–7.

National Council on Disability. (1999). *Outreach and people with disabilities from diverse cultures:* *A review of the literature.* Retrieved from http://www.ncd.gov/publications/2003/nov302003

Manley, J., & Mayeux, R. (2004). Ethnic differences in dementia and Alzheimer's disease. In N. B. Anderson, R. A. Bulatao & B. Cohen (Editors). *Critical perspectives on racial and ethnic differences in health in late life.* National Research Council (US) Panel on Race, Ethnicity, and Health in Later Life (2004). Washington (DC): National Academies Press (US) Retrieved from http://www.ncbi.nlm.nih.gov/books/NBK25535/

Nicholas, L. E., Brookshire, R. H., MacLennan, D. L., Schumacher, J. G., & Porrazzo, S. A. (1988). The Boston Naming Test: Revised administration and scoring procedures and normative information for non-brain-damaged adults. *Clinical Aphasiology* (pp. 103–115). Boston, MA: College-Hill Press.

Office of Minority Health. (n.d.). *National Standards for Culturally and Linguistically Appropriate Services (CLAS) in health and health care.* U.S. Department of Health and Human Services. Retrieved from https://www.thinkcultural-health.hhs.gov/Content/clas.asp

Office of Minority Health. (2013). *Cultural competence.* Retrieved from http://www.omhrc.gov

O'Neil-Pirozzi, T. M., Strangman, G. E., Goldstein, R., Katz, D. I., Savage, C. R., Kelkar, K., . . . Glenn, M. B. (2010). A controlled treatment study of internal memory strategies (I-MEMS) following traumatic brain injury. *Journal of Head Trauma Rehabilitation, 25*, 43–51.

Parette, P., & Huer, M. B. (2002). Working with Asian American families whose children have augmentative and alternative communication (AAC) needs. *Journal of Special Education Technology, 17*, 5–13.

Paul-Brown, D., & Ricker, J. (2003). *Evaluating and treating communication and cognitive disorders: Approaches to referral and collaboration for speech-language pathology and clinical neuropsychology [Technical report].* Retrieved from http://www.asha.org/docs/html/TR2003-00137.html

Payne, J. C. (1997). *Adult neurogenic language disorders: Assessment and treatment. An ethnobiological approach* (pp. 37–75). San Diego, CA: Singular.

Payne, J. C. (2011, November 1). *Cultural competence in treatment of adults with cognitive and language disorders.* Retrieved from http://www.asha.org/Publications/leader/2011/111101/Cultural-Competence-in-Treatment-of-Adults

-with-Cognitive-and-Language-Disorders .htm

Pedraza, O., Graff-Radford, N. R., & Lucas, J. A. (2009). Differential item functioning of the Boston naming test and cognitively normal African American and Caucasian older adults. *Journal of International Neuropsychological Society, 15,* 758–768.

Pfeiffer, D., Sam, A. A., Guinan, M., Ratliffe, K. T., Robinson, N. B., & Stodden, N. J. (2003). Attitudes toward disability in the helping professions. *Disability Studies Quarterly, 23,* 132–149.

Riquelme, L. F. (2004, April 13). *Cultural competence in dysphagia.* Retrieved from http://www .asha.org/Publications/leader/2004/040413/ f040413b3/

Riquelme, L. F. (2006). Working with limited-English-speaking adults with neurological impairment. *Perspectives on Gerontology, 13,* 3–8.

Riquelme, L. F. (2013). Cultural competence for everyone: A shift in perspectives. *Perspectives on Communication Disorders and Sciences in Culturally and Linguistically Diverse Populations, 19,* 71–76.

Ross-Swain, D. (1996). *Ross Information Processing Assessment* (2nd ed.). Austin, TX: Pro-Ed.

Ruoff, J. (2002). Cultural-linguistic considerations for speech-language pathologists in serving individuals with traumatic brain injury. *Perspectives on Communication Disorders and Sciences in Culturally and Linguistically Diverse Populations, 8,* 2–5. doi:10.1044/cds8.3.2

Salas-Provance, M. B. (2012). Counseling in a multicultural society: Implications for the field of communication disorders. In L. Flasher & P. Fogle (Eds.), *Counseling skills for speech-language pathologists and audiologists* (2nd ed., pp. 159–160). Clifton Park, NY: Delmar Cengage Learning.

The Joint Commission. (2010). *Advancing effective communication, cultural competence, and patient- and family-centered care: A roadmap for hospitals.* Oakbrook Terrace, IL: Author.

Threats, T. (2005). Cultural sensitivity in healthcare settings. *Perspectives on Communication Disorders and Sciences in Culturally and Linguistically Diverse Populations, 12,* 3–6.

Tomoeda, C. K., & Bayles, K. A. (2002, April 2). *Cultivating cultural competence in the workplace, classroom, and clinic.* Retrieved from http://www.asha.org/Publications/leader/ 2002/020402/020402d.htm

Ulatowska, H. K., Wertz, R. T., Chapman, S. B., Hill, C. L., Thompson, J. L., Keebler, M. W., . . . Auther, L. L. (2001). Interpretation of fables and proverbs by African Americans with and without aphasia. *American Journal of Speech-Language Pathology, 10,* 40–50.

Westby, C., & Vining, C. B. (2004). *Cultural variables affecting research with Native American populations.* Retrieved from http://div14perspectives.asha.org/content/11/1/3.full.pdf+html

Williams, S. W., & Harvey, S. (2013). Culture, race and SES: Application to end of life decision making for African American caregivers. *Perspectives on Gerontology, 18,* 69–76.

Wilson, B. (2002). Neurologic-based communication disorders: Cultural issues in providing services to clients and their families. *Perspectives on Communication Disorders and Sciences in Culturally and Linguistically Diverse Populations, 8,* 5–9. doi:10.1044/cds8.3.5

Wolf, K. E. (2004, April 13). *Cultural competence in audiology.* Retrieved from http://www.asha .org/Publications/leader/2004/040413/ f040413b2.htm

Wright-Harp, W. (2005, February). *Clinical management of traumatic brain injury among culturally diverse populations.* Invited speech at the Winter workshop sponsored by the DC Speech and Hearing Association.

Wright-Harp, W. (2006, March). *Traumatic brain injury in diverse populations: Issues in assessment and intervention.* Seminar in the Department of Biobehavioral Sciences Program in Speech and Language Pathology at the Teacher's College Columbia University, New York, NY.

Wright-Harp, W., Mayo, R., Martinez, S., Payne, J., & Lemmon, R. (2012, November). *Addressing health disparities in minority populations with communication disorders.* Mini-seminar presented at the annual convention of the American Speech-Language-Hearing Association, Atlanta, GA.

Wyatt, T. A. (1998). Speech-language pathology in children and adults. Language intervention for linguistically different learners. In C. M. Seymour & E. H. Nober (Eds.), *Introduction to communication disorders: A multicultural approach.* Boston, MA: Butterworth-Heinemann.

SECTION II

The Disorders

CHAPTER 3

Neurology Basics

INTRODUCTION

Since the early discoveries of Gall, Broca, and Wernicke and the more contemporary research of Geschwin (1975) and Luria (1977), advances in neuroimaging technologies, such as computerized axial tomography (CT), positron emission tomography (PET), single photon emission computerized tomography (SPECT), magnetic resonance imaging (MRI), and functional magnetic resonance imaging (fMRI), have allowed scientists to see the interconnectedness of brain structures previously thought to function independently for language and cognition. What has emerged from neuroimaging studies is that language and cognition are complex functions of the central nervous system in humans. In addition, a number of structures are implicated in neurogenic disorders such as dementia, aphasia, and traumatic brain injury. In order to understand the dynamics of neurogenic disorders as these affect language and cognition and the literature on these disorders, this chapter is intended to be a review of basic neurology.

It is important to study cortical structures in the left hemisphere of the cerebrum because: (1) research has held that these structures actively participate in language comprehension, formulation, and expression and (2) these structures are most often implicated in neurogenic disorders of language and cognition. Before any discussion of the cerebrum, a review of embryonic brain development is necessary first to see how the fetal brain divides into functional and structural divisions, followed by a review of the structure of the neuron and the process of synaptic transmission.

The neuron is the smallest unit of the brain with interconnections to other neurons that are both electrical and chemical. The neuron, synaptic transmission, and the role of neurotransmitters are important to understand in order to appreciate what pathologic effects are created by dementia, stroke, and traumatic brain injury. Because of advancements in the study of neurotransmitters, those that are critical for cognition and learning are identified.

Neurons make up the tissue of the cerebrum, which is the largest component of the central nervous system. Three of the lobes of the left cerebral hemisphere house important structures for language and cognition. The structures to be reviewed are Broca's area in the left frontal lobe, Wernicke's area in the left temporal lobe, and the angular and supramarginal gyri in the left parietal lobe. The neocortex of the cerebrum, the most recent proliferation of cortical tissue, is not found in lower animals and is the highest level of control, housing areas for language, personality, executive functioning and memory, problem solving, judgment, and centers for motor schema.

Under the gray mantle of the cerebrum are subcortical structures that interact with cortical structures through ascending and descending pathways. Subcortical structures, specifically the thalamus and basal ganglia, play significant roles in language (Robin & Schienberg, 1990). The left basal ganglia are thought to play a role in the expression of highly automatized language. The thalamus is responsible for four major functions: sensation, motor control, regulation of rhythmic cortical activity, and higher order processes such as language and emotion (Larson, 1989). When both cortical and subcortical structures are damaged, the effects on language and cognition are more severe than from damage to the cortical structures alone. The subcortical structures discussed in this chapter are the basal ganglia, thalamus, hippocampus in the limbic system, and the brainstem.

The limbic system, considered a part of the older, instinctual brain, the archicortex, has significant roles in drives, emotional responses, aggression, fight or flight, smell (olfaction), and reproductive cycles. Within the limbic system is the hippocampus, which is located in the medial temporal lobes of the brain. The hippocampus is actively involved in learning and auditory memory. Horner and his associates (2012) note that the hippocampus is also critical for the ability to recollect contextual details of past auditory memories.

The brainstem, part of the oldest part of the brain, the paleocortex, has structures that are responsible for attention and wakefulness. The reticular formation, also found in the midbrain, is critical for cognition. The ability to be conscious and focus on external stimuli (perception) depends upon the reticular formation in the brainstem and midbrain.

The cerebrum and spinal cord have two circulatory systems, which protect the delicate structures of the central nervous system (CNS) and provide oxygen-rich blood to nervous tissue. These circulatory systems include the meninges, the ventricular system, and the vascular system. The vascular system and the meningeal/ventricular system are described because of their vulnerability to cerebrovascular accidents and traumatic brain injuries. The meninges and ventricular system contain cerebrospinal fluid (CSF), a blood derivative, which cushions and protects the brain and can be compromised by closed or penetrating head injuries. The cerebrovascular integrity (vascular system), of the cerebrum is the site of cerebrovascular accidents.

Specific structures in cholinergic and noradrenergic systems and the cerebellum are discussed to prepare the reader for the research on dementia and cerebrovascular accidents. Recent investigations have shown that these pathways contribute to cognition, particularly memory, and transfer information to the neocortex of the cerebrum. Recent research also shows that the cerebellum, which contributes to fine motor movement and coordination, plays a significant role in language functioning.

The right hemisphere, originally thought to be passive in language, is now acknowledged to be active in integrating language functions, including emotional expression, prosody, lower order perceptual skills, linguistic, and higher cognitive skills. Functions of the right hemisphere in linguistic, nonlinguistic, and extralinguistic functioning are covered extensively in Chapter 6.

Embryonic brain development, the neuron as the building block of the nervous system, synaptic transmission, and types of neurotransmitters begin the discussion of the CNS.

EMBRYONIC BRAIN DEVELOPMENT

The brain begins to develop early in the gestational period. Stiles and Jernigan (2010) describe embryonic brain development as "a protracted process that begins in the third gestational week (GW) with the differentiation of the neural progenitor cells and extends at least through late adolescence, arguably throughout the lifespan." Furthermore, it is "a complex series of dynamic and adaptive processes that operate throughout the course of

development to promote the emergence and differentiation of new neural structures and functions" (p. 328).

The first step in brain development involves the formation of the first well-defined neural structure, the neural tube, which is seen in Figure 3–1.

The neural tube forms during the third week of gestation from specialized cells (progenitor cells) that arise from a neural plate. The initial sign of neural tube development is the appearance of two ridges that form along the two sides of the neural plate. Over the course of several days, the ridges rise, fold inward, and fuse to form a hollow tube. Fusion begins in the center of the developing neural tube and then proceeds until the last segments of the tube close. When the neural tube is complete, specialized cells, called the neural progenitors, form a single layer of cells that line the center of the neural tube immediately adjacent to its hollow center. In the embryo, the hollow center of the neural tube is cylindrical, like the center of a straw.

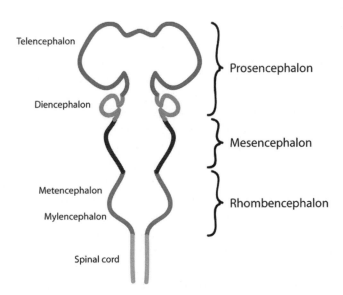

Figure 3–1. The neural tube (User: Nretz / Wikimedia Commons / CC-BY-SA-3.0).

The neural tube is, however, never a straight, simple cylinder (Nolte, 2002). But as the brain becomes larger and more complex, the shape of the hollow cavity also changes, eventually forming the ventricular system of the brain. Progenitor cells found in the brain are early descendents of stem cells that can differentiate to form one or more kinds of cells; but have limited reproducibility (Boston Children's Hospital, 2013; Goldman & Sim, 2005). Because the neural progenitors are located in the region that will become the ventricles, the region is called the ventricular zone (VZ), which will become the lateral ventricles, the third ventricle, the cerebral aqueduct, the fourth ventricle, and the central canal. The neural progenitor cells in the most rostral region of the neural tube will give rise to the brain, while more caudally positioned cells will give rise to the hindbrain and spinal column (Stiles & Jernigan, 2010). Even before the rostral and caudal cells close, bulges begin to appear in the rostral end of the neural tube in the region of the future brain, and bends begin to appear as well (Nolte, 2002).

As the neural tube develops, during the fourth and fifth weeks, the primary and secondary bulges, or vesicles, appear. These definite areas can be identified as the prosencephalon (forebrain), the mesencephalon (midbrain), and the rhombencephalon (hindbrain) of the three primary vesicles, which appear during the fourth week. By the fifth week, the primary vesicles subdivide further into the five secondary vesicles that will become the mature brain at birth. The prosecephalon divides into the telencephalon (end-brain) and the diencephalon (in-between brain). The mesencephalon remains undivided. The rhombencephalon divides to become the metencephalon and myencephalon.

Neural tube subdivisions each eventually develop into distinct regions of the central nervous system by the division of neuroepithelial cells:

- The *prosencephalon* further goes on to develop into the telencephalon (the forebrain or cerebrum) and the diencephalon (the optic vesicles, thalamus, and hypothalamus).
- The *mesencephalon* develops into the midbrain.
- The *rhombencephalon* develops into the metencephalon (the pons and cerebellum) and the myelencephalon (the medulla oblongata).

The telencephalon becomes the cerebral hemispheres and the underlying basal ganglia of the adult brain. The diencephalon gives rise to the thalamus (ovoid-shaped gray matter between the basal ganglia and the cortex), the hypothalamus (an autonomic control center), and the retina. The metencephalon becomes the pons (part of the brainstem) and the cerebellum. The myencephalon becomes the medulla (brainstem structure that becomes the spinal cord). Neurons of the developing embryonic brain's forebrain extend axons to communicate with other parts of the nervous system. These axons bundle together to form three major white matter systems: the cortical white matter, the corpus callosum, and the internal capsule.

The developed or mature brain is shown in Figures 3–2 and 3–3. Figure 3–2 shows the four lobes of the brain: frontal, temporal, parietal, and occipital. Figure 3–3 gives a medial view of the mature brain and shows the cerebrum, diencephalon, brainstem, cerebellum, and spinal cord.

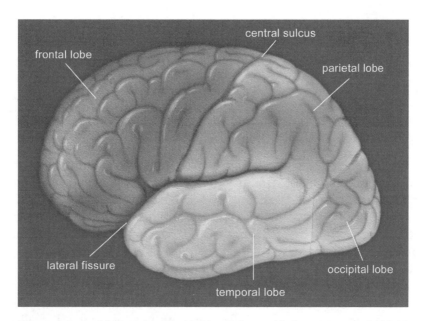

Figure 3–2. Mature brain showing lobes of left cerebrum. © 2013 Medical Art Studio. Reprinted with permission.

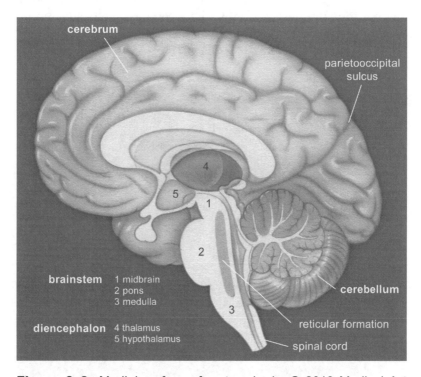

Figure 3–3. Medial surface of mature brain. © 2013 Medical Art Studio. Reprinted with permission.

THE NEURON

The smallest unit in the nervous system is the neuron. The most numerous types of neurons are the multipolar neurons, which have a cell body that contains a soma, dendrites, and an axon. See Figure 3–4 for an illustration of a neuron and a synapse. Dendrites and axons are long, narrow extensions designed to carry information to and from the cell body. Multipolar neurons have at least two dendrites and usually more and carry information to and from the cell body. There is a single axon that arises from the cell body from an axon hillock. Axons are usually much longer and less branched than the dendrites. Branches of the axon are called collaterals.

Dendrites have numerous branches that form a dendritic tree. The dendritic tree form has traditionally been thought to be the main information receiving network for the neuron. However, information outflow (i.e., from dendrites to other neurons) can also occur. The axon, a much finer, cable-like projection, may extend tens, hundreds, or even tens of thousands of times the diameter of the soma in length. This is the structure that carries nerve signals away from the neuron.

Neurons receive and send information both electrically (action potentials) and chemically (neurotransmitters). In order to minimize metabolic expense yet maintain a rapid conduction velocity, many neurons have insulating sheaths of myelin around their axons. The sheaths are formed by glial cells: oligodendrocytes in the CNS and Schwann cells in the peripheral nervous system. The axon is encased in a myelin sheath, which enables the action potential to move swiftly down the axon to the terminal bouton. Breaks between the myelin sheaths are called the nodes of Ranvier.

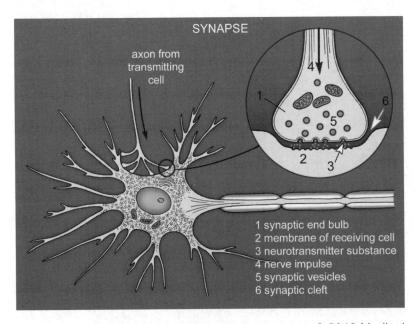

SYNAPSE

axon from transmitting cell

1 synaptic end bulb
2 membrane of receiving cell
3 neurotransmitter substance
4 nerve impulse
5 synaptic vesicles
6 synaptic cleft

Figure 3–4. Schematic of a neuron and a synapse. © 2013 Medical Art Studio. Reprinted with permission.

At the end of the axon is the terminal bouton, within which there are numerous tiny, smooth, hollow spheres called synaptic vesicles. Neurotransmitters, or specialized chemicals designed to propagate an electrical signal, are contained within these vesicles. Terminal boutons are adjacent to another neuron's plasma membrane, and the space between them is called the synaptic cleft. The terminal bouton and postsynaptic membrane together form the synapse.

SYNAPTIC TRANSMISSION

The human brain has a gigantic number of synapses. Each of 100 billion neurons has on average 7,000 synaptic connections to other neurons. Most authorities estimate the total number of synapses at 1,000 trillion for a 3-year-old child. This number declines and with age stabilizes by adulthood. Estimates vary for an adult from 100 to 500 trillion synapses.

Neurons have excitable membranes, which allow them to generate and propagate electrical signals. The cell membrane in the axon and soma contains voltage-gated ion channels, which allow the neuron to generate and propagate an electrical impulse known as an action potential. Electrical activity can be produced in neurons by a number of stimuli. Pressure, stretch, chemical transmitters, and electrical current passing across the nerve membrane as a result of a potential difference in voltage all can initiate nerve activity.

A neuron's dendritic tree is connected to a thousand neighboring neurons. When one of those neurons fire, a positive or negative charge is received by one of the dendrites. The strengths of all the received charges are added together through the processes of spatial and temporal summation. Spatial summation occurs when several weak signals are converted into a single large one, whereas temporal summation converts a rapid series of weak pulses from one source into one large signal. Once a neuron fires, it keeps on triggering all the neurons in the vicinity.

When the neuron is in a state of resting potential, electrically charged ions are at homeostasis. In order for the neuron to be charged, the cell membrane begins to allow large, positively charged ions like sodium (Na+) and potassium (K+) to enter the intracellular space. The sodium-potassium pump is a mechanism that allows these positively charged ions to enter the intracellular space rapidly in order to trigger an action potential.

When the intracellular voltage is great enough (−65 mV), an action potential is generated. The electrical impulse traveling down the axon stimulates the vesicles to open, releasing a neurotransmitter to communicate with target neurons. Neurotransmitters are chemicals that are used to relay, amplify, and modulate electrical signals between a neuron and another cell (Nolte, 2002). Figure 3–4 shows the terminal bouton, synaptic vesicles, the synaptic cleft, and postsynaptic side.

Changing the constitution of various neurotransmitter chemicals can increase or decrease the amount of stimulation that the firing axon imparts on the neighboring dendrite. Altering the neurotransmitters can also change whether the stimulation is excitatory or inhibitory.

TYPES OF NEUROTRANSMITTERS

A chemical can be classified as a neurotransmitter under the following conditions:

1. It is synthesized endogenously, that is, within the presynaptic neuron.
2. It is available in sufficient quantity in the presynaptic neuron to exert an effect on the postsynaptic neuron.
3. Externally administered, it must mimic the endogenously released substance.
4. A biochemical mechanism for inactivation must be present.

It is important to understand neurotransmitters because they facilitate communication between the neurons in synaptic transmission. Further, neurotransmitters help to regulate brain mechanisms that control cognition, language, speech, hearing, moods, attention, memory, personality, motivation, and physiological tuning of the brain (Bhatanagar, 2002). While there are many neurotransmitters in the human nervous system, five are most often implicated in neurological pathologies that compromise language and cognition. These are acetylcholine, gamma aminobutyric acid (GABA), dopamine, norepinephrine, and glutamate.

Acetylcholine

Acetylcholine is a neurotransmitter at all autonomic ganglia, at many autonomically innervated organs, at the neuromuscular junction, and at many synapses in the CNS. It is found at the neuromuscular junction between the motor nerve and skeletal muscles. It is degraded by acetylcholinesterase, an enzyme that breaks up acetylcholine into acetic acid and choline at the postsynaptic side. In Alzheimer's disease (AD), there is a marked decrease in acetylcholine concentration in the cerebral cortex and caudate nucleus (Waymire, 2013).

Dopamine

Dopamine is a neurotransmitter that helps to control the brain's reward and pleasure centers and to regulate movement and emotional responses. Dopaminergic neurons of the midbrain, specifically, the substantia nigra, are the main source of dopamine in the brain. Dopamine has been shown to be involved in the control of movements, in the signaling of error in prediction of reward, in motivation, and in cognition. Loss of dopamine in the caudate nucleus of the basal ganglia, as seen in Parkinson's disease, results in cognitive disorders (Ostrosky-Solis, Madrazo, Drucker-Colin, & Quintanar, 1989).

Gamma Aminobutyric Acid

An inhibitory transmitter in the mature brain, in the developing brain it is excitatory. GABA regulates the proliferation of the neural progenitor cells and the growth of embryonic and neural stem cells (Ganguly, Schinder, Wong, & Poo, 2001).

Norepinephrine

Norepinephrine is released from the adrenal medulla into the blood as a hormone and is a neurotransmitter in the CNS and sympathetic nervous system, where it is released from noradrenergic neurons in the locus coeruleus (LC). The noradrenergic neurons in the brain form a neurotransmitter system that, when activated, exerts effects on large areas of the brain. Norepinephrine may play a significant role in synchronizing cortical activity in response to a decision process (Nieuwenhuis, Aston-Jones, & Cohen, 2005).

Glutamate

Glutamate is considered to be the major mediator of excitatory signals in the mammalian CNS and is involved in most aspects of normal brain function, including cognition, memory, and learning. Glutamate transporters may modify the time course of synaptic events, the extent and pattern of activation, and desensitization of receptors outside the synaptic cleft and at neighboring synapses (intersynaptic cross-talk). Furthermore, the glutamate transporters provide glutamate for synthesis of, for example, GABA, glutathione, and protein, and facilitates energy production (Danbolt, 2001).

THE CEREBRUM

The cerebrum, the largest structure of the telencephalon, appears as gray in color because of the profusion of cell bodies and blood supply, and has six layers of cortical tissue in which there are large pyramidal cells of Betz. These large cells constitute the motor areas in the frontal lobe. On the outside of the brain are bumps (gyri), folds (sulci), and deep folds (fissures) that provide the landscape of the brain. The cerebrum is the largest and most highly developed part of the human brain. It encompasses about two-thirds of the brain mass and lies over and around most of the structures of the brain. The outer portion (1.5 mm to 5 mm) of the cerebrum is covered by a thin layer of gray tissue called the cerebral cortex.

The cerebrum is composed of two cerebral hemispheres. Each hemisphere has gray matter on its surface (cerebral cortex), white matter deep to the cortex, and large masses of gray matter deeper still (basal ganglia, amygdala, and claustrum). In addition, each hemisphere contains a lateral ventricle that extends into all four lobes: frontal, parietal, occipital, and temporal (Webster, 1999).

Figure 3–5 shows the primary language areas on the lateral surface of the left hemisphere with Brodmann classifications.

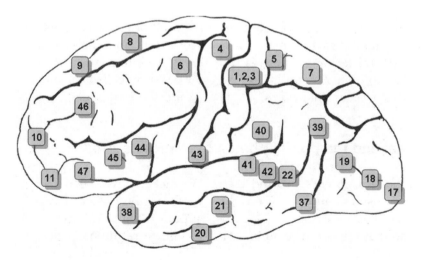

Figure 3–5. Brodmann areas on lateral surface of cerebrum (User: Pngbot / Wikimedia Commons / CC-BY-SA 3.0.).

As can be seen, Broca's and Wernicke's areas can be readily identified as areas 44/45 and 22, respectively, in the frontal and temporal lobes. Three of the four lobes of the left hemisphere of the cerebrum are directly involved in language and cognition: frontal, temporal, and parietal. The parietal lobe contains the angular (reading) and supramarginal (writing) gyri. The fourth lobe, occipital, is responsible for deciphering graphemes for reading and for providing visual feedback necessary to modify language expression.

Brodmann Areas

Along the lateral surface of the brain, specific structures are important for spoken language, auditory comprehension, reading, and writing. These areas are designated by numbers, using the Brodmann area classification developed in 1909 by Korbinian Brodmann, who numbered regions based upon their cytoarchitectonic (histological) characteristics (Bear, Connors, & Paradiso, 2001). See Figure 3–5 for Brodmann areas on the lateral surface of the cerebrum. For the study of language and cognition, the critical Brodmann areas are areas 22 (Wernicke's area), areas 44 and 45 (Broca's area), area 39 (angular gyrus), and area 40 (supramarginal gyrus).

The Frontal and Temporal Lobes

Although the terms *Broca's area* and *Wernicke's area* are still commonly used, the boundaries of these areas are not clearly defined, and they appear to be quite variable from one person to the next. In addition, each area may be involved in more than one language function (Bear et al., 2001). Tanner (2007) suggests that a more

accurate definition of Wernicke's area, for example, is "a region in the temporal-parietal lobe of the cerebrum important to understanding oral language; a cortical conduit corresponding approximately to Brodmann's areas 22, 39, 40, 41, and 42" (p. 66). It is with this understanding that Broca's area and Wernicke's area are described in the following sections.

Broca's Area

Broca's area lies in the third frontal convolution of the neocortex just behind the left eye. For Broca's area, the debate focuses on specialization for language versus domain-general functions such as hierarchical structure building aspects of action processing, working memory, or cognitive control. There is evidence that both ideas are right: Broca's area contains two sets of subregions lying side by side, one quite specifically engaged in language processing, surrounded by another that is broadly engaged across a wide variety of tasks and content domains (Federenko, Duncan, & Kanwisher, 2012). Figure 3–6 shows Broca's area and its relationship to Wernicke's area. Broca's and Wernicke's areas are interconnected by a white matter pathway called the arcuate fasciculus (Anderson et al., 1999).

Wernicke's Area

Wernicke's area, seen in Figure 3–6, is found in the posterior two-thirds of the superior temporal gyrus. Although it has been traditionally designated as the center for comprehension of spoken language, research models demonstrate that comprehension may extend to the parietal lobe as well (Musiek et al., 2011; Tanner,

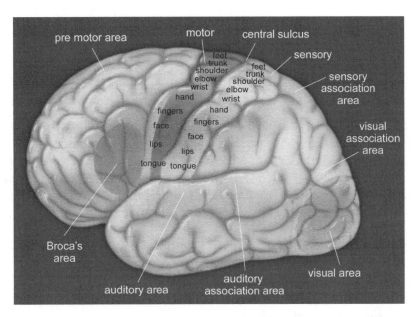

Figure 3–6. Lateral cerebrum showing Broca's and Wernicke's areas. © 2013 Medical Art Studio. Reprinted with permission.

2007). Other researchers (Naeser, Helm-Estabrooks, Hass, Auerbach, & Srinivasan, 1987) argue that comprehension of spoken language may rest largely within Wernicke's area, as demonstrated by the severity of the comprehension deficit and the amount of damage to that area and adjacent temporal lobe areas.

In a study of lesion size and comprehension deficits, Naeser and his colleagues (1987) noted that there was a highly significant correlation between comprehension and the extent of temporal lobe lesions in Wernicke's area. There was no significant correlation between comprehension and the total temporoparietal lesion size. Patients with damage in only half or less than half of Wernicke's area had good comprehension at 6 months after the onset of stroke. Patients with damage in more than half of Wernicke's area had poor comprehension even 1 year after the onset of stroke. Additional anterior-inferior tem-

poral lobe lesion extension into the middle temporal gyrus area was associated with particularly poor recovery.

Although comprehension is still largely localized to Wernicke's area, thanks to developments in neuroimaging, the traditional view of an isolated area for auditory comprehension of language and spoken language has undergoing significant change. Areas outside of the classical models of Broca's and Wernicke's are now being seen in brain activation during tasks for auditory comprehension. Binder and his associates (1997), for example, found that with MRI mapping, activity in areas surrounding the classical Broca's and Wernicke's areas can be identified. From their research, cortical activation associated with language processing was strongly lateralized to the left cerebral hemisphere and involved a network of regions in the frontal, temporal, and parietal lobes. Less consistent with classical models were:

(1) the existence of left hemisphere temporoparietal language areas outside the traditional "Wernicke's area," namely, in the middle temporal, inferior temporal, fusiform, and angular gyri; (2) extensive left prefrontal language areas outside the classical "Broca's area"; and (3) clear participation of these left frontal areas in a task emphasizing "receptive" language functions.

Further corroboration for a larger network for language function that extends beyond the classical models, specifically for auditory comprehension tasks, was identified by Démonet and colleagues (1992), who used PET to find that phonological processing was associated with activation in the left superior temporal gyrus (mainly Wernicke's area) and, to a lesser extent, in Broca's area and in the right superior temporal regions. In their view, lexical-semantic processing was associated with activity in the left middle and inferior temporal gyri, the left inferior parietal region, and the left superior prefrontal region, in addition to the superior temporal regions. No difference in activation was found in Broca's area and superior temporal areas, which suggests that these areas are activated by the phonological component of both tasks, but activation was noted in the temporal, parietal, and frontal multimodal association areas.

Working memory necessary for language refers to a brain system that provides temporary storage and manipulation of the information necessary for such complex cognitive tasks as language comprehension, learning, and reasoning. Explicit memories (remembered events or facts) and implicit (subconsciously generated responses to events or stimuli) memories, conditioned reflexes, and automatized memories are distributed throughout the CNS presumably as sets of connections in neocortical association areas (Nolte, 2002). Categories of working memory, so necessary for cognition, are dispersed throughout the frontal lobes of the cerebrum.

The definition of working memory has evolved from the concept of a unitary short-term memory system. Working memory has been found to require the simultaneous storage and processing of information (Baddeley, 1992). The central executive portion of working memory necessary for attention is particularly vulnerable to AD.

The Parietal Lobe

The parietal lobes can be divided into two functional regions. One involves sensation and perception and the other is concerned with integrating sensory input, primarily with the visual system. The first function integrates sensory information to form a single perception (cognition). The second function constructs a spatial coordinate system to represent the world around us. Individuals with damage to the parietal lobes often show striking deficits, such as abnormalities in body image and spatial relations (Kandel, 1991).

Damage to the left parietal lobe can result in Gerstmann's syndrome. Gerstmann's syndrome is a cognitive impairment that results from damage to the left parietal lobe in the region of the angular gyrus. It may occur after a stroke or in association with damage to the parietal lobe. It is characterized by four primary symptoms: a writing disability (agraphia or dysgraphia), a lack of understanding of the rules for calculation or arithmetic (acalculia or dyscalculia), an inability to distinguish right from left, and an inability to identify fingers (finger agnosia).

The syndrome can also produce aphasia (National Institute of Neurological Disorders and Stroke, 2013).

Damage to the right parietal lobe can result in neglecting part of the body or space (contralateral neglect), which can impair many self-care skills, such as dressing and washing. Right-side damage can also cause difficulty in making things (constructional apraxia), denial of deficits (anosagnosia), and drawing ability. Special deficits (primarily to memory and personality) can occur if there is damage to the area between the parietal and temporal lobes. Left parietal-temporal lesions can affect verbal memory and the ability to recall strings of digits (Warrington & Weiskrantz, 1970). The right parietal-temporal lobe is concerned with nonverbal memory. Right parietal-temporal lesions can produce significant changes in personality.

Angular Gyrus

Designated as Brodmann's area 39 and located in the posterior part of the inferior parietal lobule, the angular gyrus has been shown in numerous meta-analysis reviews to be consistently activated in a variety of tasks, including reading. Seghier (2012) noted in his review of the literature on the angular gyrus that it may function as a hub where converging multisensory information is combined and integrated to comprehend and give sense to events, manipulate representations, solve familiar problems, and reorient attention to relevant information. In summary, the role of the angular gyrus cannot comprehensibly be identified in isolation but needs to be understood in parallel with the influence from other regions, like the supramarginal gyrus. Figure 3–7 shows the angular and supramarginal gyri.

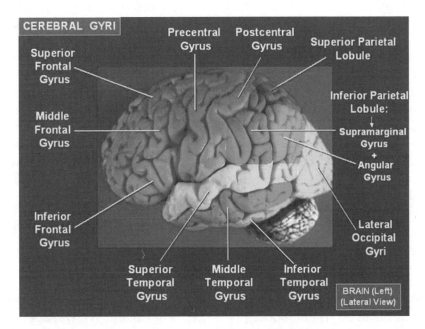

Figure 3–7. Lateral view of cerebrum showing angular and supramarginal gyri (© John A. Beal / http://www.healcentral.org/healapp/showMetadata?metadataId=40566 / CC-BY-SA-3.0).

In a large study using PET to track cerebral blood flow in normal men during reading tasks (Horwitz, Rumsey, & Donohue, 1998), the angular gyrus was found to have interconnections with the areas of visual association cortex in the occipital and temporal lobes known to be activated by words and word-like stimuli. During pseudoword reading, the left angular gyrus also was functionally linked to a region in the left superior and middle temporal gyri that is part of Wernicke's area, and to an area in frontal cortex in or near Broca's region.

Supramarginal Gyrus

A portion of the parietal lobe, lying just above the temporal lobe, is called the supramarginal gyrus (SMG). Located near other brain regions involved in language and hearing, this area plays a role in processing heard and spoken language, as well as written words. Alternate classifications of the brain based on cell structures consider this area to be a part of Brodmann's area 40, and it is sometimes referred to by this name. SMG contributes to reading regardless of the specific task demands, which suggests that this may be due to automatically computing the sound of a word even when the task does not explicitly require it (Stoeckel, Gough, Watkins, & Devlin, 2009). The angular gyrus works closely with the supramarginal gyrus to process linguistic information. Processing the meaning and semantics of words seems to be the domain of the angular gyrus, whereas the supramarginal gyrus acts to determine their sound. These two gyri are connected to parts of the brain involved in emotional processing, such as the amygdala, and this connection may mediate the emotional response to language.

The supramarginal gyrus seems to be involved in phonological and articulatory processing of words, whereas the angular gyrus (together with the posterior cingulate gyrus) seems more involved in semantic processing. The SMG contributes to reading regardless of the specific task demands, which suggests that this may be due to automatically computing the sound of a word even when the task does not explicitly require it (Stoeckel et al., 2009).

The right angular gyrus appears to be active as well as the left, thus revealing that the right hemisphere also contributes to semantic processing of language. Together, the angular and supramarginal gyri constitute a multimodal associative area that receives auditory, visual, and somatosensory inputs. The neurons in this area are thus very well positioned to process the phonological and semantic aspect of language that enables us to identify and categorize objects. Bilateral reactions of the SMG may facilitate enactment of a verbal message. Russ, Mack, Grama, Lanfermann, and Knopf (2003) observed activation on fMRI when study participants were asked to enact "Cut the bread" in the bilateral inferior parietal areas covering the SMG. This finding suggests that the SMG may be a central structure in what the researchers referred to as a neurofunctional explanation of the enactment effect.

SUBCORTICAL STRUCTURES

The Thalamus

The thalamus, located in the diencephalon, is an ovoid (egg)-shaped structure that forms a large part of the third ventricle (Wallesch & Papagno, 1988). Each thalamus consists of more than 30 anatomically and functionally separate nuclei, which are separated by white matter sheets (internal medullary laminae) into five major nuclei groups. The groups are the anterior, medial, ventral, posterior, and nonspecific intralaminar and midline nuclei. The ventral anterior, the ventral lateral nucleus, and pulvinar, the largest of the posterior nuclei, participate in language processes (Wallesch & Papagno, 1988). The pulvinar has widespread reciprocal relationships with the parieto-occipital association and visual association cortex. As such, the pulvinar collaborates closely with the cerebral cortex in many important cognitive functions, including complex visual and language functions (Heimer, 1983; Hebb & Ojemann, 2012). Figure 3–8 provides a schematic medial view of the thalamus.

Thalamic nuclei transmit incoming information from the special senses and multiple subcortical structures to the cortex. As the nuclei are interconnected with each other, they act as relays and also integrate and transform information passing through. This modification of outgoing information, according to Luria (1977), involves blocking of already evoked or extraneous associations. Topographical organization of the thalamic afferents and efferents is contralateral, and the lateralization of the thalamic functions affects both sensory and motoric aspects. Symptoms of lesions located in the thalamus are closely related to the function of the areas involved (Herrero, Barcia, & Navarro, 2002).

Without the integration of the thalamus, the selectivity of speech breaks down. Paraphasia and disturbances of lexical processes are caused by lesions in the thalamus and anterior limb of the internal capsule, which provide evidence of thalamic gating in language production and

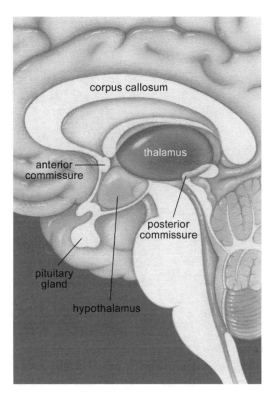

Figure 3–8. Medial view showing the thalamus. © 2013 Medical Art Studio. Reprinted with permission.

coordination of the cognitive and motoric aspects of language production (Johnson & Ojemann, 2000; Ojemann, 1979; Ozeren, Sarica, & Efe, 1994). Wallesch and Papagno (1988) propose that the basal ganglia and the ventral thalamus are integrated into a frontal lobe system. These nuclei together integrate response selection and are involved in gating a number of possible lexical alternatives. Figure 3–9 shows the nuclei of the thalamus.

The Basal Ganglia

The basal ganglia are a collection of nuclei found on both sides of the thalamus, outside and above the limbic system but

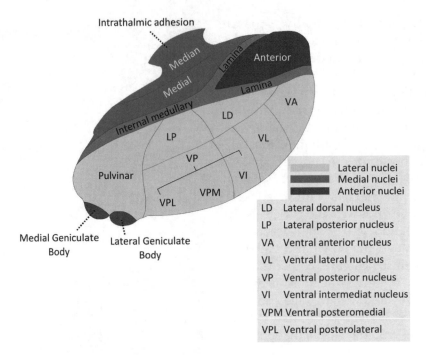

Figure 3–9. Thalamic nuclei (User: Madhero88 / Wikimedia Commons / CC-BY-SA-3.0).

below the cingulate gyrus and within the temporal lobes. See Figure 3–10 for a lateral view of the basal ganglia.

The inhibitory neurotransmitters GABA and dopamine play the most important roles in the basal ganglia. The telencephalic structures that comprise the ganglia are collectively called the corpus striatum (striped body), made up of the caudate nucleus (tail), the putamen (shell), and the globus pallidus (pale globe). All of these structures appear as one set on each side of the central septum. The main components of the basal ganglia are the striatum and the lentiform nucleus. The lentiform nucleus consists of the putamen and the globus pallidus, also called the pallidum. The corpus striatum can be further subdivided into the striatum and global pallidus.

Basal Ganglia Components (Payne, 1997)

Corpus striatum = striatum and pallidum (globus pallidus, putamen, caudate nucleus)

Striatum = caudate nucleus and putamen

Lentiform nucleus = putamen and globus pallidus

Pallidum = globus pallidus

The globus pallidus and putamen are lateral to the internal capsule (Baumgartner & Bentley, 1989). The caudate nucleus, which is continuous with the lateral wall of the lateral ventricle, is shaped like a tadpole (Wallesch & Papagno, 1988). The inner medial division of the globus pal-

Basal Ganglia and Related Structures of the Brain

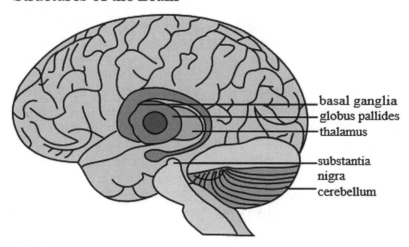

basal ganglia
globus pallides
thalamus
substantia nigra
cerebellum

Figure 3–10. Lateral view of the cerebrum showing the basal ganglia (John Henkel, from the Food and Drug Administration / Wikimedia Commons / Public Domain).

lidus is continuous caudally with the substantia nigra, a darkly colored band on each side of the midline in the cerebral peduncle of the midbrain (Heimer, 1983). The substantia nigra, found in the midbrain, is considered to be part of the basal ganglia (Nolte, 2002). There is evidence that the cholinergic activity of the caudate nucleus plays a major role in the acquisition and early maintenance stages of learning. According to Prado-Alcalá (1989), interconnections between the caudate nucleus and the midbrain substantia nigra are possibly implicated in recent memory and in the retention and storage of overtrained tasks using multiple training sessions and reinforcement. Moreover, inasmuch as dopamine, GABA, and acetylcholine are the major neurotransmitters for the nigrostriatum system, it is reasonable to conclude that this system is critical for memory and language functions (Cappa, Cavallotti, Guidotti, Pap-

agno, & Vignolo, 1983; D'Esposito & Alexander, 1993; Kennedy & Murdoch, 1993; Larson, 1989; Mega & Alexander, 1992; Okuda, Taneka, Tachibana, Kawabata, & Sugita, 1994).

The Limbic System

Descriptions of the limbic lobe or limbic system include the historical perspectives of Paul Broca, who in 1878 first identified a great horseshoe-shaped rim of cortex surrounding the junction between the diencephalon and each cerebral hemisphere, and of Paul MacLean, a pioneering neurophysiologist who is credited with identifying the limbic system (MacLean, 1985, 1988, 1990; Newman & Harris, 2009). The ends of the arc are joined by olfactory areas at the base of the brain so that a complete loop is formed (Nolte, 2002). While the limbic system is comparatively small in reptiles, it is large in all mammals and also of similar relative size across different mammalian species.

The limbic system is described by Webster (1999) as a functional rather than a structural arrangement that includes all three-layered regions (septal region, cingulate gyrus, parahippocampal gyrus, uncus, and hippocampus), the amygdala, the mammillary bodies of the hypothalamus, and the anterior, dorsomedial, and lateral dorsal nuclei of the thalamus. Figure 3–11 shows the limbic system. Although all limbic structures are important, the hippocampus is particularly critical for memory.

The Hippocampus

The hippocampus and nearby cortical areas are important for some forms of memory. In particular, the hippocampus seems to be significant for laying down or consolidating new memories as well as memory for remembering events (episodic memory) and knowing facts (semantic memory). These forms of memory are referred to as explicit or declarative memories, meaning that items stored are accessible to consciousness and can be declared as remembered events or facts. The hippocampus also acts as a memory indexer for long-term storage and retrieval by sending memories out to the appropriate parts of the cerebral hemisphere. Bilateral destruction of the hippocampus results in the inability to acquire new factual memories (Webster, 1999).

THE MENINGES AND VENTRICULAR SYSTEM

The Meninges

The cerebrum and the spinal cord are both encased in bone. The cerebrum sits within the bony cranial vault; the spinal

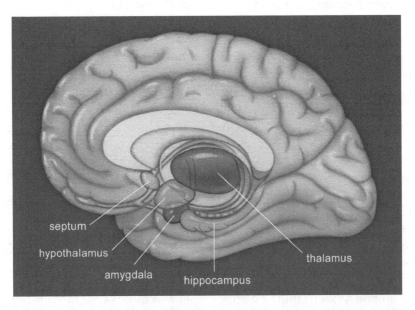

Figure 3–11. Medial view showing the limbic system. © 2013 Medical Art Studio. Reprinted with permission.

cord is protected by the spinal vertebrae, or spinal column. Neither comes in direct contact with bone. Rather, the soft tissue of the brain and spinal cord are protected and cushioned by three membranes known collectively as the meninges, or coverings. The three membranes are the dura mater (hard mother), arachnoid (spider), and the pia mater (gentle mother). Figure 3–12 shows the meninges.

The pia mater is a thin membrane that adheres closely to the surface of the brain. Along the pia mater run many blood vessels that provide blood supply to the underlying brain tissue. The pia mater is separated from the arachnoid by a fluid-filled space, the subarachnoid space, which is filled with CSF, a clear colorless bodily fluid produced in the choroid plexus of the brain. The choroid plexus is composed of many capillaries that filter CSF. Five functions are ascribed to CSF (Sorokin, 2009):

1. **Protection:** CSF protects the brain from damage by "buffering" the brain. In other words, the CSF acts to cushion a blow to the head and lessen the impact. CSF is produced and secreted by epithelial cells in choroid plexus (specialized blood cells) of the meninges, the ventricles, and the spinal cord. CSF is reabsorbed by the arachnoid villi and within the sagittal sinuses.

2. **Excretion of waste products:** The one-way flow from the CSF to the blood takes potentially harmful metabolites, drugs, and other substances away from the brain.

3. **Endocrine medium for the brain:** The CSF serves to transport hormones to other areas of the brain. Hormones released into the CSF can be carried to remote sites of the brain where they may act.

4. **Buoyancy:** Because the brain is immersed in fluid, the net weight of the

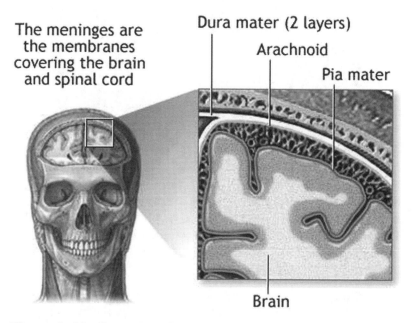

The meninges are the membranes covering the brain and spinal cord

Dura mater (2 layers)

Arachnoid

Pia mater

Brain

Figure 3–12. Illustration of the meninges (© Grook de Oger, 2011 / http://medlineplus.gov / CC-BY-SA-3.0).

brain is reduced from about 1,400 g to about 50 g. Therefore, pressure at the base of the brain is reduced.

5. **Barrier:** The CNS is tightly sealed from the changeable environment of blood by the blood–brain barrier and the blood–CSF barrier established by the epithelial cells in the choroid plexi. The barrier and secretory function of the choroid plexus epithelial cells are maintained within numerous transport systems that flow into the CSF and remove toxic agents out of the CSF. In the event of CNS pathology, barrier characteristics of the blood–CNS barriers are altered. Once the barrier characteristics are changed, edema (swelling) can form and inflammatory cells can invade the CNS.

The Ventricular System

Inside of the brain is hollow space. The fluid-filled cavities and canals inside the brain constitute the ventricular system. The ventricular system includes five cavities in the core of the brain that also contain choroid plexi, including: (1) two lateral ventricles, (2) one third ventricle, (3) one aqueduct, called the aqueduct of Sylvius, and (4) one fourth ventricle.

Figure 3–13 shows a coronal view of the lateral and third ventricles in the ventricular system. Figures 3–14 and 3–15 show a lateral and a dorsal view of the ventricles in relation to the four lobes of the brain. CSF flows from the paired lateral ventricles of the cerebrum to the third ventricle through the aqueduct to the

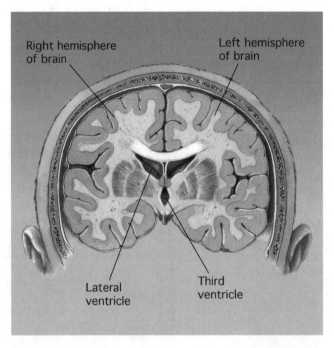

Figure 3–13. Coronal view of the lateral and third ventricles. © 2013 Medical Art Studio. Reprinted with permission.

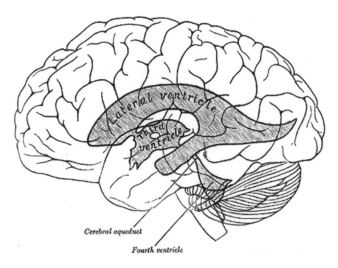

Lateral ventricle

Third ventricle

Cerebral aqueduct

Fourth ventricle

Figure 3–14. Lateral view of the ventricular system within the cerebrum (From *Anatomy of the Human Body, Twentieth Edition* by Henry Gray / Wikimedia Commons / Public Domain).

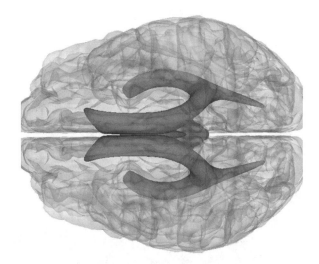

Figure 3–15. Dorsal view of ventricular system within the cerebrum (Life Science Databases / Wikimedia Commons / CC-AS-2.5 Generic).

fourth ventricle. CSF exits the ventricular system and enters the subarachnoid space by way of small openings, or apertures near where the cerebellum attaches to the brainstem. In the subarachnoid space, CSF is absorbed by the blood vessels at special structures called the arachnoid villi (Bear, Connors, & Paradiso, 2001).

BLOOD SUPPLY TO THE BRAIN

Maintenance and function of the neurons depend on arterial blood supply. Blood supply arrives to the frontal, medial, and posterior brain through two arterial systems, which make up the anterior carotid and the vertebrobasilar circulatory systems. Together, these two systems supply blood to the anterior, middle, and posterior cerebrum, as seen in Figure 3–16. These arteries converge in the arterial circle of Willis on the base of the cerebrum and are interconnected through communicating arteries that allow arterial blood to circulate in both directions, as seen in Figure 3–17. Within the circle of Willis, if an artery is obstructed, this arrangement provides for continued blood flow from another corresponding artery. This system does not, however, apply to blood supply systems outside of the circle of Willis (Potagas, Kasselimis, & Evdokimidis, 2013).

THE BRAINSTEM

The brainstem, also the hindbrain, consists of the pons and medulla. Within the brainstem and the midbrain, the reticular formation is ventral to the cerebral aqueduct. It contains neurons not occupied by prominent nuclei or tracts and is a diffusely organized area that forms the central core of the brainstem. The brainstem has several functions of primary

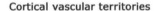

Cortical vascular territories

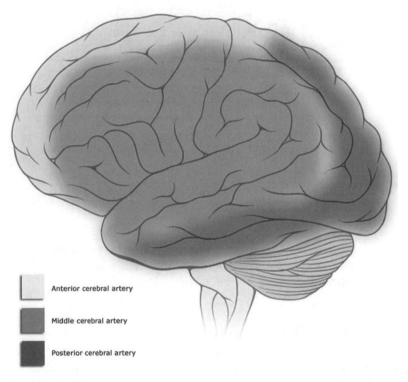

Anterior cerebral artery

Middle cerebral artery

Posterior cerebral artery

Figure 3–16. Blood supply to the brain (© Dr. Frank Gillard, 2008 (CEO of Radiopedia) / http://radiopaedia.org / GFDL 1.3; CC-BY-SA-3.0).

importance, including influencing levels of consciousness and degrees of alertness through the ascending reticular activating system. The brainstem also functions in control of movement (cranial nerves and spinal cord) and is a contributor to respiration and cardiovascular centers through the autonomic nervous system (Barr & Kiernan, 1983).

The reticular formation is only a part of the reticular activating system. The system includes a large part of the reticular formation as well as parts of the diencephalon and telencephalon (Barr & Kiernan,

1983). Neurons in the ventricular formation of the midbrain and rostral pons collect information about multiple sensory modalities. The intralaminar nuclei in turn project to widespread areas of the cortex, causing heightened arousal in response to sensory stimuli or attention-demanding tasks. The thalamus is also involved in mediating the interaction of attention and arousal in humans (Portas et al., 1998). Reticulothalamic projections are essential for the maintenance of a normal state of consciousness. Bilateral damage to neurons in the midbrain reticular

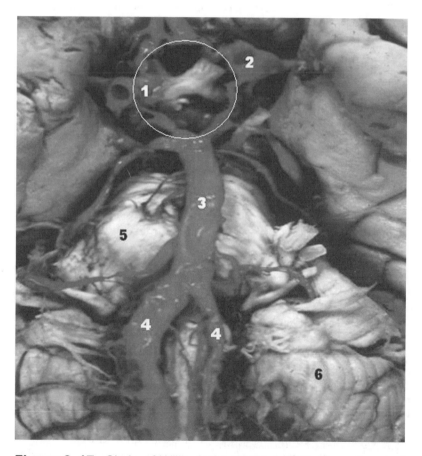

Figure 3–17. Circle of Willis (John A. Beal, PhD, Department of Cellular Biology & Anatomy, Louisiana State University Health Sciences Center Shreveport / Wikimedia Commons / CC-A-2.5 Generic). Legend: 1. Arterial Circle of Willis; 2. Internal Carotid Artery; 3. Basilar Artery; 4. Vertebral Arteries; 5. Pons; 6. Cerebellum.

formation and fibers passing through it results in prolonged coma (Nolte, 2002).

The ascending reticular system sends information to the cortex. The cortex, in turn, is stimulated with a profound effect on levels of consciousness and on alerting reactions to sensory stimuli. Cutaneous stimuli appear to be especially important in maintaining consciousness, whereas visual, acoustic, and mental stimuli have a special bearing on alertness and attention (Barr & Kiernan, 1983).

Within the brainstem is the locus coeruleus (LC), the major noradrenergic reticular nucleus. The LC, as seen in Figure 3–18, is located in the posterior area of the rostral pons in the lateral floor of the fourth ventricle. Adrenergic neurons synthesize epinephrine or nonepinephrine. Noradrenergic projections have a profound influence on brain function and are known to regulate brain tone by inhib-

iting background activity and enhancing the signal-to-noise ratio in the brain. Along with other nonadrenergic neurons, the LC is also thought to mediate attention and vigilance (Bhatanagar, 2002).

The projections of this nucleus reach long distances. For example, they innervate the spinal cord, brainstem, cerebellum, hypothalamus, thalamic relay nuclei, amygdala, basal telencephalon, and cortex. The norepinephrine from the LC has an excitatory effect on most of the brain, mediating arousal and priming the brain's neurons to be activated by stimuli. The LC is affected in many forms of neurodegenerative diseases: genetic and idiopathic Parkinson's disease, progressive supranuclear palsy, Pick's disease, and AD. There is up to a 70% loss of LC neurons in AD, according to Samuels and Szabadi (2008), who found that both AD and PD have significant neuronal loss in the LC. In AD, neuronal loss was most severe and best correlated with the duration of illness in the LC (Zarow, Lyness, Mortimer, & Chui, 2003).

Together with other nuclei located in the anterodorsal part of the brainstem, the LC belongs to what used to be described as the "ascending reticular activating system," an area critical for arousal and wakefulness. LC neurons have extremely wide projections, and they are innervated by only a few brainstem nuclei and forebrain areas. Activity of LC neurons varies not only with arousal but also with specific cognitive processes, resulting in concerted release of noradrenaline in multiple target areas, with very complex effects. The LC is thought to be critical for numerous functions, including stress response, attention, emotion, motivation, decision making, and learning and memory (Bouret & Sara, 2010).

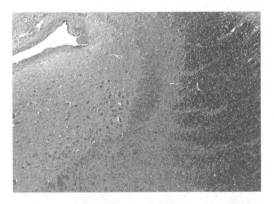

Figure 3–18. Low magnification micrograph of the locus coeruleus. The locus coeruleus is a nucleus found in the rostral pons in the lateral floor of the fourth ventricle. It literally means *blue spot*, based on its gross appearance. It is a center of norepinephrine (noradrenaline) production (User: Nephron / Wikimedia Commons / CC-A-SA-3.0 Unported; GFDL 1.2).

THE CEREBELLUM

The cerebellum in adult humans is a 150-g brain structure approximately the size of an adult fist. It is located beneath and behind the cerebrum at the base of the skull in the posterior fossa (Highnam & Bleile, 2011). Its role is to help regulate muscle tone, maintain balance, and coordinate skilled movements. Figure 3–19 provides two lateral views of the cerebellum.

The cerebellum is attached to the back of the brainstem by three peduncles (superior, inferior, middle) and lies just below the occipital lobe of the cerebrum. Figure 3–20 shows the cerebellum with peduncles.

The most important to speech is the superior peduncle. The cerebellum receives an enormous amount of information from the highest level of the human brain, the cerebrum. The cerebrum is connected to the human cerebellum by approximately 40 million nerve fibers. The superior cerebellar peduncle is the major output pathway of the cerebellum. Most of the

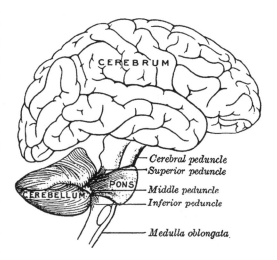

Figure 3–20. Lateral view of the cerebellum with peduncles (From *Anatomy of the Human Body, Twentieth Edition* by Henry Gray / Wikimedia Commons / Public Domain).

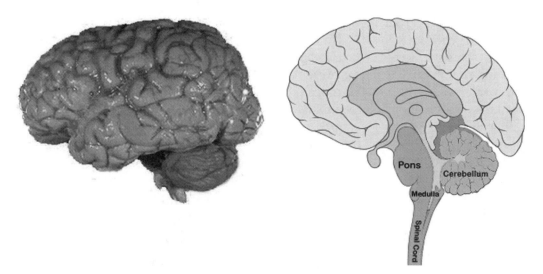

Figure 3–19. Two lateral views of the cerebellum (National Institutes of Health, part of the United States Department of Health and Human Services / Wikimedia Commons / Public Domain; Patrick J. Lynch, Medical Illustrator, http://patricklynch.net / Wikimedia Commons / CC-A-SA-2.5 Generic).

efferent fibers originate within the dentate nucleus, which in turn project to various midbrain structures, including the red nucleus, the ventral lateral/ventral anterior nucleus of the thalamus, and the medulla. The dentatorubrothalamocortical (dentate nucleus > red nucleus > thalamus > premotor cortex) and cerebellothalamocortical (cerebellum > thalamus > premotor cortex) pathways are two major pathways that pass through this peduncle and are important in motor planning.

The cerebellum receives input from the vestibular system and all other sensory receptors. Although the cerebellum has been described as important for monitoring voluntary motor activity, increasingly the cerebellum has been implicated in language and cognition. Highnam and Bleile (2011) reported on the clinical and neuroimaging literature that confirms the existence of multiple, independent cerebrocerebellar loops that "provide a neural substrate for modulation of cognition in primates as well as language in the human species" (p. 343). From their investigations, the cerebellum is involved in verbal fluency, semantic access, word completion, and oral naming. Clinical presentations of persons with cerebellum lesions may include mild anomia, agrammatism, simplification of syntactic structures, substitution or omission of grammatical morphemes, and reduced auditory verbal comprehension. The cerebellum also has a role in cognition and has been shown to function in the modulation of affect, working memory, attention, and executive functioning.

Patients with cerebellar lesions may evidence unremarkable changes in language. Standardized aphasia batteries may not reveal clinical deficits because the impairments are too subtle. Highnam and Bleile (2011) recommend that language examinations administered to persons with cerebellar lesions include tests of verbal fluency using multiple semantic categories and phonemic requests. Other testing should include an assessment of verbal working memory and confrontational naming using timed picture-naming tasks.

CHOLINERGIC PATHWAYS

The basal forebrain is the area at and near the inferior surface of the telencephalon, between the hypothalamus and the orbital cortex. The basal forebrain reaches the surface of the brain in the anterior perforated substance and extends superiorly into limbic regions near the rostrum of the corpus callosum. The corpus callosum is a collection of white matter tissue that connects the two cerebral hemispheres.

Acetylcholine is one of the most important neurotransmitters in the CNS. Receptors that synthesize acetylcholine and that use acetylcholine as their neurotransmitter are called cholinergic receptors. Within the basal forebrain there are an abundance of cholinergic receptors. Cholinergic neurons are concentrated in the reticular formation, the basal forebrain, and the striatum. Within the forebrain (nucleus basalis of Meynert), the cholinergic neurons supply the neocortex, hippocampus, and amygdala.

NUCLEUS BASALIS OF MEYNERT AND SUBSTANTIA INNOMINATA

The nucleus basalis of Meynert, or just nucleus basalis, is a group of neurons in the substantia innominata of the basal forebrain, inferior to the globus pallidus, which has wide projections to the neo-cortex and is rich in acetylcholine and choline acetyltransferase. The nucleus basalis is the major source of cholinergic innervation of the cerebral cortex (Teipel et al., 2005).

The substantia innominata (literally "unnamed substance") of Meynert is a stratum in the human brain consisting partly of gray and partly of white matter, which lies below the anterior part of the thalamus and lentiform nucleus (Berridge & Waterhouse, 2003). The gross anatomical structure is called the anterior perforated substance because, to the naked eye, it appears to be perforated by many holes, which are actually blood vessels (Hanyu et al., 2002). Figure 3–21 shows the area of location of the substantia innominata. The cholinergic pathways of the nucleus basa-lis of Meynert and the pedunculopontine nucleus (composed of cholinergic and noncholinergic neurons) are known to play a role in the functional organization of the basal ganglia and in the modulation of the thalamocortical neuronal system.

Many of the auditory pathways receive innervation from the pedunculopontine and laterodorsal tegmental nuclei, two nuclei referred to collectively as the pontomesencephalic tegmentum (Definitions.net, 2013). The PMT provides the major source of acetylcholine to the auditory thalamus and the midbrain and is a substantial source (in addition to the superior olivary complex) of acetylcholine in the cochlear nucleus (Schofield, Mott, & Mellott, 2011).

Both the nucleus basalis of Meynert and substantia innominata are important

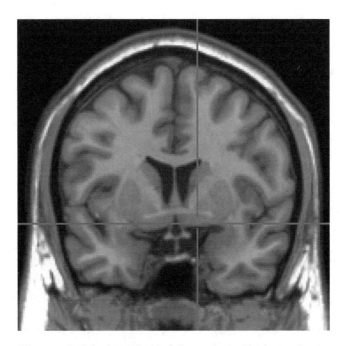

Figure 3–21. Location of the substantia innominata. The coronal MRI slice of the brain shows the location of the substantia innominata with the cross hairs (User: Genesis 12 / Wikimedia Commons / Public Domain).

because these structures undergo significant neuronal loss in dementia (Berridge & Waterhouse, 2003). Overall activity of nucleus basalis neurons is severely decreased in AD, which means that there is a decrease in cholinergic activity throughout the cortex. In addition, Hanyu and colleagues (2002) found that the thickness of the substantia innominata in patients with AD and in those with vascular dementia, frontotemporal dementia, or Parkinson's disease with dementia decreased more significantly than that in elderly control subjects. Although the thickness of the substantia innominata is seen to decrease with age in normal, healthy subjects, the substantia innominata has been found to be atrophied not only in patients with AD but also in patients with non-AD dementia, compared with age-matched control subjects. As the substantia innominata contains mainly the nucleus basalis of Meynert, atrophy of this structure is probably due to loss of neurons in the nucleus basalis of Meynert and a reduction in neuropils. Neuropils are found in the neocortical gray matter and are dense tangles of axon terminals, dendrites, and glial cell processes. It is a dense network of interwoven nerve fibers and their branches and synapses, together with glial filaments where synaptic connections are formed between branches of axons and dendrites (Cajigas et al., 2012).

NEUROIMAGING

Recent technological advances have made it possible to see the brain in several dimensions and provide accurate analyses of both structure and function. Neuroimaging includes the use of various techniques to either directly or indirectly image the structure and function/pharmacology of the brain. Cerebral structures can be examined using CT scans, MRI, fMRI, MR spectroscopy, PET, and SPECT. Regional blood flow, transcranial Doppler, and MR angiography provide clear and accurate information on the arterial systems of the brain. Refer to Table 3–1 for a complete description of these brain imaging techniques.

SUMMARY

Several key findings emerge from this chapter. In particular, the roles of the cerebrum, hippocampus, thalamus, and reticular activating system in memory add to an understanding of how memories are formed and stored. This has saliency for the discussion of how traumatic brain injuries and dementia affect the varieties of memory necessary for language and cognition. Furthermore, interconnections among the language centers of the frontal, temporal, and parietal lobes are vast and complex. Research has shown how widespread these areas actually are for both spoken language and auditory comprehension. Although Broca's and Wernicke's areas remain the primary areas for distinguishing types of aphasia, it is helpful to understand that lesions are not often neatly confined to these areas. Rather, severity of aphasia is dependent in part on the size of lesion and the number of areas affected, on subcortical structure involvement, such as the thalamus and the basal ganglia, and on lesions in the cortical areas surrounding both Broca's and Wernicke's areas.

The complexity of the reticular activating system is that it transports sensory information to the ascending pathways that pass through the diencephalon to the cortex for attention and arousal. The implications of this system are seen in

Table 3–1. Neuroimaging Techniques

Type	Name	Technique	Purpose
Stuctural and metabolic	Computed tomography (CT)	Uses a narrow x-ray beam to examine the brain in 1 to 2-mm slices. Detectors pick up beam from the head and send to computer for analysis.	Identifies space-occupying lesions of the brain.
	Magnetic resonance imaging (MRI)	Uses radiowaves, which interact with certain nuclei in brain tissue.	Detects myelinating disease, metabolism and blood flow, white matter lesions, edema, atrophy, and hematomas.
	Functional MRI (fMRI)	Measures change in magnetism between oxygen-rich and oxygen-poor blood.	Measures brain activity by detecting associated changes in blood flow
	Positron emission tomography (PET)	Uses PET scanner or camera to produce pictures of how positron emitting radiation is distributed in the scanner opening. Assesses physiological changes in brain cells.	Assesses physiological changes in brain cells. Measures glucose metabolism and blood flow. Detects neuronal changes in Alzheimer's disease.
	Single photon emission computed tomography (SPECT)	Uses radiotracer substance to emit a single x-ray.	Measures regional blood flow (rCBF) using gamma rays.
Metabolic	Transcranial doppler (TCD)	Blood flow measure-ments are taken from probes placed over the orbit of eye, temporal bones, and foramen magnum.	Measures velocity of blood flow.
	Magnetic resonance angiography (MRA)	Measures large extracranial and intracranial arteries and veins using contrast injection.	Screens for sizable aneurysms, arterial occlusions, and vascular malformations.
	Regional blood flow (rCBF)	Monitors a radioactive tracer to measure blood flow.	Assesses dynamics of brain activity.

Source: Bhatnagar, S. (2002) and Filler, A. G. (2009).

coma duration in traumatic head injury in that the brainstem cannot be injured in isolation from other structures above it.

To understand the pathophysiology of brain trauma and dementia, it is critical to acknowledge the impact on synaptic transmission in diffuse axonal injuries associated in closed head injuries and in the dissolution of cortical tissue in dementia. Not only are important connections lost in cerebral damage and atrophy, but critical interconnections important for language and cognition are lost as well. Severity of brain injuries can best be envisioned when the protective functions of the meninges and vestibular system are well understood. Finally, the circulatory system is designed to provide blood to collateral areas in cases where an artery is blocked. This explains, in part, how spontaneous recovery occurs after cerebrovascular accidents.

STUDY QUESTIONS

1. What is working memory? How is problem solving and working memory configured in the cerebrum?

2. What is synaptic transmission? How does it occur?

3. What are the neurotransmitters commonly associated with disorders that compromise language and cognition?

4. What are major divisions in the embryonic brain? What elements of the mature brain emerge from the primary vesicles?

5. Where and what is Broca's area?

6. Where and what is Wernicke's area? How are Broca's and Wernicke's connected?

7. What are the white matter areas in the cerebrum?

8. What are the effects on language when the basal ganglia and thalamus are damaged?

9. What are the roles of the angular and supramarginal gyri?

10. How does the hippocampus participate in memory?

11. What is the triune brain?

12. What are the functions of the meninges and ventricular system?

13. How does the brain receive its blood supply?

14. What is the reticular activating system? How does it differ from the reticular formation?

15. What neuroimaging techniques provide information about brain structures?

16. Where are the angular and supramarginal gyri? What are their functions?

17. What is norepinephrine?

18. How does the cerebellum participate in cognition and language?

19. What types of testing should be given to persons with cerebellar lesions?

20. What and where is the substantia innominata?

21. What and where is the nucleus basalis of Meynert? What is its relationship to the substantia innominata?

22. What happens to the nucleus basalis of Meynert in Alzheimer's disease?

23. What roles do the nucleus basalis of Meynert and the locus coerulus play in cognition?

24. What is a cholinergic pathway?

25. What are the structures of the basal ganglia? Which structure is most important for language?

26. What role does the pontomesencephalic tegmentum play in the integrity of the auditory pathway?

27. Which structures function to mediate attention and vigilance in the central nervous system?

28. Which structure functions to consolidate new memories as well as memory for remembering events and knowing facts?

29. What is the function of the postsynaptic enzyme?

30. What and where are the four ventricular structures?

REFERENCES

Anderson, J. M., Gilmore, R., Roper. S,, Crosson, B., Bauer, R. M., Nadeau, S., Beversdorf, D.Q., . . . Rogish, M. (1999). Conduction aphasia and the arcuate fasciculus: A reexamination of the Wernicke-Geschwind model. *Brain and Language, 70,* 1–12.

Baddeley, A. (1992). Working memory. *Science, 255,* 556–559.

Barr, J. J. A., & Kiernan, M. L. (1983). *The human nervous system* (4th ed.). Philadelphia, PA: Harper & Row.

Baumgartner, J. M., & Bentley, W. H. (1989). Basic neuroanatomy. In D. P. Kuehn, M. L. Lemme, & J. M. Baumgartner (Eds.), *Neural bases of speech, hearing and language* (pp. 25–45). Boston, MA: College-Hill Press.

Bear, M. F., Connors, B. W., & Paradiso, M. A. (2001). *Neuroscience: Exploring the brain* (2nd ed., pp. 140–239). Philadelphia, PA: Lippincott, Williams & Wilkins.

Berridge, C. W. & Waterhouse, B. D. (2003). The locus coeruleus-noradrenergic system: Modulation of behavioral state and state-dependent cognitive processes. *Brain Research Review, 42,* 33–84.

Bhatnagar, S. (2002). *Neuroscience for the study of communicative disorders* (2nd ed., pp. 1–150). Philadelphia, PA: Lippincott Williams & Wilkins.

Binder, J. R., Frost, J. A., Hammeke, T. A., Cox, R. W., Rao, S. M., & Prieto, T. (1997). Human brain language areas identified by functional magnetic resonance imaging. *Journal of Neuroscience, 17,* 353–362.

Boston Children's Hospital. (2013). *Adult stem cells 101.* Retrieved from http://stemcell.ChildrenHospital.org

Bouret, S., & Sara, S. J. (2010). Locus coeruleus. *Scholarpedia, 5,* 2845.

Cajigas, I. J., Tushev, G., Will, T. J., tom Dieck, S., Fuerst, N., & Schuman, E. M. (2012). The local transcriptome in the synaptic neuropil revealed by deep sequencing and high-resolution imaging. *Neuron, 74,* 453–466.doi:10.1016/j.neuron.2012.02.036

Cappa, S. F., Cavallotti, G., Guidotti, M., Papagno, G., & Vignolo, L. A. (1983). Subcortical aphasia: Two clinical CT scan correlation studies. *Cortex, 19,* 227–241.

Danbolt, N. C. (2001). Glutamate uptake. *Progress in neurobiology, 65,* 1–105.

Démonet, J-F., Chollet, F., Ramsay, S., Cardebat, D., Nespoulous, J-L., Wise, R., . . . Frackowiak, R. (1992). Anatomy of phonological and semantic processing in normal subjects. *Brain, 115,* 1753–1768.

D'Eposito, M., & Alexander, M. P. (1995). Subcortical aphasia: Distinct profiles following left putamenal hemorrhage. *Neurology, 45,* 279–293.

Federenko, E., Duncan, J., & Kanwisher, N. (2012). Languge-selective anddomain-general regions lie side by side within Broca's area. *Current Biology, 22,* 2059–2062.

Filler, A. G. (2009). The history, development and impact of computed imaging in neurological diagnosis and neurosurgery: CT, MRI, and DTI. *Nature Proceedings.* Retrieved from http://dx.doi.org/10.1038/npre.2009.3267.5

Ganguly, K., Schinder, A. F., Wong, S. T., & Poo, M. (2001). GABA itself promotes the developmental switch of neuronal GABAergic responses from excitation to inhibition. *Cell 105,* 521–532.

Geschwin, N. (1975). Language and cerebral dominance. In T. N. Chase (Ed.), *The nervous system, Volume 2, The clinical neurosciences* (pp. 433–440). New York, NY: Raven Press.

Goldman, S. A., & Sim, F. (2005). Neural progenitor cells of the adult brain. *Novartis Foundation Symposium, 265*, 66–80.

Hanyu, H., Asano, T., Sakurai, H., Tanaka, Y., Takasaki, M., & Kimihiko, A. (2002). MR analysis of the substantia innominata in normal aging, Alzheimer's disease, and other types of dementia. *American Journal of Neuroradiology, 23*, 27–32.

Hebb, A. O., & Ojemann, G. A. (2012). The thalamus and language revisited. *Brain and Language*. Retrieved on May 23, 2013, from http://dx.doi.org/10.1016/j.bandl.2012.06.010

Heimer, L. (1983). *The human brain and spinal cord.* New York, NY: Springer-Verlag.

Herrero, M. T., Barcia, C., & Navarro, J. M. (2002). Functional anatomy of thalamus and basal ganglia. *Child's Nervous System, 18*, 386–404.

Highnam, C. L., & Bleile, K. M. (2011). Language in the cerebellum. *American Journal of Speech-Language Pathology, 20*, 337–347. doi:10.1044/1058-0360(2011/10-0096)

Horner, A. J., Gadian, D. G., Fuentemilla, L., Jentschke, S. Vargha-Khadem, F., & Duzel, E. (2012). A rapid, hippocampus-dependent, item-memory signal that initiates context memory in humans. *Current Biology, 22*, 2369–2374.

Horwitz, B., Rumsey, J. M., & Donohue, B. C. (1998). Functional connectivity of the angular gyrus in normal reading and dyslexia. *Proceedings of the National Academy of Sciences USA, 95*, 8939–8944.

Johnson, M. D., & Ojemann, G. A. (2000).The role of the human thalamus in language and memory: Evidence from electrophysiological studies. *Brain and Cognition, 42*, 218–230.

Kandel, E. R. (1991). Cellular mechanisms of learning and the biological basis of individuality (3rd ed.). In E. Kandel, J. Schwartz, & T. Jessell (Eds.), *Principles of neural science* (pp. 1009–1031). Norwalk, CT: Appleton & Lange.

Kennedy. M., & Murdoch, B. E. (1993). Chronic aphasia subsequent to striato- capsular and thalamic lesions in the left hemisphere. *Brain and Language, 44*, 284–295.

Larson, C. R. (1989). Basic neurophysiology. In D. P. Kuehn, M. L. Lemme, & J. M. Baumgartner (Eds.), *Neural bases for speech, hearing, and language* (pp. 46–86). Boston, MA: College-Hill Press.

Luria, A. R. (1977). On quasi-aphasic speech disturbances in lesions of the deep structures of the brain. *Brain and Language, 4*, 432–459.

MacLean, P. D. (1985). Evolutionary psychiatry and the triune brain. *Psychological Medicine, 15*, 219–221.

MacLean, P. D. (1988). Evolution of audiovocal communication as reflected by the therapsid-mammalian transition and the limbic thalamocingulate division. In J. D. Newman (Ed.), *The physiological control of mammalian vocalization* (pp. 185–201), New York, NY: Plenum Press.

MacLean, P. D. (1990). *The triune brain in evolution: Role in paleocerebral functions.* New York, NY: Plenum Press.

Mega, M. S., & Bernard, M. A. (1992). Subcortical aphasia: The core profile of capsulostriatal infarction. *Neurology, 44*, 1824–1829.

Musiek, F., Mohanani, A., Wierzbinski, E., Kilgore, G., Hunter, J., & Marotto, J. (2011). Pathways: Will Wernicke's area ever be defined? *Hearing Journal, 64*, 6.

Naeser, M. A., Helm-Estabrooks, N., Haas, G., Auerbach, S., & Srinivasan, M. (1987). Relationship between lesion extent in 'Wernicke's area' on computed tomographic scan and predicting recovery of comprehension in Wernicke's aphasia. *Archives of Neurology, 44*, 73–82.

National Institute of Neurological Disorders and Stroke. (2013). *NINDS Gerstman syndrome information page*. Retrieved from http://www.ninds.nih.gov/disorders/gerstmanns/gerstmanns.htm

Newman, J. D., & Harris, J. C. (2009). The scientific contributions of Paul D. MacLean (1913–2007). *Journal of Nervous and Mental Diseases, 197*, 3–5.

Nieuwenhuis, S., Aston-Jones, G., & Cohen, J. D. (2005). Decision making, the P3, and the locus coeruleus-norepinephrine system. *Psychological Bulletin, 131*, 510–532.

Nolte, J. (2002). *The human brain: An introduction to its functional anatomy* (5th ed.). St. Louis, MO: Mosby.

Ojemann, G. A. (1979). Subcortical language mechanisms. In H. Whitaker & H. A. Whitaker (Eds.), *Studies in neurolinguistics* (Vol. 1, pp. 292–328). New York, NY: Academic Press.

Okuda, B., Tanaka, H., Tachibana, H., Kawabata, K., & Sugita, M. (1994). Cerebral blood flow in subcortical global aphasia. Perisylvian cortical hypoperfusion as a crucial role. *Stroke, 25,* 1495–1499.

Ostrosky-Solis, F., Madrazo, I., Drucker-Colin, R., & Quintanar, L. (1989). Cognitive effects of adrenal autografting in Parkinson's disease. In A. Ardila & F. Ostrosky-Solis (Eds.), *Brain organization of language and cognitive processes.* New York, NY: Plenum Press.

Ozeren, A., Sarica, Y., & Efe, R. (1994). Thalamic aphasic syndrome. *Acta Neurologyica Belgium, 94,* 205–208.

Payne, J. C. (1997). *Adult neurogenic language disorders: Assessment and treatment. An ethnobiological approach* (pp. 272–278). San Diego, CA: Singular.

Pedunculopontine tegmental nucleus. (2013, May 22). Definitions.net. Retreived from http://www.definitions.net/definition/pedunculopontine tegmental nucleus

Portas, C. M., Reed, G., Howseman, A. M., Josephs, O., Turner, R., & Frith, C. D. (1998). A specific role for the thalamus in mediating the interaction of attention and arousal in humans. *Journal of Neuroscience, 18,* 8979–8989.

Potagas, C., Kasselimis, D. S., & Evdokimidis, I. (2013). Elements of neurology essential for understanding the aphasias. In I. Papathanasiuou, P. Coppens, & C. Potagas (Eds.), *Aphasia and related neurogenic communication disorders* (pp. 25–48). Burlington, MA: Jones & Barlett Learning.

Prado-Alcalá, R. A. (1989). The striatum as a temporary memory store. In A. Ardila & F. Ostrosky-Solis (Eds.), *Brain organization of language and cognitive processes.* New York, NY: Plenum Press.

Robin, D. A., & Schienberg, S. (1990). Subcortical lesions and aphasia. *Journal of Speech and Hearing Disorders, 55,* 90–100. doi:10.2174/157015908785777229 PMCID: PMC2687936

Russ, M. O., Mack, W., Grama, C. R., Lanfermann, H., & Knopf, M. (2003). Enactment effect in memory: Evidence concerning the function of the supramarginal gyrus. *Experimental Brain Research, 149,* 497–504.

Samuels, E. R., & Szabadi, E. (2008). Functional neuroanatomy of the noradrenergic locus coeruleus: Its roles in the regulation of arousal and autonomic function part i: principles of functional organisation. *Current Neuropharmacology, 6,* 235–253.

Schofield, B. R., Mott, S.D., & Mellott, J.G. (2011). Cholinergic cells of the pontomesencephalic tegmentum: Connections with auditory structures from cochlear nucleus to cortex. *Hearing Research, 279,* 85–95.

Seghier, M. (2012). The angular gyrus: Multiple functions and multiple subdivisions. *Neuroscientist, 19,* 43–61.

Sorokin, E. B. (2009). The blood-brain and the blood-cerebrospinal barriers: Function and dysfunction. *Seminars in Immunopathology, 4,* 497–511. doi:10.1007/s00281-009-0177-0

Stiles, J., & Jernigan, T. L. (2010). The basics of brain development. *Neuropsychology Review, 20,* 327–348.

Stoeckel, C., Gough, P.M., Watkins, K. E., & Devlin, J. T. (2009). Supramarginal gyrus involvement in visual word recognition. *Cortex, 45,* 1091–1096.

Tanner, D. C. (2007). Redefining Wernicke's area: Receptive language and discourse semantics. *Journal of Allied Health, 36,* 63–66.

Teipel, S. J., Flatz, W. H., Heinsen, H., Bokde, A. L. W., Schoenberg, S.O., Stockel, S., . . . Hampel, H. (2005). Measurement of basal forebrain atrophy in Alzheimer's disease using MRI. *Brain, 128,* 2626–2644.

Wallesch, C-W., & Papagno, C. (1988). Subcortical aphasia. In F. C. Rose, R. Whurr, & M. A. Wyke (Eds.). *Aphasia* (pp. 256–287). London, UK: Whurr.

Warrington, E. K., & Weiskrantz, I. (1970). Amnesic syndromes: Consolidation or retrieval? *Nature, 228,* 628–630.

Waymire, J. C. (2013). *Chapter 11: Acetylcholine neurotransmission.* Retrieved from http://neurosciences.uth,tmc.edu

Webster. D. B. (1999). *Neuroscience of communication* (2nd ed., pp. 317–343.). San Diego, CA: Singular.

Zarow, C., Lyness, S. A., Mortimer, J. A., & Chui, H. C. (2003). Neuronal loss is greater in the locus coeruleus than nucleus basalis and substantia nigra in Alzheimer's and Parkinson's diseases. *Archives of Neurology, 60,* 337–341.

CHAPTER 4

The Dementias

DEFINITION AND PREVALENCE OF DEMENTIA

Dementia is characterized by abnormal changes in memory, behavior, language, cognition, and the ability to perform daily living tasks caused by a number of diseases and conditions (Alzheimer's Association, 2012). Dementia, often defined by criteria from the *Diagnostic and Statistical Manual of Mental Disor*ders, Fourth Edition (DSM-IV; American Psychiatric Association, 2000a), includes a decline in memory and a deficit severe enough to interfere with daily life in at least one of the following cognitive abilities:

1. Ability to generate coherent speech or understand spoken or written language.
2. Ability to recognize or identify objects, assuming intact sensory function.
3. Ability to execute motor activities, assuming intact motor abilities and sensory function and comprehension of the required task.
4. Ability to think abstractly, make sound judgments, and plan and carry out complex tasks.

Dementia is a growing national problem affecting millions of persons. Recent estimates suggest that 13.9% of persons aged 71 and older in the United States have some form of dementia (Plassman et al., 2007). Although previous observations of a leveling off of incidence among the oldest old have been reported, it is anticipated that dementia incidence may continue to increase because of the aging and the expected longer life expectancies of baby boomers.

Alzheimer's disease (AD) is the most prevalent of the dementias. More than five million Americans, or one in eight older Americans, are living with AD, which is the sixth-leading cause of death in the United States and the only cause of death among the top 10 in the United States that cannot be prevented, cured, or even slowed (Alzheimer's Association, 2012).

Establishing a definitive diagnosis of dementia includes ruling out conditions that can be reversed with treatment or surgery, specifically depression, delirium, side effects from medications, metabolic conditions like thyroid problems, vitamin deficiencies, infections, intracranial masses, arteriosclerotic complications, speech and hearing disorders, epilepsy, neurosyphilis, normal pressure hydrocephalus, chemo brain, or alcohol abuse (American Psychiatric Association, 2000b; Kean & Locke, 2008; Tonkovich, 1988). By contrast, dementia is irreversible and is caused by permanent damage to neurons and their connections.

EARLY SIGNS OF DEMENTIA

Dementia affects the patient, the family, and community health service providers. These dynamics may intrude upon when and how an evaluation of dementia will be sought, whether treatment for dementia complications will be initiated, and whether a patient will comply with treatment. A definitive diagnosis is often not made until the person is well into the course of dementia for a variety of reasons. One possible reason is that family members, who have not been alarmed by the subtle changes in memory or reasoning they have observed for many years, may not fully understand the ramifications of dementia symptoms or what constitutes nonpathological aging changes. Many of the observed behavioral and cognitive changes of dementia are, therefore, dismissed as normal aging.

Another possibility is that the interplay of cultural dynamics, discussed in Chapter 1, may prolong the time when family members actively seek treatment because of a perceived stigma of mental illness or distrust of the health care system. Still another possible explanation is that families may not have access to routine health care or to specialists who can diagnose dementia.

Memory loss alone is an insufficient criterion for dementia; however, an early diagnosis of AD is critically important to developing appropriate interventions. Given recent innovations in the diagnosis and treatment of dementia in the areas of diagnostics using positron emission tomography PET scans with amyloid-imaging agent Pittsburgh Compound B and retinal vascular biomarkers, and therapies using deep brain stimulation and new drug regimens (Lyketos, 2012; Rabin, 2012a), there is promise for early diagnoses and treatment.

Distinguishing between mild cognitive decline and other forms of dementia may still be difficult and may require an interdisciplinary evaluation for both cognitive and functional status. Santacruz and Swagerty (2001) provide five broad categories of signs and symptoms that should prompt an evaluation for dementia, which are:

- **cognitive changes**, such as new forgetfulness and disorientation
- **psychiatric symptoms**, such as withdrawal and apathy
- **personality changes**, such as inappropriate friendliness or flirtatiousness
- **problem behaviors**, such as agitation and wandering
- **changes in day-to-day functioning**, such as difficulty driving and getting lost.

In addition to these changes and behaviors, there are several risk factors that will need to be taken into consideration when evaluating dementia.

RISK FACTORS FOR DEMENTIA

Although many of the irreversible dementing illnesses either are rare or have no established etiology, there are several risk factors that should become part of the case history intake for a diagnosis of dementia.

Advancing Age

The greatest risk factor for AD and other dementing illnesses or conditions is advancing age. Most people with AD are diagnosed at age 65 or older. These individuals are said to have late-onset Alzheimer's disease. However, people younger than age 65 can also develop the disease. When AD develops in a person younger than age 65, it is considered as younger-onset or early-onset Alzheimer's disease.

Family History

Individuals who have a parent, brother, or sister with AD are more likely to develop the disease than those who do not have a first-degree relative with AD. Those who have more than one first-degree relative with Alzheimer's are at even higher risk of developing the disease. Heyman and his colleagues (1984) found that first-degree biological relatives of others with AD are more likely to develop the disease because it may be an autosomal dominant trait. In an investigation of Down syndrome patients (Yates, Simpson, Maloney, Gordon, & Reid, 1980) found that those persons who lived to middle age developed neuritic tangles and neurofibrillary tangles characteristic of AD. Although the data were inconclusive and are still under investigation, it does appear that there may be a chemical relationship between the two syndromes through the cerebrovascular amyloid protein.

Differences in thinking skills among twins may reflect a genetic risk for dementia (Gatz, Reynolds, Finkel, Pederson, & Walters, 2010). However, cognitive changes and elevated genetic risk do not always predict that twins or siblings of people with dementia will eventually develop dementia themselves. When diseases run in families, heredity (genetics), shared environmental/lifestyle factors, or both may play a role.

Traumatic Brain Injury

Traumatic brain injury (TBI) is associated with an increased risk of AD and other dementias. Moderate head injuries are associated with twice the risk of developing AD compared with no head injuries, and severe head injuries are associated with 4.5 times the risk (Lye & Shores, 2000). Moderate head injury is differentiated from mild head injury by the loss of consciousness or posttraumatic amnesia that lasts more than 30 minutes; if either of these lasts more than 24 hours, the injury is considered severe. These increased risks have not been shown for individuals experiencing mild head injury.

Of the several studies that have been conducted (Adle-Bassette et al., 1996; Chandra, Kokmen, Schoenberg, & Beard, 1989; Heyman et al., 1984; Katzman et al., 1996; Mortimer, 1983; Plassman et al., 2007; Rudelli, Strom, & Ambler, 1982; Tang et al., 1996; Vickrey et al., 2006), the consensus is that a history of head injury, particularly with loss of consciousness, may damage the blood–brain barrier, among other structures, which allows the pathological changes of AD to occur.

Groups that experience repeated head injuries, such as boxers, football players, and combat veterans, may be at increased risk of dementia, late-life cognitive impairment, and evidence of tau tangles at autopsy. Tau is an important protein found in neurons (Roberts, Allsop, & Bruton, 1990). Others suggest that carriers of apolipoprotein E–epsilon 4 (ApoE-e4) who experience moderate or severe head injury are at higher risk of developing AD than ApoE-e4 carriers who do not have a history of moderate or severe head injury. The ApoE gene encodes a protein that helps regulate the levels and distribution of cholesterol and other lipids in the body (Alzheimer's Association, 2012).

Cardiovascular Disease

The health of the brain is closely linked to the overall health of the heart and blood vessels. The brain is nourished by one of the body's richest networks of blood vessels, as seen in Chapter 3. A healthy heart helps ensure that enough blood is pumped through these blood vessels to the brain, and healthy blood vessels help ensure that the brain is supplied with the oxygen- and nutrient-rich blood it needs to function normally.

Some data show that cardiovascular disease risk factors, such as physical inactivity, high cholesterol (especially in midlife), hypertension, diabetes, smoking, and obesity, are associated with a higher risk of developing AD and other dementias (Anstey, von Sanden, Salim & O'Kearney, 2007; Kramer et al., 1999; Kramer & Erickson, 2007; Lorenzen & Murray, 2008; Pendlebury & Rothwell, 2009; Rusanen, Kivipelto, Quesenberry, Zhou, & Whitmer, 2010; Whitmer et al., 2008; Yaffe et al., 2011). Small-vessel cerebrovascular disease, visualized as white matter hyperintensities or white matter lesions on magnetic resonance imaging (MRI) scans, may be a key factor independently predictive of AD. Furthermore, among persons with mild cognitive impairment, the appearance of white matter hyperin-

tensities may be predictive also of a later diagnosis of AD (Provenzano et al., 2013). Unlike genetic risk factors, many of these cardiovascular disease risk factors can be changed or modified to decrease the likelihood of developing cardiovascular disease and, possibly, the cognitive decline associated with AD and other forms of dementia.

Genetic Mutations

The only risk factor gene identified so far for late-onset AD is a gene that makes ApoE. Everyone has ApoE, which helps carry cholesterol in the blood. Only about 15% of people have the form that increases the risk of AD. It is likely that other genes also may increase the risk of AD or protect against AD, but they remain to be discovered. ApoE-e4 is one of three common forms (e2, e3, and e4) of the ApoE gene, which provides the blueprint for a protein that carries cholesterol in the bloodstream (Alzheimer's Association, 2012).

Everyone inherits one form of the ApoE gene from each parent. Those who inherit one ApoE-e4 gene have increased risk of developing AD and of developing it at an earlier age than those who inherit the e2 or e3 forms of the ApoE gene. Those who inherit two ApoE-e4 genes have an even higher risk. Unlike inheriting a known genetic mutation for AD, inheriting one or two copies of this form of the ApoE gene does not guarantee that an individual will develop Alzheimer's disease.

Another known cause of AD is a genetic mutation for genes that enable cells to digest unwanted proteins. This action is essential for brain cell survival. Mutations disrupt this cellular protein-recycling process, killing nerve cells.

A small percentage of AD cases, probably less than 1%, are caused by three known genetic mutations that interfere with cellular protein recycling. Persons with an inherited form of AD carry mutations in the presenilin proteins (PSEN1 and PSEN2) or the amyloid precursor protein (APP). These disease-linked mutations result in increased production of the longer form of amyloid-beta (main component of amyloid deposits found in AD brains). Presenilins are thought to regulate APP processing. Inheriting any of these genetic mutations guarantees that an individual will develop AD. Mutations in PSEN1 and PSEN2 genes account for the majority of cases of early-onset familial AD. In such individuals, the disease tends to develop before age 65, sometimes in individuals as young as age 30. There may also be a link between PSEN1 and a familiar form of frontotemporal dementia (Alzheimer's Association, 2012; Vetrivel, Zhang, Xu, & Thinakaran, 2006).

Huntington's disease (HD) is an example of a progressive neurological disorder with dementia that has a genetic profile. Huntington's disease is an autosomal dominant disease, meaning that in affected individuals, one gene of the gene pair (the HD gene) is not functioning correctly and expresses itself more strongly, or dominates, the other working gene. Since the gene pair is not on one of the sex chromosomes, the HD gene can affect both males and females, and each gender has the same chance of having affected children (Stipe et al., 1979). A variation in the genetic code for a gene on chromosome 4 was found among persons affected with HD. Normally, the genetic code for this gene has three DNA bases, CAG, which are repeated several times. In HD, the gene sequence appears as a triplet (Indiana University School of Medicine, 1995).

Mild Cognitive Impairment

Mild cognitive impairment (MCI) is a condition in which an individual has mild but measurable changes in thinking abilities that are noticeable to the person affected and to family members and friends but does not affect the individual's ability to carry out everyday activities (Rabin, 2012b). People with MCI, especially MCI involving memory problems, are more likely to develop AD and other dementias than people without MCI. Approximately 10% to 15% of persons with MCI develop AD, and 10% to 30% of persons with MCI have less cortical gray matter compared with healthy controls in areas known to be affected by AD pathology (Prestia et al., 2010).

Petersen (2004) identified three distinct types of MCI based on specific effects on cognition and language. In his opinion, amnestic MCI (a-MCI), characterized by memory loss, is the most common type of MCI and the most likely to convert to AD. A second subtype of MCI is single non-memory domain MCI (sd-MCI), in which the predominant features are significant deficits in language and executive and visuospatial functions. The third subtype is a multiple-domain MCI (md-MCI) that is characterized by multiple cognitive deficits and may occur with or without significant memory loss.

Mild cognitive impairment can be reversed in some patients when caused by certain medications. However, compared with normal older adults, those with MCI with memory and those with MCI with language deficits were significantly more likely to develop some form of dementia within a 4-year period from the onset of symptoms (Roundtree et al., 2007).

TYPES OF DEMENTIAS

The Cortical/Subcortical Dichotomy

Among the irreversible dementias, there are those that are predominantly cortical and others that are predominantly subcortical. Those dementias that affect both neocortical and subcortical areas have elements of both levels of neurological impairment.

Cortical dementias occur in diseases with predominant degeneration in neocortical association areas, with relative sparing of subcortical structures. Subcortical dementias have pathologic alterations that affect deep structures such as the basal ganglia, thalamus, and brainstem, with relative sparing of the cerebral cortex. The most prevalent of the cortical dementias is Alzheimer's disease.

The cortical/subcortical dichotomy has detractors who argue that the characteristics of each type of dementia are not exclusive to that type (Damasio, Damasio, Rizzo, Varney, & Gersh, 1982). Whitehouse and colleagues (1981) criticized the dichotomization for its implied lack of interdependence between cortical and subcortical structures. However, Cummings and Benson (1984) emphasized that subcortical dementia is a clinical rather than an anatomical concept, distinct from that of the cortical dementias. In their view, subcortical dementia, unlike cortical dementia, has a clinical presentation of forgetfulness, slowing of mental processes, impairment of manipulation of acquired knowledge, and personality and affective changes, including apathy and depression. Cortical dementia, in contrast, presents with deterioration of both verbal expression and auditory comprehension, indifference, disinhibition, and severe memory problems.

Newer technologies have provided a window into the brain that was not available at the time of the writing of these observations by Cummings and Benson (1984). However, both the detractors of the dichotomy and those who argued for it appear to be right in their judgments. Interdependence exists between subcortical and cortical structures, and there are those distinct manifestations of behaviors that are dependent on the type of dementia. The subcortical disorders, for example, may be more similar to one another than they are to Alzheimer's dementia in that they are characterized by cognitive slowness, concomitant motor abnormalities, and a relatively low frequency of aphasias and apraxias. However, any classification of the dementias must be sensitive to the fact that they seem to lie along a continuum involving a greater or lesser degree of cortical and subcortical pathology (Turner, Moran, & Kopelman, 2002). Table 4–1 gives the characteristics of all the dementias to be discussed in this chapter.

ALZHEIMER'S DISEASE

Prevalence

As of 2012, 4.5 to 5.4 million Americans are living with AD, a disease someone develops every 69 seconds. One in eight older Americans has AD (Alzheimer's Association, 2012). Alzheimer's disease is the most prevalent of the dementias and is expected to grow in proportion to the aging population. As 78 million American baby boomers turn 65, cases of AD are expected to increase exponentially.

Table 4–1. Types of Dementia and Characteristics

Type of Dementia	Characteristics
Alzheimer's disease (AD)	Primarily cortical. Most common type of dementia; accounts for an estimated 60% to 80% of cases. Difficulty remembering names and recent events is often an early clinical symptom; apathy and depression are also often early symptoms. Later symptoms include impaired judgment, disorientation, confusion, behavior changes, and difficulty speaking, swallowing, and walking.
	New criteria and guidelines for diagnosing AD were proposed and published in 2011, which recommend that AD disease be considered a disease that begins well before the development of the disease. Hallmark abnormalities are deposits of the protein fragment beta-amyloid (plaques) and twisted strands of the protein tau (tangles) as well as evidence of nerve cell damage and death in the brain.
Vascular dementia (VaD)	Cortical and subcortical. Previously known as multi infarct or post-stroke dementia, VaD is less common as a sole cause of dementia than is AD. Impaired judgment or ability to make plans is more likely to be the initial symptom, as opposed to the memory loss often associated with the initial symptoms of AD. Often the result of microscopic bleeding and blood vessel blockage in the brain. Brain changes of both AD and VaD can occur simultaneously.
Dementia with Lewy bodies (DLB)	Cortical and subcortical. People with DLB have some of the symptoms common in AD, but are more likely than people with AD to have initial or early symptoms such as sleep disturbances, well-formed visual hallucinations, and muscle rigidity or other Parkinsonian movement features. Lewy bodies are abnormal aggregations (or clumps) of the protein alpha-synuclein. When they develop in a part of the brain called the cortex, dementia can result. Alpha-synuclein also aggregates in the brains of people with Parkinson's disease, but the aggregates may appear in a pattern that is different from DLB. The brain changes of DLB alone can cause dementia, or they can be present at the same time as the brain changes of AD and/or vascular dementia, with each entity contributing to the development of dementia. When this happens, the individual is said to have "mixed dementia."
Mixed dementia	Characterized by the hallmark abnormalities of AD and another type of dementia most commonly, vascular dementia, but also other types, such as dementia with Lewy bodies. Recent studies suggest that mixed dementia is more common than previously thought.

continues

Table 4–1. *continued*

Type of Dementia	Characteristics
Parkinson's disease (PD)	Primarily subcortical. As Parkinson's disease progresses, it often results in a severe dementia similar to DLB or AD (PD-d). Problems with movement are a common symptom early in the disease. Alpha-synuclein aggregates are likely to begin in an area deep in the brain in the substantia nigra. The aggregates are thought to cause degeneration of the nerve cells that produce dopamine. The incidence of Parkinson's disease is about one-tenth that of AD disease.
Frontotemporal degeneration (FTD)	Cortical and subcortical. Includes dementias such as behavioral-variant FTD, primary progressive aphasia, Pick's disease, and progressive supranuclear palsy. Typical symptoms include changes in personality and behavior and difficulty with language. Nerve cells in the front and side regions of the brain are especially affected. No distinguishing microscopic abnormality is linked to all cases. The brain changes of behavioral-variant FTLD may be present at the same time as the brain changes of AD, but people with behavioral variant generally develop symptoms at a younger age (at about age 60) and survive for fewer years than those with AD.
Creutzfeldt–Jacob disease (CJD)	Subcortical. Rapidly fatal disorder that impairs memory and coordination and causes behavior changes. Results from an infectious misfolded protein (prion) that causes other proteins throughout the brain to misfold and thus malfunction. Variant Creutzfeldt–Jakob disease is believed to be caused by consumption of products from cattle affected by mad cow disease.
Korsakoff's disease (KD)	Subcortical. Also called Korsakoff's syndrome. Caused by a dietary deficiency of thiamin (vitamin B-1), which the body uses to convert carbohydrates into energy. Over time, thiamin deficiency can cause damage to several brain areas critical for memory: including the thalamus, hippocampus, mammillary bodies, and basal forebrain. In rare cases, this damage culminates in KD. Symptoms of the dementia associated with KD are either nonprogressive or slowly progressive. Another term for KD is alcohol amnestic syndrome, meaning loss of memory. Alcohol can inflame the stomach lining and impede the body's ability to absorb the key vitamins it receives. Korsakoff's syndrome may also occur in other conditions where there is severe malnutrition, but this is extremely rare.

Table 4–1. *continued*

Type of Dementia	Characteristics
Human immunodeficiency virus dementia (HIV-D)	Subcortical. Occurs in 20% to 30% of diagnosed with AIDS. More than half of all patients infected by HIV develop central of peripheral neurologic complications. The majority of those who develop AIDS also develop dementia. The criteria for HIV dementia include seropositivity, history of progressive cognitive, and behavioral decline, CNS opportunistic processes. The clinical features are: demonstrated deficits in frontal lobe tasks and nonverbal memory and slowed limb and eye movement when major psychiatric and metabolic disorders and substance abuse are excluded. Age is a risk factor for survival from HIV infection. Advanced age at AIDS onset is a predictive risk for dementia because of age-related decline in immune status.
Huntington's disease (HD)	Subcortical. Also called Huntington's chorea. A chronic,degenerative inherited brain disease caused by a deficiency of the neurotransmitter gamma aminobutyric acid and acetylcholine in the basal ganglia. Results from genetically programmed degeneration of neurons which causes uncontrolled movements, loss of intellectual faculties, and emotional disturbance. HD is a familial disease, passed from parent to child through a mutation in the normal gene. As HD is autosomal dominant, this means the gene involved is on an autosomal and recently has been localized on the fourth autosomal chromosome pair (the #4 chromosome). Symptoms generally appear between 30 and 50 years of age but have appeared as young as 2 and as old as 70 years of age.
Multiple sclerosis (MS)	An immune-mediated motor disease in which the myelin sheaths that protect the axons become damaged. Symptoms generally appear between 20 and 50 years of age, but disease can appear in older adults and children. The etiology is unknown, but several possible causes have been suggested, including environmental, familial, and viral causes. The disease has a highly variable clinical profile and persons diagnosed with MS go through several stages, including remissions. Higher cognitive functions and higher order language abilities appear to deteriorate during the course of the disease.

Source: Adapted from Alzheimer's Association. (2012). AD disease facts and figures. *AD Disease and Dementia, 8*(2), 133.

Some experts expect that the number of Americans with AD will triple, perhaps even quadruple by 2050 if there is no workable solution to this medical crisis (Rabin, 2012c).

Pathophysiology of AD

Alzheimer's disease was first reported in 1907 by Alois Alzheimer, who described postmortem findings in the brains of patients who suffered intellectual and cognitive decline, behavioral changes, and, in the terminal stages, complete dependency. Although there are numerous theories on the causes, including infectious agents, toxic substances, and genetic or familial transmission, it is generally accepted that AD is a progressive atrophic neurological syndrome with a gradual and steady deterioration and course.

During the course of AD, both neurons and the number of dendritic branches decrease, which reduces the efficiency of the brain as a communication system. The intricate process of communication between nerve cells breaks down. Alzheimer's disease has specific biomarkers which are anatomic, physiologic, biochemical or molecular parameters associated with the presence and severity of a disease (Albert, 2012). In AD, the biomarkers are neurofibrillary tangles, areas of granulovacuolar degeneration, and amyloid plaques in the brain.

Neurofibrillary tangles are twisted fibers inside neurons. Normally, every brain cell or neuron contains long fibers made of protein, which act as scaffolds, holding the neuron in its proper shape and also helping transport nutrients within the neuron. In AD, these fibers begin to twist and tangle. The neuron loses its shape, becomes unable to transport nutri-

ents properly, and eventually dies. The fiber tangles remain in the brain long after the dead neuron has been cleared away. The chief component of neurofibrillary tangles is a protein called A68, a form of tau. In AD, tau is twisted into paired helical filaments, two threads wound around each other. These paired helical filaments are the major components of neurofibrillary tangles and are most common in the temporal lobe structures, such as the hippocampus and amygdala (Davies, 1991).

Granulovacuolar degeneration from progressive neuronal loss occurs from the primary to the association cortices (Hamos, DeGennaro, & Drachman, 1989). Figure 4–1 shows a comparison of a normal brain with that of a person with AD. Figure 4–2 shows the progressive neuronal loss by severity of AD. Compared with their age cohorts, the brains of persons with AD are approximately 10% smaller by weight. The greatest loss is found in the medial temporal structures.

Greater proportional neuron loss is associated with more rapid decline in older patients (Double et al., 1996). Atrophy can be seen also in the lateral ventricular dilation, sunken gyri, and widened sulci. Cortical degeneration in AD leads to progressive dementia with prominent amnesia, aphasia, apraxia, and anosmia (loss of smell). Alzheimer's disease is also characterized by a loss of neurotransmitters, which may account for the severity of the cognitive impairment in dementia (Perry & Perry, 1985).

Plaques contain dense deposits of an amyloid protein and other associated proteins. They are found outside and around neurons and proliferate in brain areas important for memory. Small numbers of plaques, called senile plaques, develop in the brain with age, but large numbers of senile plaques are found almost exclu-

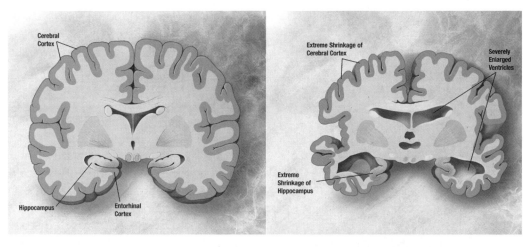

Figure 4–1. Comparison of normal brain and brain of patient with Alzheimer's disease (User: Garrondo / Wikimedia Commons / Public Domain).

sively in patients with AD (Hsaio et al., 1996). Senile plaques consist of beta-amyloid mixed with dendritic debris from surrounding cells. Beta-amyloid is a protein fragment clipped from a larger protein, APP, during metabolism. Beta-amyloid segments join up with other beta-amyloid filaments and fragments of dead and dying dendrites. Together these form the dense and insoluble plaques that characterize AD (Braak & Braak, 1991; Williamson, Rossor, Owen, & Hardy, 1991).

Within the medial temporal lobe, the hippocampus and the entorhinal cortex (EC) of the limbic system are particularly vulnerable to the pathological changes associated with AD. The EC plays a crucial role as a gateway connecting the neocortex and the hippocampal formation. The name *entorhinal* ("inside rhinal") derives from the fact that it is partially enclosed by the rhinal (olfactory) sulcus. Together with the hippocampal formation and neighboring portions of the parahippocampal region, it forms a major substrate mediating conscious (declarative) memory (Witter, 2011). Layer II of

the EC gives rise to a pathway that is the major source of the excitatory input to the hippocampus.

Gomez-Isla and her colleagues (1996) found that the neuronal population in the EC remained stable in healthy controls between the ages of 60 and 90 years of age. However, they also observed very severe neuronal loss in the EC even in very mild AD cases at the threshold for clinical detection of dementia. This neuronal loss was so marked that it must have started well before onset of clinical symptoms. As the clinical severity of dementia progressed, all of the EC was affected. Results indicated that the degree of neuronal loss in the EC paralleled the incidence of neurofibillary tangles and neuritic plaques but not of diffuse plaques without neuritic changes.

Stages of Alzheimer's Disease

Historically, the stages of AD have been classified as mild/early, moderate/middle, and severe/late stage. New criteria and guidelines established in 2011 for the

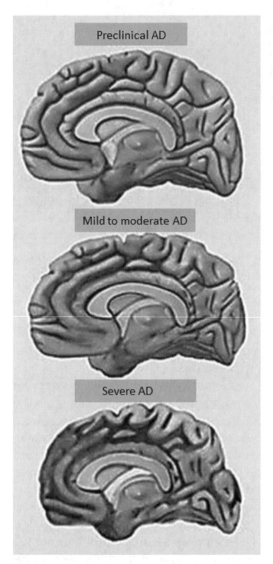

Figure 4–2. Stages of progressive Alzheimer's disease (National Institute on Aging / Wikimedia Commons / Public Domain).

are identified, an individual with a diagnosis using the new criteria would be said to have preclinical AD or MCI due to AD. The third stage of the new criteria, dementia due to AD, encompasses all stages of AD as described today, from mild/early stage to severe/ late stage (Voysey, 2009; Alzheimer's Association, 2012).

Staging has also been described according to the deterioration of the brain as AD unfolds. Braak and Braak (1991) identified six stages of dissolution associated with AD. The six stages of disease propagation can be distinguished with respect to the location of the tangle-bearing neurons and the severity of changes. These stages are: I–II = clinically silent cases; limbic stages III–IV = incipient AD; neocortical stages V–VI = fully developed AD. The Braak staging corresponds to the staging of AD dementia stages.

Three stages have been identified for the dementia classification in AD:

◆ **Early or mild stage:** Memory problems are more severe than those seen in normal aging adults. Patient may become disoriented in unfamiliar locations, may not be able to recall recent events, and may begin to be unable to remember the names of persons just met.

◆ **Middle or moderate stage:** More functional decline appears in the middle or moderate stages of AD. Orientation to time and place and memory for recent events are affected. Complex tasks become more difficult to perform with accuracy and efficiency. Social withdrawal, flat affect, and loss of initiative, tact, and judgment occur.

◆ **Final or severe stage:** In the final stage, patient is bedridden

stages of AD are: (1) preclinical AD, (2) mild cognitive impairment due to AD, and (3) dementia due to Alzheimer's AD. The new criteria propose that AD begins before the mild/early stage and that new technologies have the potential to identify Alzheimer-related brain changes that occur before mild/early stage disease. When these very early changes in the brain and incontinent. Primitive reflexes such as grasp and suck responses may appear, and involuntary movements become severe. Alzheimer's disease patients usually die from pneumonia or heart failure (Overman & Geoffrey, 1987).

Disorders of Cognition Associated With AD

Dissolution of cognitive abilities corresponds with the functional stages of intellectual, behavioral, and language deterioration associated with AD. In the early or mild stages, memory problems appear that are more severe than those seen in normal aging adults. Persons with AD at this stage may become disoriented in unfamiliar locations, may not be able to recall recent events, and may begin to be unable to remember the names of persons just met (Overman & Geoffrey, 1987). More functional decline occurs in the middle or moderate stage of AD dementia. Orientation to time and place is affected, as is memory for recent events. In the middle stage, complex tasks become increasingly difficult to perform with accuracy and efficiency, like managing personal finances, grocery shopping, and food preparation. In addition, there are symptoms of social withdrawal, flat affect, and loss of initiative, tact, and judgment. In the severe stage, the patient withdraws and becomes mute (Bayles, 1984).

Language Disorders in AD

Semantic Dissolution

Semantic dissolution is progressive throughout AD. Semantic memory stores the individual's knowledge of the world and manipulates that knowledge through the processing of association, ideation, and inferencing (Bayles, 1988). Semantic memory is responsible for categorization, visual imagery, and conceptualization of steps needed to prepare a meal, get ready for bed, or plan a family reunion. This ability to conceptualize and order associated concepts and propositions is what Bayles (1988) refers to as a schema. Communication is more affected in cortical dementia patients because the conceptual system for semantic memory and discourse cohesion become increasingly impaired as the disease progresses (Bayles, 1988; Ripich & Terrell, 1988).

Decreased Idea Density

Problems with idea density and use of grammatical complexities in adolescence may be associated with decreased cognitive and language scores in later life (Snowdon et al., 1996). Two measures of linguistic ability in early life—idea density and grammatical complexity assessed from early autobiographical writings—were studied in older persons diagnosed with AD. The most significant correlation with decreased cognitive performance was paucity of idea density (Snowdon et al.,1996).

Disturbed Naming

Naming is extremely disturbed in AD because of progressively deteriorating cognitive function (Ripich, 1991). Patients with AD are, however, more likely to be successful in word frequency when compared with patients suffering from transient acute confusional states (Wallesch & Hundsalz, 1994). In the mildest stages of AD dementia, which typically last 1 to 3 years, patients produce some errors on naming tasks but use compensatory measures, such as pauses and word substitutions. In the early stages also, patients will often correct their naming errors. As the disease progresses, more errors are observable on naming tasks, such as circumlocution and semantic and literal paraphasias. In the moderate stages, which range from 2 to 10 years, patients cannot correct their errors, and cueing will not enable the patient to produce the target word. In the severe stages, patients present with severely impaired naming or the inability to perform naming tasks at all (Bayles & Kaszniak, 1987).

Decreased Verbal Coherence

Verbal output becomes increasingly difficult for the listener to follow. Initially, patients can engage in relatively intact and coherent discourse, can initiate automatic speech, and can repeat more frequently occurring words in sentences. Errors can be detected in repetition with increasing sentence length and in some omissions in a series during automatic speech. In the moderate stages, the patient cannot tell a coherent story, needs prompting to begin a series, and has difficulty repeating both frequently and less frequently occurring words. In the most severe stages, the patient becomes unable to use meaningful verbal expression but may produce jargon and rambling, incoherent discourse.

Comprehension Deficits

Comprehension becomes increasingly affected in AD. Patients with early AD evidence little difficulty in attending to sentences but may begin to show problems in attending to longer materials with understanding. Moderately involved patients with AD cannot answer questions when asked or will give irrelevant answers. Given structured tasks, patients may perform moderately well but may have problems in understanding information when the length and complexity of material increases. In the severe stages, the patient with AD shows no evidence of understanding verbal requests for information and is unable to attend to structured tasks.

Disorders of Reading and Writing

Similar patterns of deterioration are seen for reading and writing. Mildly impaired patients with AD can write a paragraph with some spelling errors and can read aloud. In the moderate stages, patients cannot write more than one sentence but may be able to write names. The patient may produce spelling and grammatical errors but is unable to recognize them. Reading is most affected in the moderate stages. Patients cannot read paragraphs and will substitute one word for another or produce a nonsense word. Patients also cannot answer questions about what has been read. In the severe stages, patients are unable to read, write, or attend to structured tasks.

Summary

Cognitive and language disorders that have been reported for AD are:

- Semantic dissolution
- Problems with idea density
- Problems with grammatical complexity
- Disturbed naming
- Incoherent discourse
- Impaired comprehension
- Impaired reading and writing

- ◆ Impaired memory
- ◆ Impaired orientation
- ◆ Impaired attention and focus.

VASCULAR DEMENTIA

Prevalence

Formerly referred to as multiple infarct dementia, vascular dementia (VaD) is the second most prevalent dementia, after AD, accounting for 20% to 30% of all persons with dementia diagnosis (Alzheimer's Association, 2012).

Pathophysiology

The term *vascular cognitive impairment* represents a syndrome that takes into account the spectrum of cognitive severity, from mild to severe, which often includes executive dysfunction and the various types of brain vascular disease that could underlie cognitive symptoms, including subclinical vascular brain injury (Gorelick et al., 2011). The most severe form of vascular cognitive impairment is VaD, which refers to the subtly progressive worsening of memory and other cognitive functions that is presumed to be due to vascular disease within the brain.

Patients with VaD often present with similar symptoms as patients with AD; however, the related changes in the brain are not due to AD pathology but to chronic reduced blood flow in the brain from one or more strokes, which can occur as silent infarcts that eventually result in dementia. Vascular dementia occurs when blood clots block small blood vessels in the brain and destroy brain tissue.

The course of the dementia is stepwise and variable. Cognitive problems may begin as mild changes that worsen gradually as a result of multiple minor strokes or other conditions that affect smaller blood vessels, leading to cumulative damage. Probable risk factors are high blood pressure, arteriosclerosis, and advanced age.

VaD presents with both cortical and subcortical involvement. Three clinical subgroups have been identified: (1) those with large cerebral infarctions or chronic ischemia caused by large, vessel thrombotic strokes or multiembolic strokes; (2) those with numerous small, subcortical lacunar infarctions often involving the middle cerebral artery; and (3) those with Binswanger's disease, a subcortical atherosclerotic encephalopathy of the penetrating cerebral arteries (Rogers, Meyer, Mortel, Mahurin, & Judd, 1986). Lacunes are small cavities of infarcted brain tissue.

Binswanger's disease is a rare form of VaD characterized by cerebrovascular lesions in the deep white matter of the brain, loss of memory and cognition, and mood changes. Patients usually show signs of abnormal blood pressure, stroke, blood abnormalities, disease of the large blood vessels in the neck, and disease of the heart valves. Other prominent features of the disease include urinary incontinence, difficulty walking, clumsiness, slowness of conduct, lack of facial expression, and speech difficulty. These symptoms, which tend to begin after age 60, are not always present in all patients and may sometimes appear only as a passing phase (Bayles & Kaszniak, 1987). Table 4–2 provides a summary of the effects of large vessel occlusion, lacunae state, and Binswanger's disease.

An inherited form of VaD is cerebral autosomal dominant arteriopathy with subcortical infarcts and leukoencephalopathy (CADASIL). This is a recently

Table 4–2. Language and Related Disorders Associated with VaD Large Vessel Occlusion, Lacunae State, and Subcortical Infarcts (Binswanger's Disease)

Disorder	Language or Related Deficit
Large vessel occlusion	
Left anterior arteries	Transcortical motor aphasia
Bilateral anterior artery	Decreased initiative, loss of motivation
Left middle cerebral artery	Aphasia, apraxia, dementia
Right middle cerebral artery	Visuospatial disorders, disturbed prosody
Posterior middle artery	Fluent aphasia, alexia with agraphia
Posterior cerebral artery	
Right side	Visual hallucinations, abnormal facial recognition, spatial orientation
Left side	Hemisensory loss, anomia, alexia with agraphia
Bilateral	Severe permanent amnesia, cortical blindness, visual agnosia, difficulty recognizing familiar faces (prosopagnosia)
Lacunar state	Dementia, pseudobular palsy, dysarthria, dysphagia
Binswanger's disease	Memory impairment

Source: From Bayles, K. A., & Kaszniak, A. W. (1987). The brain and age-related dementing diseases. In K. A. Bayles & A. W. Kaszniak (Eds.), *Communication and cognition in normal aging and dementia* (pp. 27–31) Boston, MA: Pro-Ed. Reprinted with permission.

described neurovascular disease that affects young to middle-age individuals. The disease is caused by a mutation on the Notch3 gene on chromosome 19 (LaPoint, Patel, & Rubio, 2000; Ruchoux & Maurage, 1997). Clinically, CADASIL is characterized by migrainous headaches (with or without aura), mood disturbances, focal neurological deficits, transient ischemic attacks, strokes, and dementia. Pathologically, the disease is characterized by a stereotypic degeneration of the arterial walls. Gradual destruction of vascular smooth muscle cells leads to progressive wall thickening and fibrosis and luminal narrowing in small and medium-sized penetrating arteries. The reduced cerebral blood flow finally causes lacunar infarcts, mainly in the basal ganglia and frontotemporal white matter, which lead to cognitive deficits and dementia of the subcortical vascular type (Kalimo et al., 1999; Kalimo, Ruchoux, Viitanen, & Kalaria, 2002).

The Notch3 gene provides instructions for producing the Notch3 receptor protein located on the surface of the muscle cells that surround blood vessels (vascular smooth muscle cells). The Notch3 receptor protein is specific to arteries, which are blood vessels that carry blood from the heart to the rest of the body. The protein is not present in veins, which return blood to the heart. When certain molecules attach (bind) to Notch3 receptors, the receptors send signals to the nucleus of the cell. These signals then turn on (activate) particular genes within vascular smooth muscle cells. Notch3 receptors play a key role in the function and survival of vascular smooth muscle cells. These receptors are thought to be essential for the maintenance of healthy muscle cells in the brain's arteries (Federico, Bianchi, & Dotti, 2005).

Cognitive Disorders Associated with VaD

Symptoms of VaD, which often develop in a stepwise manner, include confusion, problems with recent memory, wandering or getting lost in familiar places, loss of bladder or bowel control (incontinence), emotional problems such as laughing or crying inappropriately, difficulty following instructions, and problems handling money (Myer, Bishop, & Murray, 2012).

In some cases, a sudden loss of cognitive function (such as language, memory, complex visual processing, or organizational skills) can occur after a stroke. Strokes are usually diagnosed easily with modern brain imaging techniques. Cognitive problems are usually worse at the time of the stroke and improve over time. Such cases are not usually diagnosed as dementia, but rather as residual cognitive impairment from a stroke. As is the case with AD, the cognitive changes in VaD can remain quite mild for a substantial period of time. Patients with more advanced VaD experience severe disruption in their personal, social, and vocational functioning (UCSF Memory and Aging Center, 2012).

Onset of VaD is rapid, with over 50% of cases occurring acutely in the form of a sudden attack of confusion. There is usually a gradual intellectual loss. Memory impairment tends to be inconsistent. Patients may be unable to remember one minute and then regain total capacity the next (Shadden, 1990). In addition to focal neurological signs, cognitive functions such as abstract thinking, judgment, impulse control, and personality are nearly always affected (Tonkovich, 1988).

Patients with VaD are more heterogeneous in their signs and symptoms than patients with AD and display a wider range of symptoms. Clinical characteristics vary because of differences in locus of pathology. Patients with deep hemispheric infarctions differ from those with superficial cortical infarctions or those with both deep and superficial infarctions (Shadden, 1988).

Language Disorders Associated with VaD

Bayles and Kaszniak (1987) provided insight into the types of language deficits that can be expected from VaD patients who suffer multiple, bilateral large vessel occlusions, lacunar state, and Binswanger's disease. Table 4–2 gives a summary of their observations. The large vessel occlusions are likely to predominate in brain regions supplied by the anterior, middle, or posterior cerebral arteries.

A diagnosis of lacunar state is applied to patients who have large numbers of lacunar infarctions in the small, deep cavities of the basal ganglia, thalamus, brainstem, and deep cerebral white matter. Binswanger's disease is caused by multiple infarcts in the subcortical white matter. Depending on the involved vessel, language disorders can include aphasia, alexia with agraphia, and anomia. Other disorders that can impair communication are dysarthria and dysphagia.

Summary

Patients with VaD are likely, given the site and size of the lesion(s), to present with the following cognitive and language disorders:

- ◆ Memory loss
- ◆ Emotional lability
- ◆ Transcortical motor aphasia
- ◆ Apraxia
- ◆ Fluent aphasia
- ◆ Anomia
- ◆ Alexia with or without agraphia
- ◆ Problems with abstract reasoning
- ◆ Impaired judgment and impulse control
- ◆ Personality changes
- ◆ Visuospatial disorders
- ◆ Disturbed prosody
- ◆ Visual agnosia
- ◆ Visual hallucinations.

DEMENTIA WITH LEWY BODIES

Prevalence

Dementia with Lewy bodies (DLB) is the third most common form of dementia, accounting for about 10% to 25% of dementia cases, following AD, which accounts for about 60%, and VaD. Dementia with Lewy bodies tends to affect males more than females, and the age of onset typically falls between 50 and 80, with a duration of illness of about 6 years. It is considered to have a more rapid progres-

sion than pure AD (NINDS, 2012b; Lewy Body Dementia Association, 2013).

Pathophysiology

The Lewy body was identified as the neuropathologic hallmark of Parkinson's disease (PD) in 1912. The hallmark brain abnormalities linked to DLB are named after Frederick H. Lewy, M.D., the neurologist who discovered them while working in Dr. Alois Alzheimer's laboratory during the early 1900s. Alpha-synuclein protein, the chief component of Lewy bodies, is found widely in the brain, but its normal function is not yet known. In 1961, Dr. Okazaki first described a relationship between the presence of cortical Lewy bodies and dementia, later confirmed by others (Alzheimer's Association, 2012).

The defining neuropathologic biomarkers of DLB are Lewy bodies, Lewy neurites, and spongiform encephalopathy in the amygdala, entorhinal cortex, and temporal gyrus. Lewy bodies are rounded intracytoplasmic neuronal inclusions, and Lewy neurites are diffuse and filamentous inclusions (Figure 4–3). Lewy bodies and Lewy neurites largely comprise alpha-synuclein 25, a protein normally expressed in neuronal synapses with a possible role in synaptic vesicle release.

The symptoms of DLB are caused by the build-up of Lewy bodies—accumulated bits of alpha-synuclein protein —inside the nuclei of neurons in areas of the brain that control particular aspects of memory and motor control. It is not yet known why alpha-synuclein accumulates into Lewy bodies or how Lewy bodies cause the symptoms of DLB, but there is evidence that alpha-synuclein accumulation is also linked to PD, multiple sys-

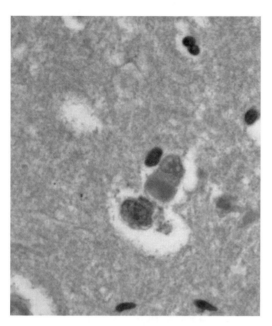

Figure 4–3. Pattern of neuronal loss in DLB: Braak staging (Naomi P. Visanji, Patricia L. Brooks, Lili-Naz Hazrati, and Anthony E. Lang / Wikimedia Commons / CC-A-2.5 Generic).

tem atrophy, and several other disorders, which are referred to as the synucleinopathies. Whitwell and colleagues (2007) found decreased midbrain, hypothalamus, and substantia innominata regions in DLB and suggest that there is an ascending pattern of neuronal loss from the brainstem to the basal areas of the brain. Figure 4–4 shows the progression of neuronal deterioration according to Braak staging. Braak staging is named after the work of Braak and Braak (1991;1995). According to this model, neuronal loss begins in the brainstem and ascends to the neocortex. The disease initiates in the periphery, gaining access to the CNS through retrograde transport along projection neurons from the gastrointestinal tract. As the disease progresses, the severity of lesions in susceptible regions increases. The neurons of the substantia innominata, located just under the thalamus and lenticular

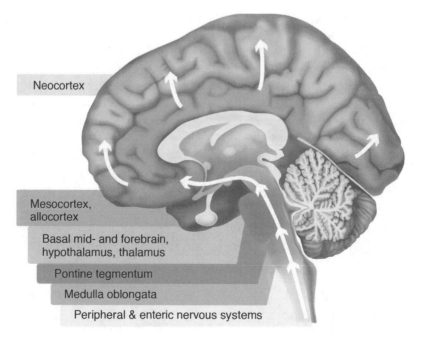

Neocortex

Mesocortex, allocortex

Basal mid- and forebrain, hypothalamus, thalamus

Pontine tegmentum

Medulla oblongata

Peripheral & enteric nervous systems

Figure 4–4. DLB frontal Lewy bodies (User: Jensflorian /Wikimedia Commons / CC-A-SA-3.0 Unported; GFDL 1.2).

nucleus, provide the major source of cholinergic innervation for the entire neocortical surface (Mesulam, Mufson, Wainer, & Levey, 1983).

Lewy bodies are also found in other brain disorders, including AD and PD dementia (PD-d). Many people with Parkinson's eventually develop problems with thinking and reasoning, and many people with DLB experience movement symptoms, such as hunched posture, rigid muscles, a shuffling walk, and trouble initiating movement (Alzheimer's Association, 2012).

Cognitive Disorders Associated with DLB

The central feature required for a diagnosis of DLB is a progressive cognitive decline of sufficient magnitude to interfere with normal social or occupational function. Two of the following core features are essential for a diagnosis of probable DLB, and one is essential for possible DLB:

◆ Fluctuating cognition with pronounced variations in attention and alertness
◆ Recurrent visual hallucinations that are typically well formed and detailed
◆ Spontaneous motor features of Parkinsonism.

In addition, there are clinical presentations that distinguish DLB from other forms of dementia, specifically:

◆ Changes in thinking and reasoning
◆ Confusion and alertness that varies significantly from one

time of day to another or from one day to the next
◆ Parkinson's symptoms, such as a hunched posture, balance problems, and rigid muscles
◆ Visual hallucinations
◆ Delusions
◆ Trouble interpreting visual information
◆ Acting out dreams, sometimes violently, a problem known as rapid eye movement (REM) sleep disorder
◆ Malfunctions of the autonomic nervous system
◆ Memory loss that may be significant but less prominent than in Alzheimer
◆ Unexplained loss of consciousness, frequent falls.

Dementia with Lewy bodies shares many features with AD. There are, however, key differences between AD and DLB:

◆ **Memory loss** tends to be a more prominent symptom in early AD than in early DLB, although advanced DLB may cause memory problems in addition to its more typical effects on judgment, planning, and visual perception.
◆ **Movement symptoms** are more likely to be an important cause of disability early in DLB than in AD, although AD can cause problems with walking, balance, and getting around as it progresses to moderate and severe stages.
◆ **Hallucinations, delusions, and misidentification** of familiar

people are significantly more frequent in early-stage DLB than in AD.

◆ **REM sleep disorder** is more common in early DLB than in AD.

◆ **Disruption of the autonomic nervous system**, causing a blood pressure drop on standing, dizziness, falls, and urinary incontinence, is much more common in early DLB than in AD.

Use of cholinesterase inhibitors in DLB has been examined in a series of small studies. Results indicate a reduction in the frequency and intensity of hallucinations, confusion, and agitation in AD and DLB; and in some cases of DLB, the results may be rather dramatic. This benefit of cholinesterase inhibitors in DLB may be related to the depleted levels of choline acetyltransferase in DLB. Research to date indicates that avoiding medications with anticholinergic properties and providing cholinergic replacement should be a primary consideration when treating the cognitive and behavioral symptoms of DLB (Gomez-Isla et al., 1996).

Language Disorders Associated with DLB

Confabulation, perhaps a function of paranoia and hallucinations, appears to be a significant feature of the language of DLB patients. The neuropathological basis of Lewy body dementia includes neuronal loss and the presence of Lewy bodies in subcortical nucleus and in frontal, temporal, and parietal lobes, which may explain the predominantly attentional, executive, and visuospatial dysfunction found in this disease (Gómez-Isla et al., 1999).

However, persons with DLB also have impaired verbal fluency, naming, comprehension, and visual-language problem-solving skills. Noe and colleagues (2004) compared the performance on neuropsychological and language tests of patients with AD, DLB, and PD-d. Compared with the other two groups of subjects, patients with DLB scored better on verbal memory tests and worse on attentional, visuoperceptual, visuoconstructive, and visual memory tests. Contrastively, AD, DLB, and PD-d patients shared similar deficits on encoding/acquisition, orientation, naming, verbal fluency, language comprehension and repetition, and verbal-visual reasoning. The DLB and AD groups exhibited similar degrees of language impairment in naming, comprehension, fluency, repetition, orientation, and categorizing similarities.

Patients with PD-d and DLB also have significant difficulty organizing narrative speech. Narrative impairment was found to be associated with reduced cortical volume in the inferior frontal and anterior cingulated regions (Ash et al., 2007). Frontal involvement also causes impairment in the ability to process sentences with increasing working memory demands (Gross et al., 2012).

Summary

Persons diagnosed with DLB may present with the following symptoms of impaired cognition and language:

◆ Memory loss
◆ Impaired comprehension
◆ Poor verbal fluency

◆ Confabulation
◆ Visual hallucinations
◆ Paranoia
◆ Impaired repetition
◆ Disordered thinking
◆ Variable attention and alertness
◆ Impaired narrative discourse
◆ Impaired orientation
◆ Impaired sentence processing.

MIXED DEMENTIA

Prevalence

No definitive prevalence is available. However, it is suspected that mixed dementia is more common than is presently known.

Pathophysiology

Mixed dementia is a condition in which abnormalities characteristic of more than one type of dementia occur simultaneously. This type of dementia is also referred to as dementia-multifactorial. In the most common form of mixed dementia, the abnormal protein deposits associated with AD coexist with blood vessel problems linked to VaD. Alzheimer's brain changes also often coexist with Lewy bodies. In some cases, a person may have brain changes linked to all three conditions—AD, VaD, and DLB. Although mixed dementia is infrequently diagnosed during life, many researchers believe it deserves more attention because the combination of two or more types of dementia-related brain changes may have a greater impact on the brain than one type alone (Alzheimer's Association, 2012).

Autopsy findings from the Memory and Aging Project study (Bennett et al.,

2005) involving long-term cognitive assessments followed by eventual brain autopsy confirmed that:

◆ 94% of participants with a diagnosis of dementia had AD—the autopsies of those diagnosed with AD showed that 54% had coexisting pathology;
◆ the most common coexisting abnormality was previously undetected blood clots or other evidence of vascular disease; and
◆ Lewy bodies were the second most common coexisting abnormality.

Summary

Compared with persons who have one type of dementia, persons with mixed dementia, that is, persons presenting with two or more types of dementia, may have more severe manifestations of cognitive and language disorders associated with each of the dementia types. The most common types of mixed dementia are AD and VaD, AD and DLB, and a combination of all three types: AD, VaD, and DLB.

FRONTOTEMPORAL DEMENTIA

Prevalence

Frontotemporal dementia (FTD) was once considered rare, but it is now thought to account for up to 10% to 15% of all dementia cases. It is still believed to be less common than AD, VaD, and DLB. In those younger than age 65, FTD may account for up to 20% to 50% of dementia cases. People usually develop FTD in their 50s or early 60s, making the disorder relatively more common in this younger age group. There is a strong genetic component to the disease; FTD often runs in families (Alzheimer's Association, 2012).

Pathophysiology

Frontotemporal dementia describes a group of clinical syndromes associated with shrinking of the frontal and temporal anterior lobes of the brain. Originally known as Pick's disease, FTD is marked by cell loss and scarring in the frontal lobes, parts of the temporal lobes, and the deeper brain structures that link to them. The tissue loss results from changes in the proteins that normally help cells function. When proteins change shape or quantity (either too much or too little), they no longer function normally. Consequently, the cells that depend on those proteins can no longer function normally either. If a cell

or a protein is dysfunctional, the body destroys it. When enough cells in a specific brain area are lost, then the signs and symptoms of the disease become evident (Liu, 2004; NINDS, 2012c).

Unlike AD, FTD is not characterized by amyloid plaques and neurofibrillary tangles. Instead, FTD brains show severe atrophy and specific neuronal inclusions. The brain tissue of approximately 40% of people with FTD shows tau inclusions or Pick's bodies. Pick's bodies, also called Pick's cells, are found in the outer three layers of the cortex and are characterized by silver and chromium (argentophilic) inclusions. Tau is a neuronal protein that binds to microtubules and is thought to be involved in the stabilization of the neuron's three-dimensional structure. Tau mutations can reduce the binding affinity of tau for microtubules or increase tau accumulation, both of which lead to FTD and Parkinsonism, as is seen in Figure 4–5.

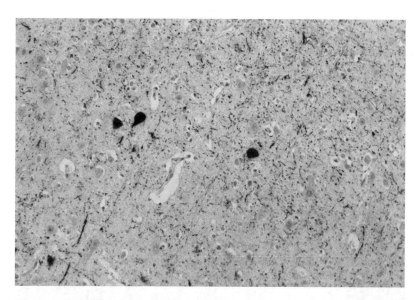

Figure 4–5. Biopsy specimen of a frontotemporal dementia and Parkinsonism showing numerous tau-positive neuronal and glial inclusions in neocortical areas (User: Jensflorian /Wikimedia Commons / CC-A-SA-3.0 Unported; GFDL 1.3).

Most patients with tau gene mutations develop an autosomal-dominantly inherited syndrome with features of FTD. However, a large pathological and clinical heterogeneity is observed both among and within FTD families, such as corticobasal or progressive supranuclear palsy syndrome. No tau mutations have so far been reported in cases with classical AD (NINDS, 2012c).

Frontotemporal dementia has long been associated with focal cortical atrophy, as seen in Figure 4–6, whereas the subcortical structures have received less emphasis.

In the behavioral variant of FTD (bvFTD) and semantic dementia (SD), however, dramatic changes in eating, sexual conduct, and compulsivity emerge, all of which may relate to striatal dysfunction. Later-stage patients often show extrapyramidal motor signs, such as rigidity and bradykinesia, which may reflect a loss of nigrostriatal projection targets (Halabi et al., 2013).

FTD Clinical Syndromes

Currently, the symptoms of FTD fall into clinical patterns that involve either: (1) changes in behavior, (2) problems with language, or (3) changes in motor function. These symptoms, however, may overlap or occur together. Based on the distinct patterns of signs and symptoms, three different clinical syndromes (Alzheimer's Association, 2012) have been grouped together under the category of FTD:

1. **BvFTD**
2. **Primary progressive aphasia (PPA):** affects language skills in early stages, but often also affects behavior as it advances. The two chief forms of PPA have somewhat different symptoms:
   ◆ In **SD**, people speak easily, but their words convey less and less meaning. They tend to use broad general terms, such as "animal" when they mean "cat."

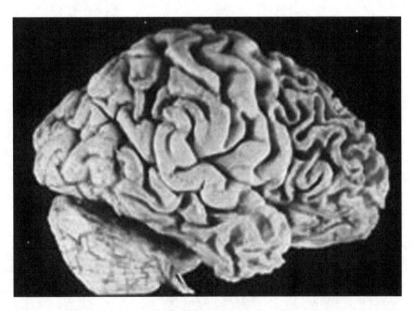

Figure 4–6. Frontotemporal degeneration (Wikipedia Commons / GFDL, 1.2; CC-A-SA-3.0 Unported).

Language comprehension also declines.

◆ In progressive nonfluent aphasia (PNFA), people lose their ability to generate words easily, and their speech becomes halting, difficult, and ungrammatical. Ability to read and write also may be impaired.

3. **Motor neuron disease (FTD-MND)**

Behavioral-Variant Frontotemporal Dementia

The first type, bvFTD, is the most prevalent, features behavior that can be either impulsive (disinhibited) or bored and listless (apathetic), and includes inappropriate social behavior; lack of social tact; lack of empathy; distractability; loss of insight into the behaviors of oneself and others; an increased interest in sex; changes in food preferences; agitation or, conversely, blunted emotions; neglect of personal hygiene; repetitive or compulsive behavior; and decreased energy and motivation (NINDS, 2012c).

Behavioral-variant frontotemporal dementia takes its greatest toll on personality and behavior. It may begin with subtle changes that may be mistaken for depression. As bvFTD progresses, people often develop disinhibition, a striking loss of restraint in personal relations and social life.

Primary Progressive Aphasia

Primary progressive aphasia affects language skills in early stages but often also affects behavior as it advances.

Semantic Dementia. Semantic dementia, which has also been called temporal variant FTD, accounts for 20% of FTD cases.

Individuals with SD present with severe and early semantic memory deficits and loss of word and object meaning despite relatively intact episodic memory. Errors on confrontational naming are often semantically related (Mahendra & Hopper, 2013). Persons have difficulty making or understanding speech, often in conjunction with the behavioral type's symptoms. Spatial skills and memory remain intact.

Progressive Nonfluent Aphasia. Progressive nonfluent aphasia accounts for only about 20% of all people with FTD. In semantic dementia, the person maintains the ability to speak but loses the meaning of the word. People with PNFA have difficulty producing language fluently even though they still know the meaning of the words they are trying to say. The person may talk slowly, having trouble saying the words, and have great trouble with the telephone, talking within groups of people, or understanding complex sentences. In recent years it has become apparent that many patients with PNFA go on to develop severe Parkinsonian symptoms that overlap with progressive supranuclear palsy and corticobasal degeneration, such as an inability to move the eyes side-to-side, muscle rigidity in the arms and legs, falls, and weakness in the muscles around the throat (NINDS, 2012c).

Motor Neuron Disease

Approximately 15% of patients with FTD also develop FTD-MND. Frontotemporal dementia movement disorders affect certain involuntary, automatic muscle functions. These disorders also may impair language and behavior. Most often, this combination occurs in patients with bvFTD, and only rarely does MND arise in patients with SD or PNFA.

Motor neuron disease affects motor nerve cells in the spinal cord, the brainstem, and the cerebral cortex. The most common type of MND is amyotrophic lateral sclerosis (ALS), also called Lou Gehrig's disease, which can occur as a purely motor disorder. More often, however, patients with ALS also have behavioral or cognitive problems similar to those seen in FTD. Motor neuron disease symptoms include slurring of speech, swallowing difficulty, choking, limb weakness, and muscle wasting. In patients with FTD-MND, there is often (but not always) a family history of the disease (Merrilees et al., 2013). The two primary FTD movement disorders are:

◆ **corticobasal degeneration**, which causes shakiness, lack of coordination, and muscle rigidity and spasms; and

◆ **progressive supranuclear palsy**, which causes walking and balance problems, frequent falls, and muscle stiffness, especially in the neck and upper body. It also affects eye movements. (Alzheimer's Association, 2012)

Cognitive Disorders Associated with FTD

One of the most significant clinical signs of FTD is apathy. Merrilees and colleagues (2013) note that patients with bvFTD typically present with apathy, disinhibition, aberrant motor behaviors, hyperorality or appetite disturbance, and loss of sympathy and empathy for others. Behaviorally, SD is also associated with apathy, mental rigidity, obsessive preoccupations, and depression.

Throughout the course of the disease, cognition, language, and memory decline. Near the end of the disease, patients become mute. Early symptoms of Pick's disease include personality aberrations, loss of tact and concern, impaired judgment, and a decline in recent memory (Cummings & Benson, 1984; Shadden, 1988). Passivity and impulsiveness in the final stages of the disease have been reported (Holland, McBurney, Moossy, & Reinmuth 1985).

Language Disorders Associated with FTD

Frontotemporal dementia used to be called Pick's disease, after Arnold Pick, a physician who in 1892 first described a patient with distinct symptoms affecting language. Some researchers still use the term "Pick's disease." Other terms used to describe FTD include frontotemporal disorder, frontotemporal degeneration, and frontal lobe disorder (Alzheimer's Association, 2012). The current classifications of language disorders under FTD PPA, including SD and PNFA, replace the designation of Pick's disease as a singular type of dementia. Pick's disease is now described as one of several types of dementias in the frontal lobe that strikes persons between the ages of 40 and 60 years and occurs more commonly among women than men (Tonkovich, 1988).

Language impairment, the predominant complaint of people with SD, is due to the disease damaging the left temporal lobe, an area critical for assigning meaning to words. In SD, people speak easily, but language comprehension declines. The language deficit is not in producing speech but is a loss of the meaning, or semantics, of words. The most salient clinical features of SD are anomia with circumlocution and semantic paraphasia, single-word comprehension deficit, and reduced category fluency. Patients with SD also show deficits on nonverbal tasks using visual, auditory, and other modalities. This suggests that the key impairment in SD is a breakdown in conceptual knowledge rather than a specific problem with language. Atrophy is seen in the anterior and inferior temporal lobe rather than in classic language areas, further distancing SD from aphasic syndromes (Knibb & Hodges, 2005). In the first stages, individuals with SD may substitute a word like "thingy" for the target word, but eventually a person with SD will lose the meaning of more common words as well. In advanced SD, patients lose the ability to categorize and recall names. Reading and spelling usually decline as well, but the person may still be able to do arithmetic and use numbers, shapes, or colors well.

Names of people, even good friends, can become quite difficult for people with SD. Like the behavioral variant, memory, an understanding of where they are, and sense of day and time tend to function as before. Muscle control for daily life and activities tends to remain good until late in the disease. Some of these skills may seem worse than they actually are because of the language difficulty people with SD have when they try to express themselves (Hodges, 2003).

When SD starts in the right temporal lobe, people in the early stages have more trouble remembering the faces of friends and familiar people. Additionally, these people show profound deficits in understanding the emotions of others. The loss of empathy is an early and often preliminary symptom of patients with this right-sided form of SD (Hodges, 2003). Eventually people with right-sided onset develop progression to the left side and then present with the classical language features of SD. Similarly, left-sided cases progress to involve the right temporal lobe and then the person experiences difficulty recognizing faces, foods, animals, and emotion. SD patients eventually develop classical bvFTD behaviors, including disinhibition, apathy, loss of empathy, and diminished insight (Liu, 2004). The time from diagnosis to the end is longer than for those with bvFTD, typically taking about 6 years.

Much has been written about PPA (Bayles & Kaszniak, 1987; Crosile, 1992; Cummings & Duchen, 1981; Graff-Radford et al., 1990; Henry, 2010; Holland et al., 1985; Jokel, Cupit, Rochon, & Leonard, 2009; Knibb & Hodges, 2005; Kesler, Artzy, Yaretzky, & Kott, 1995; Kobayashi et al., 1990; Mesulam, 2001; Rogers & Alarcon, 1998). Patients with Pick's disease experience a slowly progressive language disorder without the initial intellectual or behavioral disturbances associated with dementia. Although nonverbal cognitive functions are intact for several years, the aphasia is slowly progressive. Primary progressive aphasia is typified by slowly emerging disturbances of speech fluency, spontaneous speech, and anomia. Language comprehension and nonverbal cognition are often preserved, and significant cognitive changes do not appear until several years after the initial language impairments occur (Mesulam, 2001).

Kesler and colleagues (1995) provided evidence of PPA as a slowly progressive aphasia in which the cognitive disturbances compatible with Pick's disease appeared up to 6 years after signs of nonfluent and agrammatic aphasia. Similarly, Scheltens and associates (1990) described a patient with a temporal form of Pick's disease who suffered from progressive aphasia 9 years before developing mild cognitive disturbances.

Observations of a 59-year-old man with a diagnosis of Pick's disease found prominent disturbances with word-finding difficulties for names denoting concrete entities and actions (Graff-Radford et al., 1990). The patient was aware of his deficits and was alert and fully oriented during testing. His deficits were confined to language output. The patient was able to identify the stimuli but could not retrieve its appropriate name. Although he could retrieve proper and common nouns of verbs, he could not retrieve functor items, like conjunctions and prepositions, and he was still able to communicate verbally. Over time, the patient showed a slow but definite progression of aphasia in sentence repetition and comprehension, and verbal intellectual abilities and verbal memory became impaired. He later deteriorated significantly in visual memory for designs and in arithmetic functions.

After the patient's death, autopsy findings confirmed the presence of Pick's bodies in the insula and striatum pyramidale of the left hippocampal formation and inferior temporal. No neurofibrillary tangles or neuritic plaques were noted. The investigators concluded that this patient presented with a progressive aphasia that was largely circumscribed to anomia with an unusual left temporal variant of Pick's disease.

Many cases of FTD begin with decreased verbal output (Kertesz, Hudson, Mackenzie, & Munoz, 1994). Three cases of PPD with Pick-variant pathology were analyzed for neuronal changes and expressive language. In the first case, an 82-year-old man, the Pick's bodies were absent. Neuronal degeneration and astrogliosis were found within atrophic regions of the inferior frontal and superior parietal areas. In the second case, a 53-year-old man, cortical atrophy was found in the left middle and inferior temporal gyri. The third case was that of a 55-year-old woman whose autopsy findings revealed Pick's disease. From these cases it was determined that when a patient presents with PNFA or verbal apraxia leading to mutism in the absence of neuroplasm, Pick's disease or Pick-variant pathology is the most likely cause. However, in cases where PPA is only diagnosed on the basis of anomia or word-finding difficulty, it is most difficult to differentiate PPA from AD. In order to include other neurogenerative diseases caused by focal cortical dementia, the authors proposed the concept of a Pick's complex to include PPA, frontal lobe dementia, ALS with PPA, and other corticodentonigral and corticobasal degenerative disorders (Kertesz et al., 1994).

There is evidence that PPA symptoms show improvement during speech-language pathology therapy. Jokel, Cupit, Rochon, and Leonard (2009) found that persons with PPA may benefit from a computer-based treatment for anomia. This finding corroborates that of Murray (2008), who described three approaches to therapy with a patient with PPA, including a traditional stimulation-facilitation approach, a "back-to-the drawing board" program, and a functional communication approach using an augmentative communication device. Her patient appeared to show improvement during each form of therapy, indicating that persons with PPA may be able to benefit from long-term speech-language pathology services. Henry (2010) advocates for a treatment approach that combines restitutive, augmentative, and functional approaches to treatment, in order to maximize residual cognitive-linguistic skills in patients.

Summary

Frontotemporal dementia classifications include a behavioral, language, and motor component. The following are clinical symptoms that may be present in persons with a diagnosis of FTD:

◆ Apathy
◆ Disinhibition, particularly inappropriate sexual behaviors or appetite
◆ Loss of tact, judgment, and empathy
◆ Slowly progressive aphasia
◆ Impaired comprehension
◆ Dissolution of semantic abilities (paraphasia, reduced categorization)
◆ Memory loss
◆ Poor facial recognition
◆ Impaired verbal fluency
◆ Motor disturbances
◆ Anomia with circumlocution and semantic paraphasia
◆ Poor confrontational naming
◆ Disturbed nonverbal communication skills.

PARKINSON'S DISEASE

Prevalence

Parkinson's disease is the most common of the age-related diseases of the basal ganglia and affects 1.5 million adults in the United States, with a prevalence rate of about 1 per 1,000 in the general population. The age of onset for the majority of PD patients is 50 to 60 years for both men and women of all races and ethnicities (Shadden, 1990) but is higher for non-Hispanic whites.

Pathophysiology

Parkinson's disease is a cluster of signs resulting from a variety of causes. There are four categories of possible etiologies given for PD: (1) idiopathic or unknown etiology, (2) drug-induced postencephalitic, (3) causes such as encephalitis or influenza, and (4) arteriosclerotic PD, associated with cerebral arteriosclerosis. Idiopathic PD, or PD of unknown etiology, accounts for the majority of cases (86%). Drug-induced PD is the second most common type (Ebmeier et al., 1991).

It is well established that PD is a degenerative neurological disorder of unknown etiology, which results from a deficiency of neurochemical inhibitor substance dopamine released in the basal ganglia. There are neuronal and generative changes in the basal ganglia in the nucleus basalis of Meynert and nucleus locus coeruleus. The most conspicuous neuropathologic sign is depigmentation of the substantia nigra in the midbrain (Figure 4–7). The substantia nigra is the source of dopamine in the basal ganglia (Bayles & Kaszniak, 1987).

Parkinson's disease is a movement disorder characterized by exaggerated muscle tone, rigidity, tremor, limited range of motion, cogwheel rigidity, and a mask-like facial expression. Parkinson's disease causes dementia in 20% of diagnosed cases (Waters, 1995). Parkinson's disease dementia (PD-d), with more severe neuropsychological signs, presents as a consequence of greater involvement on the left side than on the right. Correlations

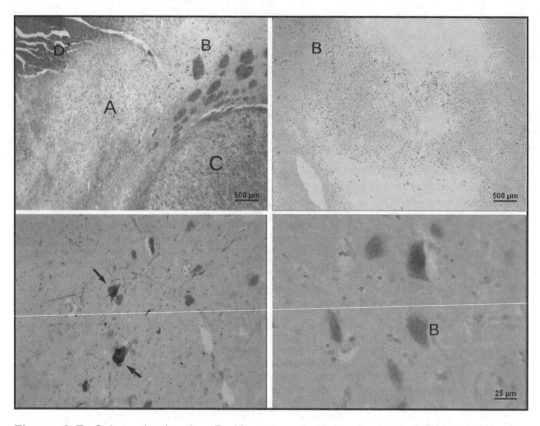

Figure 4–7. Substantia nigra in a Parkinson's patient showing loss of dopaminergic cells as well as Lewy body and Lewy neurite pathology. A = substantia nigra (pars compacta); B = neuromelanin laden cells that have dwindled in number in this Parkinson's patient; C = red nucleus; D = cerebral peduncles. (Suraj Rajan / Wikimedia Commons / CC-A-SA-3.0 Unported)

of varying types of movements in PD to intellectual decline have been reported for tremor, bradykinesia, rigidity, postural instability, and gait disturbance. Tremor at the initial stages of the disease is indicative of a more favorable outcome and preserved mental status (Zetusky, Jakovic, & Pirozzolo, 1985).

Two types of PD have been identified. One is primarily a motor disorder involving only subcortical structures without dementia; the other is a motor dysfunction involving both subcortical and corti-cal changes with dementia. Burton, Mc-Keith, Burn, Williams, and O'Brien (2004) noted that PD without dementia involves gray matter loss in frontal areas. In PD-d, this extends to temporal, occipital, and subcortical areas. Reduced gray matter volume in PD-d patients compared with controls was observed bilaterally in the temporal lobe, including the hippocampus and parahippocampal gyrus, and in the occipital lobe, the right frontal lobe, and the left parietal lobe, as well as some subcortical regions.

Cognitive Disorders Associated with PD-d

Depression is a major problem in PD. Mayeux, Stern, Herman, Greenbaum, Fahn (1986) estimate that depression occurs in 37% to 90% of the Parkinson's population. The frequency of depression in PD may be coincidental with the occurrence of depression in older persons. It may be a complex and reactive response to a chronic illness and feelings of hopelessness and despair about the financial and physical consequences of the disease (Gotham, Brown, & Marsden, 1986). Or the depression may be the result of some neurochemical aspects of the disease. The origin of depression in PD remains unclear (Yorkston, Miller, & Strand, 1995).

The striatum is considered to be critical, involved in memory and positively reinforced conditioning (Pérez-Ruiz & Prado-Alcalá, 1989; Prado-Alcalá, 1989). Cognitive and affective deficits may be attributed to degeneration of the mesocortical and mesolimbic dopamine system (Cooper, Sagar, Jordan, Harvey, & Sullivan, 1991). Those with dementia have neuropsychologic deficits that are related to degeneration of the substantia nigra and related structures (Cummings & Benson, 1984). Cognitive deficits also appear to involve extrastriatal dopamine or nondopaminergic pathology. Specifically, the predominant features of PD-d include mental slowing, poor problem solving, and deterioration of abstraction and concept formation, but exclude aphasia and agnosia.

Some investigators have queried whether patients with PD-d may actually have superimposed AD cortical changes. At least 30% of persons with PD-d develop dementia associated with both cortical and subcortical pathology (Shadden, 1990). Cortical changes, particularly neurofibrillary tangles and plaques, occur in the cerebral cortex of some patients with PD-d (Cummings & Benson, 1984). Frontal lobe–like symptomatology in PD-d may be caused by striatal dysfunction found in nigrostriatal dopaminergic degeneration and partial lesions of the ascending cholinergic and aminergic neuronal systems (Pillon, Duboic, Ploska, & Agid, 1991). The finding is partially substantiated by Cooper and his colleagues (1991), who found that the pathogenesis of cognitive deficits seen in PD-d is largely independent of frontostriatal dopamine deficiency.

Language Disorders Associated with PD-d

Persons with PD and PD-d do not demonstrate aphasia in the traditional classification of language disorders. However, Murdoch (2010) noted that several language disturbances are associated with PD-d. Specifically, language deficits are observed on those tasks that place increasing demands on the semantic and syntactical subcomponents of the linguistic system. Integrity of semantic processing may be compromised as well as verbal fluency. Verbal and semantic reasoning are also impaired.

Cummings, Darkins, Mendez, Hill, and Benson (1988) found that speech and language deficits reflect both the cognitive and motor deficits of PD-d. Decreased phrase length, impaired speech melody, and agraphia were identified in patients with PD-d. In comparison with persons with AD, patients with PD-d had more prominent writing deficits and were significantly more impaired in some aspects of language functioning than patients with PD without dementia. Bayles and Kaszniak (1987) also observed language disturbances in PD but found that deficits were demonstrated in verbal associative reasoning, linguistic disambiguation, verbal description, story retelling, and generative naming, regardless of etiology.

Syntax comprehension deficits have been identified in persons with PD with and without dementia. Persons with PD and mild dementia demonstrated high comprehension error rates for sentences with moderately complex syntax. A possible explanation for these syntactical errors is posited by Lieberman and associates (1990), who suggest that both cognitive and syntactical errors associated with PD-d may reflect the disruption of neural circuits that connect Broca's area and other areas of the frontal lobe.

Summary

Parkinson's disease is primarily a motor disturbance associated with damage to the basal ganglia. However, approximately 20% of patients develop PD with dementia, or PD-d. Cognitive and language deficits associated with the dementia include:

♦ Depression
♦ Deficits in executive functioning
♦ Memory disorders
♦ Disturbances of cognitive sequencing
♦ Mental slowing
♦ Poor problem solving
♦ Decreased phrase length
♦ Problems with writing (agraphia)
♦ Syntax comprehension deficits
♦ Impaired discourse and narrative skills
♦ Problems with generative naming.

CRUEZFELDT–JAKOB DISEASE

Prevalence

Creutzfeldt–Jakob disease (CJD) is a rare, degenerative, rapidly progressive, invariably fatal brain disorder. It affects about 1 in every 1 million people per year worldwide; in the United States there are about 200 cases per year. The disease usually appears in later life and runs a rapid course. Typically, onset of symptoms occurs at about age 60, and about 90% of individuals die within 1 year (NINDS, 2013a).

Pathophysiology

Creutzfeldt–Jakob disease belongs to a family of human and animal diseases known as the transmissible spongiform encephalopathies (TSEs). Spongiform refers to the characteristic appearance of infected brains, which become filled with holes until they resemble sponges under a microscope (Figure 4–8).

Creutzfeldt–Jakob disease is the most common of the known human TSEs. Other human TSEs include kuru, fatal familial insomnia (FFI), and Gerstmann-Straussler-Scheinker disease (GSS). Kuru, an incurable degenerative neurological disorder, was identified in people of an isolated tribe in Papua New Guinea and has now almost disappeared. FFI and GSS are extremely rare hereditary diseases, found in just a few families around the world. Other TSEs are found in specific kinds of animals. These include bovine spongiform encephalopathy, which is found in cows and is often referred to as "mad cow" disease; scrapie, which affects sheep and goats; mink encephalopathy; and feline encephalopathy. Similar diseases have occurred in elk, deer, and exotic zoo animals (NINDS, 2013a).

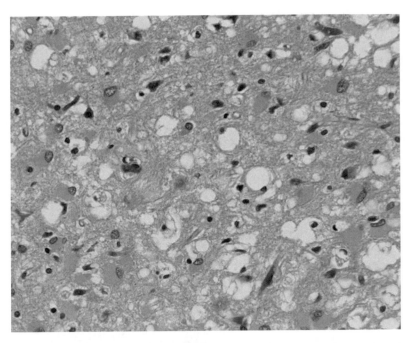

Figure 4–8. Photomicrograph of brain tissue showing prominent spongiotic changes in the cortex in CJD. (Centers for Disease Control and Prevention, part of the U.S. Department of Health and Human Services / Wikimedia Commons / Public Domain)

The disease presents as a degeneration of cortical tissues, which, in addition to dementia, is manifested in alterations in consciousness, myoclonus, cerebellar disturbances, and sensory and visual impairments (Ripich, 1991; Tonkovich, 1988). Patients experience difficulty with walking, muscle stiffness, twitches, and involuntary jerky movements.

There are diffuse cerebral pathologic changes with neuronal degeneration, glial proliferations, and, frequently, status spongiosus. Amyloid plaques are found in some patients with CJD (Kitamoto et al., 1986). Figure 4–9 illustrates amyloid plaques typical for CJD.

Mild to moderate atrophic changes are sometimes observed in the cortex, predominantly in the frontal, parietal, or temporal areas. Less consistent pathologic alterations are also seen in the basal ganglia, corticospinal tracts, motor neurons, thalamus, and cerebellum (DeJong & Pope, 1975).

There are three major categories of CJD:

◆ In sporadic CJD, the disease appears even though the person has no known risk factors for the disease. This is by far the most common type of CJD and accounts for at least 85% of cases.

◆ In hereditary CJD, the person has a family history of the disease and/or tests positive for a genetic mutation associated with CJD. About 5% to 10% of cases of CJD in the United States are hereditary.

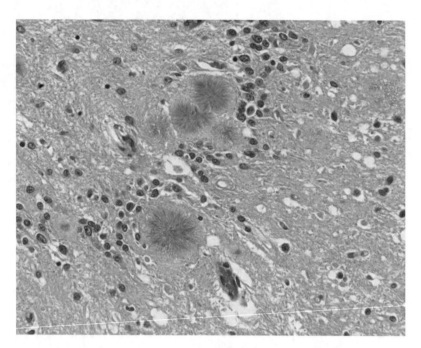

Figure 4–9. Creutzfeldt-Jakob Disease: Typical amyloid plaques. (Centers for Disease Control and Prevention, part of the U.S. Department of Health and Human Services / Wikimedia Commons / Public Domain)

◆ In acquired CJD, the disease is transmitted by exposure to brain or nervous system tissue, usually through certain medical procedures. There is no evidence that CJD is contagious through casual contact with a CJD patient. Since CJD was first described in 1920, fewer than 1% of cases have been acquired CJD (Alzheimer's Association, 2012; NINDS, 2013a).

bances. As the illness progresses, mental deterioration becomes pronounced, and involuntary movements, blindness, weakness of extremities, and coma may occur. Other indices of cognitive decline in this disease are fairly consistent. In the first stages, signs of neurological decline emerge. Among the most significant cognitive disturbances are depression, agitation, apathy, rapidly worsening confusion, disorientation, problems with memory, thinking, planning, judgment, and mood swings (Alzheimer's Association, 2012).

Cognitive Disorders Associated with CJD

In the early stages of disease, people may have failing memory, behavioral changes, lack of coordination, and visual distur-

Language Disorders Associated with CJD

In the middle stages, the neurological disturbances become overt, and aphasia, apraxia, and agnosia appear. Finally, the patient moves to a terminal vegetative stage and is mute (Cummings & Benson, 1984).

Summary

Patients diagnosed with CJD are likely to present with the following cognitive and language deficits:

- Aphasia
- Apraxia
- Agnosia
- Mutism (in terminal stages)
- Depression
- Agitation
- Apathy
- Rapidly worsening confusion
- Disorientation
- Memory problems
- Impaired thinking and planning
- Impaired judgment
- Mood swings

KORSAKOFF'S DISEASE

Prevalence

Wernicke–Korsakoff's syndrome, of which Korsakoff's disease (KD) is a major component, is diagnosed in about one in eight people with alcoholism (a dependency on, or addiction to, alcohol). Evidence shows that the condition is present in about 2% of the general population. It is more common among people in deprived communities. People affected tend to be men between the ages of 45 and 65 with a long history of alcohol misuse. However, it is possible to have Korsakoff's syndrome at an older or a younger age.

A significant proportion of women increase their alcohol consumption in their 70s. This may represent their attempts to cope with living alone or to bereavement. Widowed older women are also at a disadvantage in health and income and may adopt drinking as a way to handle stress (Arber & Ginn, 1991). Even for men who have been accustomed to regular drinking, alcohol can have a more pronounced effect in later life. If drinking is associated with poor nutritional habits, these taken together can cause cognitive changes.

Pathophysiology

Korsakoff's disease (KD) or syndrome is part of a condition known as Wernicke–Korsakoff's syndrome. This consists of two separate but related stages: Wernicke's encephalopathy is followed by Korsakoff's syndrome. However, not everyone has a clear case of Wernicke's encephalopathy before Korsakoff's syndrome develops.

Korsakoff's disease results from chronic alcohol abuse and is characterized by generalized cortical atrophy. The cognitive changes associated with KD develop as a secondary dementia that occurs after long-term alcohol abuse and vitamin B deficiency. Vitamin B deficiency is implicated in atrophy of the diencephalic and limbic structures, which affect memory for recent events. Brain lesions occur in the thalamus, particularly in the mammillary bodies that receive rich hippocampus input, the hypothalamus, and the frontal and associative areas of the neocortex (Bayles, 1984).

Cognitive Disorders Associated with KD

Symptoms of the dementia associated with KD are mild and either nonprogressive or slowly progressive. Alcohol-related dementia is caused by direct and indirect effects of alcohol on the brain. Alcohol can cause widespread damage to nerve cells and blood vessels, leading to brain shrinkage. People who misuse alcohol also tend to suffer injuries to the head—from falls or fights—and have a poor diet. These all contribute to alcohol-related dementia. *Korsakoff's disease* and *alcohol-related dementia* are terms that are often used interchangeably to refer to the neurological consequences of prolonged heavy drinking. There is evidence that the symptoms of alcohol-related dementia are broader and more numerous than those of Korsakoff's syndrome and are similar to those of AD. Symptoms include problems with:

◆ memory
◆ attention
◆ learning new tasks
◆ reasoning and problem solving
◆ semantic content
◆ empathy
◆ insight

Although not a separate disorder from alcohol-related dementia, the predominant symptoms of KD appear to be memory loss, confabulation, psychomotor retardation, circumstantiality, attention deficits, disorientation, and the inability to retain new information (Tonkovich, 1988).

Language Disorders Associated with KD

Affected individuals do not seem to use the same memory-encoding strategies and appear to rely more heavily on phonemic than semantic analysis. Verbal memory is more impaired than nonverbal

memory. With proper diet and thiamine, KD patients may become more alert, although memory problems persist (Bayles, 1988). Although there are limited data on language disorders (with the exception of reduced semantic content), memory loss, perceptual disorganization, and the inability to retain new information will have an effect on language fluency and semantics.

Summary

Persons diagnosed with KD will present with the following language and cognitive deficits:

◆ Severe memory loss
◆ Difficulty with retaining/ learning new information
◆ Deficits in semantic content
◆ Disorders of verbal fluency
◆ Attention deficits
◆ Confabulation
◆ Disorientation

HUMAN IMMUNODEFICIENCY VIRUS DEMENTIA

Prevalence

As of June 1996, the estimated prevalence of AIDS was 223,000 U.S. residents aged greater than or equal to 13 years, representing increases of 10% and 65% since mid-1995 and January 1993, respectively. Presently, it is estimated that 1 in every 200 Americans is infected with human immunodeficiency virus type 1 (HIV-1) (UNAIDS, 2000). More than half of all patients infected by HIV develop central or peripheral neurological complications and HIV dementia (HIV-D) occurs in 20% to 30% of patients diagnosed with AIDS (McArthur et al., 2003).

Pathophysiology

Most neurological illnesses occur during the later stages of HIV disease, developing concurrently with the immunodeficiency. HIV affects the nervous system in two ways: *directly*, producing distinct neurological syndromes, and *indirectly*, by causing immunodeficiency with resultant susceptibility to opportunistic infections and neoplasms (McArthur et al., 2003). The typical presentation of HIV-D includes cognitive, behavioral, and motor dysfunction. Because of these characteristics, HIV-D is characterized as a subcortical dementia.

The number of older Americans who have contracted HIV is substantial and increasing. Older age is also an important risk factor, as recent data from the Hawaii Aging with HIV cohort suggests that older HIV-positive individuals (age 50 and older) are nearly twice as likely to meet criteria for HIV-D as are younger HIV-positive individuals (Valcour, Paul, Neuhaus, & Shikuma, 2011), perhaps because of changes in the integrity of the immune system related to aging.

The criteria for HIV-D include seropositivity (a positive serum reaction especially in a test for the presence of an antibody), history of progressive cognitive and behavioral decline, and CNS opportunistic processes. The neuropathology is characterized by abnormalities of cerebral myelin, which is termed progressive leukoencephalopathy or diffuse myelin pallor. Diffuse myelin pallor is defined as reduced staining of subcortical and deep white matter by myelin-specific stains. There is a striking difference between the severity of the dementia and the inflammatory pathological changes, however (Power & Johnson, 1995).

The pathological entity that has received the most attention in relation to HIV-D is HIV encephalitis, which is defined by the presence of HIV-infected multinucleated giant cells, macrophages, and microglia, and is generally acknowledged to be the pathological result of productive HIV infection in the brain. However, AIDS patients with and without dementia may manifest HIV encephalitis (Antinori et al., 2007). Most patients with multinucleated giant cells and diffuse myelin pallor have HIV-D, although most HIV-D patients have neither multinucleated giant cells nor diffuse myelin pallor (Power & Johnson, 1995).

The introduction of highly active antiretroviral therapy (HAART) regimes in the mid-1990s has resulted in a 50% decline in the AIDS death rate, decreased maternal to infant transmission rates, reductions in incidence rates of opportunistic infections, and a 40% to 50% decrease in the incidence of HIV-associated dementia (Sacktor et al., 2002). Figure 4–10 shows PET scans of a normal control, a person with AIDS who was not taking azidothymidine (AZT), and a person with AIDS after 13 weeks of taking AZT, part of the HAART regimen. After AZT, glucose metabolism was nearly the same as that of the normal control.

Nonetheless, AIDS-associated neurological diseases, including HIV-D and sensory neuropathies, continue to be major causes of morbidity and mortality (McArthur et al., 2003). Although HAART has reduced the incidence of HIV-D, HIV-associated cognitive impairment continues to be a major clinical problem among

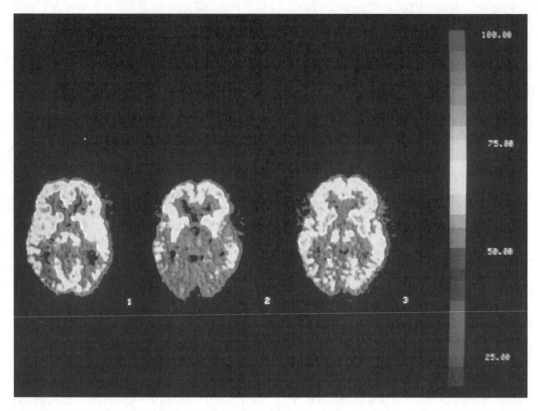

Figure 4–10. PET Scans of AIDS patient with dementia. Thirteen weeks after Patient 3 has taken AZT, the abnormal pattern of glucose metabolism has partially resolved. (National Institutes of Health, part of the U.S. Department of Health and Human Services / Wikimedia Commons / Public Domain)

individuals with advanced infection (Sacktor et al., 2002). This suggests that HAART may not provide complete protection against neurological damage in HIV/AIDS (Bouwman et al., 1998).

Cognitive Disorders Associated with HIV-D

The initial symptoms of HIV-D can be subtle and overlooked or misdiagnosed as depression. In the early stages, memory loss, mental slowing, reading and comprehension difficulties, and apathy are frequent complaints. The typical cognitive

deficits of HIV-D are characterized primarily by: (1) memory loss that is selective for impaired retrieval, (2) impaired ability to manipulate acquired knowledge, (3) personality changes characterized by apathy, inertia, and irritability, and (4) general slowing of all thought processes. However, considerable individual variability in presentation has been reported (Navia, Jordan, & Price, 1986).

Persons with HIV-D who have taken the HAART drug regimen consistently report a positive influence on their cognitive disorders (Brodt et al., 1997). Cohen and colleagues (2001) found that women who took HAART for 18 months had significant improvements in psychomotor and executive functions compared with those who did not take HAART. Others also found that taking HAART for 6 months or more resulted in improvement of cognitive performance on standardized tests (Ferrando et al., 1998; Tozzi et al., 1999). Given these findings, McArthur and associates (2003) suggest that HIV-D in the era of HAART may now have three distinct subtypes: (1) a "subacute progressive" dementia in untreated patients with a clinical syndrome of severe, progressive dementia similar to that seen in the pre-HAART era; (2) a "chronic active" dementia in patients on HAART with poor adherence or with viral resistance who are at risk for neurological progression; and (3) a "chronic inactive" dementia in patients on HAART with good drug adherence and effective virological suppression who have had some recovery from neuronal injury and remain neurologically stable.

Language Disorders Associated with HIVD

For patients in the fifth and sixth decades of life, neuropathological comorbidity from age-associated processes (e.g., vascular or neurodegenerative disease) should be considered when evaluating cognitive impairment in the older HIV-positive individual. HIV-D may be caused by primary CNS lymphomas resulting from the Epstein–Barr virus or from progressive multifocal leukoencephalopathy, although the incidence of these disorders is relative low, at 6% and 2%, respectively.

Brain inflammatory changes are common among HIV-infected individuals, whereas neuronal injury occurs predominantly in those with cognitive impairment. Despite the widespread use of HAART, HIV-associated cognitive impairment and brain injury persist in the setting of chronic and stable disease (Harezlak et al., 2011). Significantly, cognitive impairments and speech deficits related to hemiparesis are common complaints.

Patients with HIV-D should be evaluated early for auditory disorders before language or cognitive testing. Kallail, Downs, and Scherz (2008) and Khoza-Shangase (2011) noted that auditory disorders from opportunistic infections can range from mild to severe and can cause otitis media, mastoiditis in the inner ear, otorrhea, tinnitus, aural fullness, facial nerve palsy, vertigo, and central vestibular and ocular-motor disturbances. Karposi's sarcoma, the most common neoplasm in persons with HIV/AIDS, can manifest on the pinna and can also manifest in the ear canal, eardrum, or middle ear. HIV infection also may damage the cochlea, eighth nerve, or both, sometimes resulting in sensorineural hearing loss; and it also may compromise neural pathways and centers in the brain, resulting in central auditory disturbance. Although HAART has been shown to be beneficial for restoring some aspects of cognition, another consequence is that ototoxicity from some antiretroviral drugs is the most common iatrogenic source of auditory disorders (Kallail et al., 2008).

Summary

Patients presenting with HIV-D are likely to have the following cognitive and communication disturbances:

◆ Apathy
◆ Sensorineural hearing loss
◆ Conductive hearing loss

◆ Outer, middle, and inner ear pathology
◆ Memory loss
◆ Cognitive slowing
◆ Withdrawal from routine activities

HUNTINGTON'S DISEASE

Prevalence

Approximately 30,000 Americans have HD, while 150,000 persons are at risk of inheriting HD from a parent. Symptoms generally appear between 30 and 50 years of age but have appeared as early as 2 and as late as 70 years of age (Ripich, 1991).

Pathophysiology

Huntington's disease, also called Huntington's chorea, is a chronic, inherited, familial disease passed from parent to child through a mutation in the normal gene. Each child of an HD parent has a 50-50 chance of inheriting the HD gene. If a child does not inherit the HD gene, he or she will not develop the disease and cannot pass it to subsequent generations. A person who inherits the HD gene will sooner or later develop the disease. Whether one child inherits the gene has no bearing on whether others will or will not inherit the gene.

Each person is born with 46 chromosomes, which come in pairs; one member of the pair comes from each parent. Therefore, 23 chromosomes are from the mother, and 23 chromosomes are from the father. There are two types of chromosomes: (1) autosomal chromosomes, which are the first 22 pairs, and (2) sex chromosomes, which are the 23rd pair (the 23rd pair in females consists of 2 X-chromosomes, and the 23rd pair in males consists of an X-chromosome and a Y-chromosome). In affected individuals, one gene of this gene pair (the HD gene) is not functioning correctly and expresses itself more strongly, or "dominates," the other working gene. As it is not on one of the sex chromosomes, it can affect both males and females. Males and females have the same chance of having affected children. As HD is autosomal dominant, this means the gene involved is on an autosomal chromosome (not one of the sex chromosomes) and recently has been localized on the fourth autosomal chromosome pair, the #4 chromosome (NINDS, 2013b).

This is a degenerative disease of both mind and body caused by a deficiency of the neurotransmitter gamma aminobutyric acid (GABA) and acetylcholine in the basal ganglia. GABA is an inhibiting neurotransmitter that is present in neurons that leave the global pallidus and synapse in the substantia nigra. Acetylcholine occurs in neurons that originate in the caudate nucleus and synapse in the global pallidus. The basal ganglia, through their interconnections with thalamic nuclei, the cerebral hemispheres, the mesencephalon, and the cerebellum, smooth out body movements (Stipe, White, & Van Arsdale, 1979; Webb & Trzepacz, 1987; Yorkston, Miller, & Strand, 1995). Murdoch (2010) observed that neurological changes associated with HD are most marked in the head of the caudate nucleus and, to a lesser extent, the pallidus and the putamen.

Huntington's disease is characterized by personality changes, depression, mood swings, unsteady gait, involuntary movements, slurred speech, impairment judgment, difficulty in swallowing, rigidity, and an intoxicated appearance. The average duration of the disease is approximately 15 to 25 years.

Disorders of Cognition Associated with HD

Two stages of cognitive impairment are suggested by Dumas, van den Bogaard, Middelkoop, and Roos (2013). In the period before HD symptoms are obvious, patients may present with slower psychomotor speed, inability to recognize emotions in others, and, to some extent, impaired executive functioning. When HD is manifested, patients may present with these impairments and impaired recent and remote memory. In addition, persons with HD have difficulties with concentration and the acquisition of new information at all stages of the disease. Other cognitive disturbances include sudden behavioral changes, a decline in thinking and reasoning skills, including concentration, impaired judgment, and an inability to plan and organize. Smith, Mills, Epping, Westervelt, and Paulsen (2012) found that depression worsened cognitive performance in persons with HD.

Language Disorders Associated with HD

Language impairments associated with HD may result in part from nonthalamic subcortical pathology (Murdoch, 2010). Patients with HD, like those with AD, retain a considerable amount of language knowledge until the advanced stages, including phonologic and syntactic rules (Bayles, 1988). In the later stages, patients with HD present with a significant reduction in verbal fluency, syntactic complex-

ity, melodic line, phrase length, articulatory agility, and grammatical form as the disease progresses (Gordon & Illes, 1987).

Paraphasic errors, deficits in confrontational naming, and word-finding difficulty were also reported by Wallesch and Fehrenbach (1988). Semantic and pragmatic rules require conscious effortful application and are more susceptible to the effects of the disease (Bayles, 1988). Patients with HD exhibit increased visual errors and word-finding problems.

Other areas of deficit are decreased verbal fluency, syntactic comprehension, and understanding of subtle prosodic aspects during the course of the disease (Gordon & Illes, 1987; Illes, 1989; Speedie, Brake, Folstein, Bowers, & Heilman., 1990; Wallesch & Fehrenbach, 1988). Hodges, Salmon, and Butters (1991) compared naming deficits of patients with AD and HD on the Boston Naming Test (Goodglass & Kaplan, 1983). Patients with HD were significantly poorer on visual semantic tasks than were persons with AD. This finding indicated that the anomic errors of HD are primarily the result of perceptual disorders. Perceptual errors may indicate a defect at the visual analysis stage. Persons with HD have been found also to be impaired in syntactical complexity, comprehension of prosody, tonal memory, and verbal fluency (Illes, 1989; Speedie et al., 1990).

While Gordon and Illes (1987) noted that language production of patients with HD resembles various aspects of aphasic syndromes, others have not found evidence to support the aphasic nature of HD language impairments. Rather, patients with HD have been observed to produce semantic paraphasias in confrontational naming as the disease progresses owing to lesions in the left caudate and lenticular nuclei outside of the language areas.

Data from Azambuja and colleagues (2012) more closely corroborate those of Gordon and Illes (1987) in that a relationship was seen between visual organization and language disturbances in the areas of reading and verbal comprehension, which were attributed to damage to the frontostriatal and frontotemporal areas. Results from 23 persons with HD confirmed that several other language skills may be impaired as well: verbal fluency, repetition, oral agility, and narrative writing.

Summary

Persons with a diagnosis of HD are likely to produce the following cognitive and language disturbances, which increase as the disease advances:

◆ Memory loss
◆ Poor executive skills
◆ Semantic paraphasias
◆ Difficulty with concentration and attention
◆ Poor comprehension of prosody
◆ Naming disorders
◆ Verbal fluency deficits
◆ Reduced phrase length
◆ Reduced articulatory agility
◆ Impaired reading comprehension
◆ Impaired written narratives
◆ Depression

MULTIPLE SCLEROSIS

Prevalence

Currently, there are approximately 300,000 patients suffering from multiple sclerosis (MS) in North America. The age of onset peaks between 20 and 30 years. Almost 70% of patients manifest symptoms between ages 21 and 40. Disease rarely occurs prior to 10 or after 60 years of age. However, patients as young as 3 and as old as 67 have been described. MS is at least two to three times more common in women than in men, suggesting that hormones may also play a significant role in determining susceptibility to MS. The female to male ratio may be as high as three or four to one (National Multiple Sclerosis Society, n.d.).

The average person in the United States has about one chance in 750 of developing MS. For first-degree relatives of a person with MS, such as children, siblings, or non-identical twins, the risk rises to approximately 1 in 40, with the risk being potentially higher in families that have several family members with the disease (National Multiple Sclerosis Society, n.d.).

Pathophysiology

Multiple sclerosis is a highly variable disease that involves an immune system attack against the central nervous system (brain, spinal cord, and optic nerves). The disease is thought to be triggered in a genetically susceptible individual by a combination of one or more environmental factors. Multiple sclerosis is thought to be an autoimmune disease. However, as the specific target of the immune attack in MS has not yet been identified, MS is referred to as an immune-mediated disease (National Multiple Sclerosis Society, n.d.).

As part of the immune attack on the central nervous system, myelin (the fatty substance that surrounds and protects the nerve fibers in the central nervous system) is damaged, as well as the nerve fibers themselves. The damaged myelin forms scar tissue (sclerosis), which gives the disease its name. When any part of the myelin sheath or nerve fiber is damaged or destroyed, action potentials traveling to and from the brain and spinal cord are distorted or interrupted, producing the variety of symptoms that can occur (National Multiple Sclerosis Society, n.d.). Figure 4–11 shows the white matter lesions in MS.

Persons with MS often complain of weakness, lack of coordination, and impaired vision and speech. The disease is usually marked by remissions and relapses that occur over many years. Lesions develop around bundles of axons, and the sclerosis (hardening) is multiple because the disease attacks many sites in the nervous system at the same time (Bear, Connors, & Paradiso, 2001).

Cognitive Disorders

Frank dementia is an uncommon feature of MS, occurring in less than 5% of patients. It is usually only encountered in severely affected individuals. However, 34% to 65% of patients have cognitive impairment on the basis of neuropsychological testing, and cognitive impairment may be common even at the onset of MS. The most frequent abnormalities are with abstract conceptualization, recent memory, attention, and speed of information processing. The degree of cognitive decline in patients with MS correlates with the severity of cerebral pathology on MRI, and cortical atrophy on MRI correlates with cognitive impairment and cognitive reserve (Amato et al., 2013; Jongen, Ter Horst, & Brands, 2012). Acute cerebral lesions occasionally manifest as a confusional state associated with

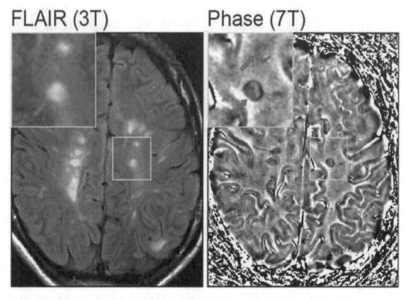

Figure 4–11. White matter lesions in MS. (Reprinted from Mehta et al. (2013). Iron is a sensitive biomarker for inflammation in multiple sclerosis lesions. *PLoS ONE 8*(3): e57573. doi:10.1371/journal .pone.0057573. Open access.)

progressive focal paralysis (Achiron & Barak, 2003; Chiaravalloti & DeLuca, 2008; Staff, Lucchinetti, & Keegan, 2009).

Language Disorders

There appears to be a relationship between severity of cognitive dysfunction and impairment of some language features in MS (Barwood & Murdoch, 2013; Jongen, Ter Horst, & Brands, 2012). Rao, Leo, Bernardin, and Unverzagt (1991) among others (Baylor, Yorkston, Barner, Brittin, & Amtmann, 2010; Mattioli, Stampeteri, Bellami, Capra, Roca & Filippi, 2010; Ruet al., 2013) found that patients with MS were more frequently impaired on measures of recent memory, sustained attention, verbal fluency, conceptual reasoning, and visuospatial perception, and less frequently impaired on measures of language and immediate and remote memory. Similarly, Fink and his associates (2010) reported that encoding and consolidation deficits as shown on the *California Verbal Learning Test* may play a major role in verbal memory impairments in persons with MS. Their findings also provide evidence for an association between degree of myelination of prefrontal fiber pathways and encoding efficiency.

Summary

Although persons with MS have a highly variable disease course, research suggests that cognitive decline can affect some individuals. Cognitive impairments have been noted as early as the first expressions of the disease, appear to worsen as the disease progresses, and reflect the severity of the disease. Patients with MS may present with the following cognitive and language impairments:

- Impaired abstract conceptualization,
- Difficulty with recent memory,
- Impaired attention
- Decreased speed of information processing
- Depression
- Reduced verbal fluency
- Deficits in visuospatial processing

ASSESSMENT

The Importance of Early Assessment

Initially, there may be few obvious language and cognitive deficits in MCI or the preclinical or even the mild stages of dementia. Major concerns for speech-language pathologists are that primary health professionals may not recommend persons suspected of dementia for assessment until the symptoms of dementia are obvious (Taylor, Kingma, Croot, & Nickels, 2009). Families, also, may not see the need for speech-language evaluations until their loved ones show irrefutable signs that they are no longer functioning as normal. However, the earlier the patient is evaluated and begins a program of intervention, the longer the patient can receive help with retaining memory and language.

Early assessments and intervention strategies are extremely important to preserve a patient's quality of life. Although there are no cures as of yet for the varieties of dementia, early intervention predicated on early assessment can prolong memory and facility with language. In addition, other cognitive impairments associated with dementia that worsen language deficits can be addressed before they become insurmountable barriers to communication.

Persons with HIV-D, for example, should be evaluated for auditory and central processing disturbances early in the HIV diagnosis to track hearing disorders. In this way, patients can be assisted with rehabilitative and compensatory strategies that will allow them to remain a part of their communities for as long as possible. As MCI may signal the onset of dementia, it is important for older adults to be screened for dementia as soon as possible in order to establish a baseline of language and cognitive competency against which to measure any changes in function should the symptoms of dementia appear at a later date. Similarly, early diagnoses of PPA can prepare patients and their families for the possible onset of changes in cognitive, motor, and functional status.

Early evaluations of dementia are extremely helpful, also, to family caregivers who are caring for the patient in the home. Dementia is extremely stressful for caregivers who can become susceptible for chronic illnesses and dementia themselves (Mason-Baughman & Lander 2012). Implementation of an early diagnosis and treatment plan by caregivers and speech-language pathologists allows: (1) a fuller understanding of the course of the dementia before the onset of the more definitive symptoms; (2) the benefit of education, counseling, and referrals for special services early in the disease, (3) work with the speech-language pathologist to develop strategies for coping with the behavioral, intellectual, and communication changes

in dementia before their frank expression, and (4) incorporation of ways to enhance the communication environment with the daily living context.

An appropriate strategy for encouraging other health care providers to recognize the value of early assessments and intervention by speech-language pathologists is to educate others within the interdisciplinary team as often as possible. In-service workshops and colloquia within the hospital or clinical setting help to underscore and reinforce the importance of the role of the speech-language pathologist on the dementia team. Reaching out to families caring for older adults to enlist their support for early referrals to speech-language pathology services can be an important goal as well. Within many communities, health fairs, places of worship, senior centers, and senior residences are places where older adults and their families often congregate and where speech-language pathologists can provide information about dementia and its early effects on language and cognition. Public service announcements in major media outlets can be used to encourage families to bring their loved ones for speech-language evaluations as soon as they suspect that something is wrong.

Goals for Assessment

Once a patient arrives for a speech-language evaluation, the first goal will be to interpret the degree of change between the patient's functioning before dementia is observed and the patient's status now that dementia is suspected. The purpose of the assessment is to ascertain the patient's remaining functional skills and how these can be incorporated into a treatment plan. The objectives of the speech-language evaluation for dementia should be to:

1. obtain the most reliable historical information from medical records and from the persons in the patient's support network about the patient and all cultural dynamics in the patient's life;
2. differentiate between the language and cognitive deficits associated with dementia from other types of language disorders associated with aging neuropathologies;
3. differentiate the language and cognitive deficits associated with dementia from other types of behavioral changes from depression or confusion and other types of treatable disorders;
4. determine the type of dementia and how it has affected cognition and language;
5. ascertain where the patient's deterioration is in relation to the progression of the dementia;
6. diagnose the patient's residual abilities as a starting point for therapy;
7. evaluate the patient's communicative needs in the daily living environment;
8. evaluate the patient's living environment for barriers to communication, for example, communication partners, lighting, privacy, to name a few;
9. determine the level of support and reinforcement that can be expected from family members and others in the support network;
10. synthesize the patient's age, gender, disease onset, severity, and presence of other confounding deficits in order to arrive at a tentative prognosis;
11. ascertain whether there are any barriers to the patient's compliance with the recommended treatment approaches;
12. evaluate the family's need for support, counseling, and education as well as their commitment to assisting their loved one during the treatment process; and,
13. target appropriate and reasonable goals for therapy.

Developing the Case History

Written reports are preferable to anecdotal accounts. The patient or the family may not be able to remember pertinent information or be able to provide information in adequate detail. Whenever feasible, the clinician should access the patient's medical records before the assessment. Because of the Health Insurance Portability and Accountability Act of 1996 (HIPAA), it will be necessary to get the patient's or the family's permission to access these records. The act's privacy rule gives patients an array of rights with respect to that information. At the same time, the privacy rule is balanced so that it permits the disclosure of personal health information needed for patient care and other important purposes (U.S. Department of Health and Human Services, n.d.). Once the medical records are obtained, the clinician can incorporate all relevant information into the case history. This medical record information is appropriate for all stages of dementia and should include:

1. **Medical diagnosis(es)**, including history of cardiovascular disease, previous surgeries, stroke(s), traumatic brain injuries, suspected cognitive, personality, intellectual, behavioral, and communication changes.
2. **ICD-9 and ICI-9-CM codes** (*International Classification of Diseases* and

International Classification of Diseases, Clinical Modification (ICD-9-CM), created by the U.S. National Center for Health Statistics and used in assigning diagnostic and procedure codes associated with inpatient, outpatient, and physician office utilization in the United States. The ICD-9-CM is based on the ICD-9 but provides for additional morbidity detail. It is updated annually on October 1 (National Center for Health Statistics, 2013)

3. **Assessments of activities of daily living (ADLs)**, as determined by physical and occupational therapists

4. **Neuropsychological assessment data** on sensory perception, constructional praxis, body schema functions, abstract reasoning, retention and memory, sensorimotor performance, and language functions (Benton, 1975; Ripich, 1991)

5. **Neuroimaging reports**, including computerized axial tomography (CAT scan), MRI, functional magnetic resonance imaging, PET, and single photon emission computerized tomography. PET amyloid imaging (Foster, Jagust, & Fox, 2013) is one of the newest procedures that allows clinicians to see amyloid plaques before autopsy.

6. **Minimum Data Set rating and related resident assessment protocols** (in Medicare-certified facilities). The Minimum Data Set (MDS) is part of the U.S. federally mandated process for clinical assessment of all residents in Medicare- or Medicaid-certified nursing homes. This process provides a comprehensive assessment of each resident's functional capabilities and helps nursing home staff identify health problems. Fifteen categories include, among others, cog-

nitive patterns, communication and hearing patterns, disease diagnosis, other health condition, medication use, and treatments and procedures.

7. **Physician and nursing long-term or acute care progress notes** for each patient encounter, which can be summarized for a specific period of time

8. **Specialist consultation reports** from, for example, nutritionists, neurologists, neurosurgeons, social workers, psychologists, and geneticists

9. **Medications and side effects**, the data for which can be accessed from the *Physicians' Desk Reference*

10. **General health and nutritional status.**

11. **HIV status and adherence to HAART or combination antiretroviral therapy regimens**, if applicable. Many physicians do not request HIV screening for mature adults; however, if this information is available, it should be included in the patient's case history together with the prescribed drug regimen for HIV and AIDS.

12. **History of alcohol or drug use**, which complicates general health status and poses threats to cognitive functioning

Dementia is a heterogeneous disorder across subtypes and stages of the disease. The case history should be guided by questions that address the nature and stage of the dementia, the way the patient's functioning with dementia is shaped by external influences; educational, cultural, and socioeconomic background; health; personality; interests; intellectual capacity; personal goals and achievements; support network; and the environment in which the patient will function along a continuum of the stages of the dementia (Payne, 2011; Ripich & Horner, 2004).

Other Important Case History Information

Additional information for the case history should include:

Demographic information (age, gender, education, literacy level, socioeconomic or employment status, living arrangements, national origin, native language and primary language spoken in home, preferred language, ethnic group identification)

Density of support networks (family, friends, neighbors, work colleagues, religious, fraternal, social or service organization members)

Cultural background and affinities (family arrangements, preferred approaches to treatment, use of alternative methods of treatment, perceptions of health status, communication style, perception of Western health care, perceptions of cause of illness, special interests).

The Patient Interview

The patient interview should include those persons who are best able to provide additional information about the patient's functional changes and abilities. Care should be taken to include the persons in the initial interview who are most appropriate for the cultural orientation of the patient. For example, non-Hispanic white patients and their families may have a more biological definition of family. Persons who are biologically related may be the most preferred persons to take care of cognitively impaired older rela-

tives and may be in the best position to know about their changing functional status. American Indian older persons may be cared for by a person assigned by the tribe as the best person who understands the history and traditions of the tribe and its members (Goins, Spencer, McGuire, Goldberg, Wen, & Henderson, 2011). African American families may have a more functional than biological definition of family, and those who are not biologically related may provide supportive caring for dementia patients (Dungee-Anderson & Beckett, 1992).

Some persons who do not speak English may prefer to speak in the language that is most comfortable for them. American Indian elders are generally bilingual, but a number of these older adults do not speak English at all (Edwards & Egbert-Edwards, 1990). Many Hispanic older persons rely on their children, grandchildren, or other kin to serve as translators and guides in negotiating the health care system. For these patients, it is preferable to have bilingual staff serve as translators. Using family members as translators can disrupt the traditional role of the elder and jeopardize patient-provider privacy and confidentiality.

Coleman, Fowler, and Williams (1995) found that a large percentage of primary caregivers report that they have tried at least one alternative therapy to improve their patients' memory in the early stages of AD, without success. Twenty percent of caregivers surveyed tried three of more unproven therapies. Among these were vitamins, health foods, herbal medicine, "smart pills," and home remedies. Another 25% tried unproven therapies for behavioral problems. Lauren-Gore and Marshall (2008), Marshall and Lauren-Gore (2008), and Hecht (2008) provide compelling evidence that acupuncture and herbal remedies have their place in dementia intervention. Although these approaches may be preferred given the high costs of health care, use of these alternative strategies may cause other problems related to side effects, increased costs, and possible exploitation. Clinicians should inquire about whether caregivers have used or are using alternative methods and whether there have been any negative results.

Most patients should be in the room if a family member is providing case history information to avoid patient anxiety or feelings of rejection. The patient and the informant, however, should not be permitted to engage in a confrontational dialogue about the information given. If a patient appears to be in denial about the nature of the illness or the cognitive and language disorders, some background information, such as demographic, language, or cultural preferences, can be obtained from the family in advance of an appointment for the initial evaluation. At all times, the clinician must convey an attitude of nonjudgmental understanding (Groher, 1988).

The Need for Observations in Assessment

Observing the patient in a variety of naturalistic settings is critical to completing a comprehensive assessment. Observations of individuals with dementia should include several communicative contexts, including the present living environment of the patient and other environments that the patient considers to be important for an optimum quality of life (church, restaurants, sporting events, care facilities, senior centers, for example). Clinicians

should observe interactions with varied communication partners who are part of the patient's social network. Information from these observations and from interviews with caregivers and standardized tests will aid clinicians in assessing change in cognitive and language functioning over time and help in setting appropriate treatment goals (American Speech-Hearing-Language Association [ASHA], 2005a, 2005b).

Selecting Appropriate Assessment Instruments

Clinicians must screen basic sensory and cognitive functions and conduct a thorough assessment of cognitive and language abilities with dementia (Hopper, 2005). Using the *International Classification of Functioning, Disability and Health* (ICF; World Health Organization, 2001) as a guide, clinicians should endeavor to evaluate the range of disability and functioning as well as the personal and contextual information that shape the individual functioning within the scope of the disability. According to the Ad Hoc Committee on Dementia (ASHA, 2005b):

> The ICF is a model that promotes evaluation of the interaction between a person's health condition (disease/disorder) and the environmental and personal factors (among them sensory functions) that serve as facilitators or barriers to functioning. Adherence to this model requires comprehensive evaluation of each individual's needs in relation to the health condition. When the dementia is caused by a progressive disease, periodic reevaluation and adjustment of care plans becomes essential to meet changing needs.

Recommended Assessment Instruments

Evaluation tools to assess language-cognitive disorders for persons with dementia should meet the following criteria: (1) validity and reliability, (2) appropriate for use with a culturally diverse patient population, (3) appropriate for use with adults with dementia, and (4) ease in administration and interpretation of results.

Several assessments are recommended for evaluating language and cognitive deficits at each of the stages of dementia: MCI or preclinical, mild to moderate dementia, and moderate to severe dementia. These assessments, seen in Table 4–3, are:

1. *Alzheimer's Quick Test (AQT) Assessment of Temporal-Parietal Function* (Wiig, Nielsen, Minthon, & Warkentin, 2002). The AQT screens for AD and other parietal impairments using rapid, automatic naming tasks. Administration time is 3 to 5 minutes.

2. *Arizona Battery for Communication Disorders of Dementia* (ABCD; Bayles & Tomoeda, 1993). The ABCD is a normed test that is intended for adults who are suspected of having AD. The test provides for screening speech discrimination, visual perception, and literacy. The ABCD is available in English, Spanish, and French. Administration time is approximately 45 to 90 minutes. Eighteen subtests evaluate mental status, immediate and delayed recall of stories, auditory comprehension, repetition, word learning, reading, naming, drawing, and figure copying. Many subtests are useful for head trauma patients, and the ABCD has norms for young adults.

3. *Burns Brief Inventory of Communication and Cognition* (Burns Brief Inventory; Burns, 1997). This test was developed to evaluate individuals with communication or cognitive deficits resulting from neurological injury. The Burns Inventory assists in selecting appropriate treatment targets and functional treatment goals. There are three subtests for persons with left hemisphere involvement, right hemisphere involvement and complex neuropathological disorders. The administration time is approximately 30 minutes for each of the three subtests.

4. *Cognitive Linguistic Quick Test* (CLQT; Helm-Estabrooks, 2001).The CLQT is appropriate for adults from 18 to 89 years of age who are suspected of neurological impairment secondary to strokes, head injury, or dementia. The CLQT is available in English and Spanish and takes 15 to 30 minutes to administer.

5. *Dementia Rating Scale-2* (DRS-2; Mattis, 2001). The DRS-2 evaluates the cognitive status of adults with cortical impairments and measures the progression of behavioral, neuropathological, and cognitive decline. The DRS-2 is appropriate for adults aged 55 and over and can be administered in an office or at a bedside.

6. *Ross Information Processing Assessment, Second Edition* (RIPA-2; Ross-Swain, 1996). The RIPA-2 is designed for persons from 15 to 90 years of age and assesses auditory processing and retention, immediate and recent memory, temporal orientation (recent and remote), information recall, environmental orientation, organization, spatial orientation, problem solving, and reasoning skills. Administration time is 45 to 60 minutes.

Table 4–3. Suggested Language-Cognitive Assessments for Persons with Dementia

Stage	Assessment	Description
MCI (preclinical)	*Alzheimer's Quick Test Assessment of Temporal-Parietal Function* (AQT: Wiig, Nielsen, Minthon, & Warkentin, 2002)	Screens for Alzheimer's disease and other temporal-parietal dementias using naming tasks (3–5 minutes)
	Burns Brief Inventory of Communication and Cognition (Burns Inventory: Burns, 1997)	Appropriate for ages 18 to 80. Complex Neuropathology Subtest appropriate for dementia and head injured patients (total test time: 30 minutes)
	Cognitive-Linguistic Quick Test (CLQT: Helm-Estabrooks, 2001)	Screens in five (5) cognitive domains: attention, memory, executive functions, language, and visuospatial skills (15–30 minutes)
Mild to moderate	*Arizona Battery for Communication Disorders in Dementia* (ABCD: Bayles & Tomoeda, 1993)	Available in English, French, and Spanish. Appropriate for all dementia stages. Eighteen subtests assess mental status, immediate and delayed recall of stories, auditory comprehension, repetition, word learning, reading, naming, drawing, and figure copying (45–90 minutes)
	Dementia Rating Scale–2 (DRS-2) (Mattis, 2001)	Measures degree of cognitive, behavioral, and neuropathological decline. Can be administered at bedside or in office (15–30 minutes)
Moderate to severe	*Functional Linguistic Communication Inventory* (FLCI: Bayles & Tomoeda, 1993)	Assessment areas include greeting/naming, answering questions, writing, comprehension of signs/pictures, following commands, conversation, reminiscing, gesture/pantomime, and word reading/comprehension (30 minutes)
	Ross Information Processing Assessment, Second Edition (RIPA-2: Ross-Swain, 1996)	Assesses auditory processing and retention, temporal/environmental, orientation, information recall, and reasoning skills (45–60 minutes)
	Ross Information Processing Assessment–Geriatric (RIPA-G: Ross- Swain & Fogle, 1996)	Measures cognitive-linguistic deficits in geriatric patients who are residents in nursing homes. Includes Geriatric Treatment Manual

7. *Ross Information Processing Assessment–Geriatric* (RIPA-G; Ross-Swain & Fogle, 1996). The RIPA-G is appropriate for adults aged 55 years and older. The RIPA-G assesses cognitive-linguistic deficits in geriatric patients who are residents in skilled nursing facilities, hospitals, and clinics and includes a Geriatric Treatment Manual. Administration time is 45 to 60 minutes.

Several of the assessments described for linguistic and cognitive deficits can be given at in a short amount of time at bedside, as can be seen in Table 4–4. In addition to the AQT, the DRS, and the CLQT, clinicians may also use the *Burns Test of Communication and Cognition* (Burns Brief Inventory; Burns, 1997) and the *Montreal Cognitive Assessment* (Nasreddine et al., 2005).

The Burns Brief Inventory of Communication and Cognition (Burns Brief Inventory; Burns, 1997). The Burns Brief Inventory consists of three inventories that each take approximately 30 minutes to administer: (a) Right Hemisphere, (b) Left Hemisphere, and (c) Complex Neuropathology. The third inventory, Complex Neuropathology, is designed to assess the cognitive skills of individuals with diffuse neurological disorders.

The *Montreal Cognitive Assessment* (MoCA; Nasreddine et al., 2005) can be administered in 10 minutes. This instrument has 11 subtests: Trail Making, Visuoconstructional Skills (Cube), Visuoconstructional Skills (Clock), Naming, Memory, Attention, Sentence Repetition, Verbal Fluency, Abstraction, Delayed Recall, and Orientation. The maximum score is 30. A score of 26 is considered normal.

A number of assessment batteries are available to measure the severity of dementia and to provide insight into general areas of cognitive and functional decline that may not be accessed in language-cognitive testing. Table 4–5 provides a listing of those instruments.

Table 4–4. Suggested Bedside Screening Protocols for Persons with Dementia

Test Name	Age Range	Administration Time in Minutes
Alzheimer's Quick Test Assessment of Temporal-Parietal Function (Wiig, Nielsen, Minthon, & Warkentin, 2002)	15–88	3–5
Burns Brief Inventory of Communication and Cognition (Burns Brief Inventory; Burns, 1997)	18–80	30 per subtest
Cognitive-Linguistic Quick Test (Helm-Estabrooks, 2001)	18–89	15
Dementia Rating Scale–2 (Mattis, 2001)	55 years and older	15–30
Montreal Cognitive Assessment (MoCA; Nasreddine et al., 2005)	18–100	30

Table 4–5. Suggested Cognitive Assessments for Persons with Dementia

Test	Author	Year
Age and Education Corrected Mini-Mental State Examination (MMSadj)	Mungas, Marshall, Weldon Haan, Reed, & Reed	1996
Blessed Orientation-Memory-Concentration Examination	Katzman et al.	1983
Clinical Dementia Rating (CDR)	Hughes et al.	1982
Comprehensive Assessment and Referral Examination (CARE)	Gurland, Golden, & Challop	1982
Functional Independence Measure, Version 4.0 (FIM)	State University of New York at Buffalo	1993
Global Deterioration Scale (GDS)	Reisberg, Feris, DeLeon, & Cook	1982
Level of Rehabilitation Scale-III (LORS III)	Carey & Posavac Parkside Associates Parkside Associates	1982
Minimum Data Set for Nursing Home Resident Assessment and Care Screening (MDS)	Hawes, Morris, Phillips, Mor, Fries, & Nonemaker	1995
Patient Evaluation and Conference System (PECS)	Harvey & Jellinek	1979, 1981
Rehabilitative Institute of Chicago Functional Assessment Scale (RIC-FAS'95)	Chicowski	1995
Repeatable Battery for the Assessment of Neuropsychological Status Update (RBANS™)	Randolph	2012
Rivermead Behavioural Memory Test, 3rd Edition (RBMT-3)	Wilson et al.	2008
Severe Impairment Battery	Saxton, McGonigle, Swihart, & Boller	1990, 1993
Subtests of the Delis-Kaplan Executive Function System (D-KEFS™)	Delis, Kaplan, & Kramer	2011
Wechsler Memory Scale, 4th Edition (WMS-4R)	Drozdick, Holdnack, & Hilsabeck	2009, 2011

Cognitive Assessments

Frattali, Thompson, Holland, Wohl, and Ferketic (1995) provided a detailed summary of the characteristics of selected functional status measures, including rehabilitation and global measures. Clinicians are referred to pages 18 and 19 of the *Functional Assessment of Communication Skills for Adults*. Two of the instruments described by Frattali and her coworkers (1995) specifically measure cognitive status or impairment and language disorders and are appropriate for older patients with cognitive-language disorders. These are the *Rehabilitation Institute of Chicago Functional Assessment Scale V* (RIC-FAS V) by Cichowski (1998), and the *Minimum Data Set for Nursing Home Resident Assessment and Care* (MDS; Hawes et al., 1995).

The RIC-FAS V is an 89-item assessment with a 7-point scale. Communication is one of the domains of this test, which measures comprehension, expression, speech production, pragmatics, and voice. The RIC-FAS V can be accessed and downloaded in its entirety at http://life center.ric.org/index.php?tray=content& tid=top1&cid=1960

The MDS is a standardized, comprehensive assessment of an adult's functional, medical, psychosocial, and cognitive status. It is commonly used in long-term care facilities and outpatient and home-based social service programs for older adults. The MDS can be administered to caregivers to assess care-recipient capacities with ADLs.

An additional instrument, the *Comprehensive Assessment and Referral Evaluation* (CARE), measures psychiatric, medical, medical, nutritional, economic, and social problems for which older persons are most at risk. Two of the CARE scales specifically assess cognitive impairments

and depression (Gurland, Golden, & Challop, 1982).

Three rehabilitation-focused instruments are the *Functional Independence Measure, Version 4.0* (FIM; State University of New York at Buffalo, 1993), the *Patient Evaluation and Conference System* (PECS; Harvey & Jellinek, 1979, 1981), and the *Level of Rehabilitation Scale–III* (LORS III; Carey & Posavac, 1982; Parkside Associates, 1986). The FIM measures self-care, sphincter control, mobility, locomotion, communication, and social cognition on a 7-point scale of independence. The communication parameters measured are auditory and visual comprehension and verbal and nonverbal expression. The PECS uses a 7-level scale of independence to measure a variety of skills in rehabilitation. Language status is determined from evaluations of receptive and expressive language, reading, writing, assistive device skill, knowledge and use, and deficits in thought processing.

The LORS III measures ADLs, mobility, cognitive ability, and the language components of auditory and reading comprehension and oral and written expression on a 5-level scale. Recent research on the LORS-III by Velozo, Magalhaes, Pan, and Leiter (1995) evaluated the construct validity of the LORS III and found that the ADL/mobility scale used at admission was most appropriately targeted to the ability level of the sample.

Other assessments include the *Repeatable Battery for the Assessment of Neuropsychological Status Update* (RBANS; Randolph, 2012), the *Rivermead Behavioral Memory Test–3rd Edition* (RBM-3; Wilson et al., 2008), the *Wechsler Memory Scale, 4th Edition* (WMS-4R; Drozdick, Holdnack, & Hilsabeck, 2009), and the *Delis Kaplan Executive Function System* (D–KEFS™; Delis, Kaplan, & Kramer, 2001).

The RBANS consists of 10 subtests, which give five scores, one for each of the five domains tested: immediate memory, visuospatial/contructional, language, attention, delayed memory. The RBM-3 assesses memory problems in everyday life—for example, remembering appointments, names, and messages as well as story recall and face and picture recognition. It also measures the ability to acquire new skills and implicit memory.

The WMS-4R (2009) has a total of seven subtests. New subtests recently added are Spatial Addition, Symbol Span, Design Memory, and General Cognitive Screener. Three subtests retained from the previous edition with modifications include Logical Memory, Verbal Associates, and Visual Reproductions.

The D–KEFS (2001) measures a variety of verbal and nonverbal executive functions for both children and adults ages 8 to 89 years on eight subtests, of which there are three that can be used to evaluate persons with dementia in the areas of cognitive and language deficits, specifically, Verbal Fluency, Twenty Questions, and the Proverb Test. Others (Trail Making Test, Design Fluency Test, Sorting Test, Word Context Test, and the Tower Test) are appropriate to measure cognitive status in the areas of thinking, problem solving, concept formation, spatial planning, and inhibition of undesired responses.

Mental Status Assessments

Assessments that evaluate intellectual or mental status primarily in mild to moderately involved dementia patients include the *Blessed Orientation-Memory-Concentration Examination*, originally developed by Blessed, Tomlinson, and Roth (1968) as the *Blessed Orientation and Memory Exami-*

nation, available online at http://www.gcrweb.com/alzheimersDSS/assess/subpages/alzpdfs/bomc.pdf (Katzman et al., 1983). A short form of the test with six items (Internet Stroke Center, n.d.) is available at http://www.strokecenter.org/wp-content/uploads/2011/08/somct.pdf

The *Short Test of Mental Status* (Kokmen, Naessen, & Offord, 1987) has eight items with a maximum score of 8. This instrument evaluates orientation, attention, immediate recall, abstraction, construction and copying, information, and delayed recall.

The *Age and Education Adjusted Mini-Mental State Examination* (MMSadj; Mungas, Marshall, Weldon, Haan, & Reed, 1996) was developed because the *Mini-Mental State Examination* was found to be biased for ethnicity and education. The MMSadj is a preferable measure of cognitive impairment for low-education and culturally and ethnically diverse individuals.

Instruments that are useful for diagnosing cognitive and intellectual decline are the *Clinical Dementia Rating* (CDR; Hughes, Berg, Danzinger, Coben, & Martin, 1982) and the *Global Deterioration Scale* (GDS; Reisberg, Feris, deLeon, & Cook, 1982). The CDR evaluates dementia from 0 to 3 across six categories of memory, orientation, judgment, community affairs, home and hobbies, and personal care. The GDS (1982) assesses seven stages of the course of dementia.

The *Severe Impairment Battery* (Saxton, McGonigle, Swihart, & Boller, 1993) focuses on patients who are beyond the moderately impaired stage of dementia and measures a range of cognitive functions in patients who are considered to be untestable. The instrument measures attention, orientation, language, memory, visuospatial perception, and construction. There are also brief assessments of social skills, praxis, and the ability to respond appropriately to one's name.

Functional Communication Assessments

The overall goal of intervention is to maintain the patient's functional communication capability for the environment in which the patient lives for as long as possible. Functional assessment measures the patient's ability to function in the daily living environment in spite of disease, disabilities, or social deprivation (Frattali & Lynch, 1989). Functional communication skills directly and significantly alter daily life (Bourgeois, 1991) and are important for the patient's ability to maintain independence.

Functional communication involving the language code occurs when people intentionally use language processing systems to undertake specific tasks that enable them to make their wants and needs known or to request information. As the intentions become more complex, functional communication is increasingly affected by disturbances of the language code and its processors. Although some patients may be able to function well in many settings, their language impairments can cause substantial and powerful limitations.

As the Patient Protection and Affordable Care Act continues to unfold, clinicians will be required increasingly to document functional changes in adults with language-cognitive disorders. According to Frattali and her colleagues (1995):

Outcomes define several behavioral, perceptual and fiscal dimensions such as clinical results, functional status, consumer satisfaction, quality and cost efficiency. Outcomes also can be measured using different tools, such as instrumental and behavioral diagnostic measures, quality of life scales, handicap inventories, and consumer satisfaction surveys. Of these, functional status measures have recently received unprecedented attention. Functional assessment has broad appeal because it is both quantitative and easy to understand. (pp. 41–42)

Since 1999, some functional communication assessments have been revised and others have been developed for adults to meet the needs for evaluating communication within the daily living context. These most recent instruments have been more inclusive of a wider variety of adults from diverse backgrounds. Table 4–6 provides summary information on the functional assessments that can be used to evaluate persons with dementia. Seven functional communication assessments are recommended for use and are described in Table 4–4.

DEVELOPING A RELEVANT CONCEPTUAL BASE FOR ASSESSING ADULTS WITH DEMENTIA

Informal Testing and Working Assumptions

Because older patients with dementia are most often seen in a therapeutic environment, it is important that clinicians use cultural knowledge and sensitivity. Ulatowska and her colleagues (2001a, 2001b, 2001c) posited that some adults from diverse cultures may not respond

Table 4–6. Suggested Adult Functional Communication Assessments for Persons with Dementia

Test Name	Author	Description
Communication Abilities of Daily Living, 2nd ed.	Holland, Frattali, & Fromm (1999)	Measures communication activities in the areas of reading, writing, using numbers, social interaction, divergent communication, contextual communication, nonverbal communication, sequential relationships, and humor/metaphor/absurdity.
Functional Activities Questionnaire	Pfeffer et al. (1982)	Assesses in 10 functional activities requiring reading, memory, attention, auditory comprehension, and writing. Levels of performance range from dependence to independence.
Functional Assessment of Communication Skills for Adults (ASHA\FACS)	Frattali, Thompson, Holland, Wohl, & Ferketic (1995)	Assesses social communication, communication of basic needs, reading, writing and number concepts, and daily planning.
Functional Assessment of Reasoning and Executive Strategies (FAVRES)	MacDonald (2005)	Assesses higher level cognitive-verbal communication disorders on 4 tasks that simulate the complex activities of daily life.
Functional Communication Profile– Revised	Keilman (2003)	Assesses communication mode of communication (verbal, sign, nonverbal, augmentative) and degree of independence.
Inpatient Functional Communication Interview (IFCI)	O'Halloran, Worrall, Toffolo, Code, & Hickson (2004)	Measures how well patients with communication difficulties in an acute hospital setting can communicate in relevant hospital situations.

well to standardized tests, which require closed responses that are odds with a more open and elaborated communication style. Rather, these researchers formulated informal assessment strategies that included storytelling and the use of familiar proverbs to stimulate conversation. Informal testing like this has a place in an assessment battery to provide more qualitative and descriptive information about residual language skills.

In keeping with the need for cultural knowledge, Valle (1988–1989) recommended that clinicians should be flexible in their expectations and working assumptions of diverse patients with dementia in order to promote greater compliance with intervention. Although designed specifically for African American patients, Valle's working assumptions are appropriate for persons from all ethnic and cultural backgrounds as well. In summary, initial clinical expectations surrounding the usefulness of mental status screenings, patient/family acknowledgement of the early signs of dementia, their timeliness in seeking formal health services at the earliest signs, and a secular rather than an enhanced role of religion in help-seeking and help-taking behaviors may need to be reexamined to take different cultural variations and world views into consideration. For example, many persons from diverse cultural groups turn to their religious beliefs in times of crisis, are less likely to be comfortable with Western health care, may prolong bringing a loved one to the doctor for fear of the stigma of mental illness, and may be uncomfortable with testing that measures mental or intellectual functioning because such testing may be viewed as an invasion of privacy. Culturally competent clinical services, therefore, are important to successful patient management (discussed in more detail in Chapter 2 of this book).

MANAGING LANGUAGE-COGNITIVE DISORDERS IN PERSONS WITH DEMENTIA

Determining Candidacy for Treatment

Dementia is a progressive disorder with no cure, and clinicians are often challenged to determine whether a patient with dementia will benefit from a program of intervention. Intervention should be guided by and appropriate for each dementia stage (Voysey, 2009).

Among the many prognostic indicators to consider are age, motivation, support networks, general health, quantity and quality of residual skills, responsiveness to cues, ability to read, orientation to time/place/person, ability to follow simple directions, and ability to converse (Bayles & Tomoeda, 1993; Hinchley, 2009). These parameters and the ASHA Code of Ethics will help to determine whether a patient has the potential to be engaged in a short- or long-term intervention program.

Some treatment programs can be used to address these concerns. Memory wallets (Bourgeois, 1992; Hopper et al., 2013), for example, can be useful in determining whether patients can recognize and name familiar persons in their environment. Establishing a calendar routine for dementia patients, as seen in Table 4–7, can assist them with orientation and enable clinicians to determine how well a patient can recall important events. Assessment findings are another source of information, as these will help to define the patient's strengths and weaknesses and are the building blocks upon which to design realistic and appropriate programs of therapy.

Direct Intervention Approaches

Direct intervention can be carried out through face-to-face group and individual therapy and structured therapy programs or by using computer and low-tech augmentative devices to facilitate memory and language. Direct intervention may include structured work on memory, social, sensory and other cognitive activities. Several programs report success with groups of

Table 4–7. Establishing a Calendar Routine for Persons with Mild Cognitive Impairment

Routines

- Routines stored in your long-term memory are an internal strategy you can use to help your memory.
- Routines can also be an external memory strategy when you use a calendar or schedule.

How To Establish a Calendar Routine

1. Set a specific time to check your calendar each day.
2. Update your calendar: cross off previous days, add any new notes, appointments, birthdays, etc.
3. Mark your calendar so that you know you checked it by using initials or check marks.
4. Check your calendar with your family member at least one time per day.

Benefits of Using Routines

- Increases organization
- Increases independence
- Increases the benefit of using a calendar
- Decreases frustration
- Helps with conversation

Routine → Habit
Short-term memory → Long-term memory

Home Practice

Establishing a calendar routine

With your family member discuss . . .

- One or two times each day that both will refer to your calendar
  - Write these two times in the blank routine form.
- One time each week you both will review the past week's activities and write all the activities, appointments, dates, meetings, etc. for the upcoming week
  - Write this day on your calendar.

Source: Reprinted with permission from Figures 1 and 2: Establishing a calendar routine for persons with mild cognitive impairment from the article "Therapy Techniques for Mild Cognitive Impairment," by M. S. Bourgeois, *Perspectives on Neurophysiology and Neurogenic Speech and Language Disorders*, 23, 23–34. © 2013. The American Speech-Language-Hearing Association. All Rights Reserved.

persons with dementia and can be easily incorporated into the home or long-term care setting.

It may be advisable to provide cognitive therapy that stimulates all five mental operations of cognition, memory, convergent thinking, divergent thinking, and evaluation in order to improve overall communication. One approach is cognitive-semantic therapy (Chapey,

1977, 1986; Chapey & Lubinski, 1979; Chapey, Rigrodsky, & Morrison, 1977). These operations should be stimulated within the context of normal discourse. In this approach, the clinician uses turn taking, cueing, modeling, and reinforcement as approaches to modify the patient's responses. In the initial stages of cognitive-semantic intervention, language therapy should focus on language-related cognition: knowing, awareness, immediate discovery, recognition, comprehension, and understanding. Chapey's principles for therapy begin with the most elemental form of the language modality, such as words that convey tangible concepts. As the patient progresses, representational concepts can be used. Application of these principles is made congruent to the patient's functional environment, as seen in Chapey's module, Use of Composite Abilities. Using this approach, the patient transfers semantic knowledge to such activities as using street and store signs and maps, using a telephone directory, a dictionary, and a television schedule, using a telephone, and using language to keep meaning going in a conversation.

Other direct intervention approaches for working with individuals and groups can include Reality Orientation (Folsom & Folsom, 1974), which encourages patients to interact about current situations; SIGnature and Reminiscence Therapies (Harris, 2012; Harris & Norman, 2002), in which topics and props can be used to encourage patients to share their long-term memories and bolster self-esteem; and Validation Therapy (Feil, 1992), which is an approach to validate patient reality and memory wallets (Bourgeois, 1992) using photographs and other functional visual information to assist with memory.

Direct intervention with individuals can also include strategies in spaced retrieval (Brush & Camp, 1998), as seen in Table 4–8, errorless learning (Arkin, 1991), Montessori-based intervention (Orsulic-

Table 4–8. Behaviors Targeted Using Spaced Retrieval with Clients at Each Stage of Dementia

Early Stage	Middle Stage	Late Stage
Important names or information	Important names or information with or without visual cues	Caregiver name
Compensatory swallow techniques	Refer to card with answer to repetitive question	One step of a motor task
External memory aid involving prospective memory	Room number and location of room	
Use of daily planner of schedule		

Source: Reprinted with permission from Figure 1: Examples of behaviors targeted using SR with clients at each stage of dementia, from the article "Effective Interventions for Persons With Dementia: Using Spaced Retrieval and Montessori Techniques," by J. A. Brush & C. J. Camp, *Perspectives on Neurophysiology and Neurogenic Speech and Language Disorders*, 9, 27–32. © 1999. The American Speech-Language-Hearing Association. All Rights Reserved.

Jeras, Schneider, & Camp, 2000), attention training (Sohlberg, Johnson, Paule, Raskin, & Mateer, 2001; Sohlberg & Mateer, 1986), vanishing cues, and graphic and written cues (Hoerster, Hickey, & Bourgeois, 2001). Of the direct approaches to therapy, among the most commonly used interventions are: (1) errorless learning, (2) spaced retrieval training, (3) vanishing cues, and (4) verbal instruction/cueing (Haslam, Moss & Hodder, 2012; Hopper et al., 2013).

Attention training: The patient is given stimulus drills to activate specific areas of attention.

Errorless learning: The patient is presented with a piece of information and asked to respond to a stimulus question without delay or penalty for an incorrect answer.

Graphic and written cues: The patient is given written information or photographs to stimulate conversation in individual or group therapy.

Montessori-based intervention: The patient is given a stimulating, structured task and encouraged to describe the task within a social interaction.

Spaced retrieval: The patient is given a piece of information or is shown a behavior that has saliency for daily living and is later asked to respond to a question about the information or behavior.

Vanishing cues: The patient is given letter fragments to put together words over a series of trials.

Computer Software and Low-Tech Augmentative and Alternative Communication

In addition to direct strategies in individual and group therapy, low-tech augmentative and alternative communication device training and use (Bourgeois, Fried-Oken, & Rowland, 2010; Gentry, Wallace, Kvarfordt, & Lynch, 2008; Yasuda, Kuwabara, Kuwahara, Abe, & Tetsutani, 2009) and computer software (Archibald, Orange, & Jamieson, 2009; Brecker, Sobel, & Schwartz, 2005; Katz & Wertz, 1997; Fink et al., 2005 provide direct stimulation through the use of technology. In this information age, computer software designed to provide therapy to persons with dementia has become available for clinicians and for patients and their families who are comfortable with using the computer. Online resources for computer software, cognitive stimulation, and games and crafts for persons with dementia can be accessed at http://www.best-alzheimer's-products.com, where interactive games like Bingo and Smartbrain can be downloaded. Smartbrain is a computer-based game that provides stimulation in cognitive skills like attention and memory. The usefulness of this game with mild to moderately impaired persons with dementia has been corroborated by research findings.

In a study of mildly impaired persons with AD, Tárraga and associates (2006) found that persons receiving therapy using an interactive multimedia Internet program–based system such as Smartbrain, incorporating 19 tasks for attention, calculation, gnosis, language, memory, and orientation, performed significantly better on standardized tests than those who received drugs alone or who received an integrated psychostimulation program of music, arts, crafts, physical activity, and training in instrumental ADLs. Sobel (2001) used the game of Bingo as a cognitive stimulation activity in subjects and reported that compared with subjects who received physical intervention only, those who were given cognitive stimulation using Bingo performed significantly better on tests measuring naming and word recognition. Bingo was considered to be of great value to the daily management of AD patients.

In addition to memory wallets and books, low-tech devices can be used to support memory and language for persons with dementia. Video phone technology and face-to-face computer messaging (Skype) can be useful in therapy (Yasuda et al., 2009). Other devices include talking photo albums and personal digital assistants (PDAs) to support memory (Gentry et al., 2008). Yasuda and colleagues (2009) have reported success in reducing behavioral disturbances in persons with dementia by using personalized reminiscence photo videos (personal photos with narration and background music) and video phone technology. As the proficient computer and technology users get older, it is anticipated that there will be an increase in the use and modification of computers, cell phones, PDAs, and other electronic devices to support memory (Gentry et al., 2008).

Digital voice output, which works well for persons with aphasia, has not been as successful with persons with dementia (Bourgeois, Fried-Oken, & Rowland, 2010). However, voice output as digital speech reminders for daily tasks for persons with dementia may help them remain independent for a longer time.

Table 4–9 shows the direct intervention strategies for both groups and individuals and the appropriate stages for each technique.

Indirect Strategies

Indirect intervention can include environmental modifications, group work on a life skill, like mealtime preparation, and caregiver training. Changing the lighting and acoustics can enhance cognitive awareness and communication during mealtimes (Brush, 2008). The number and variety of environmental stimuli can be

Table 4–9. Direct Intervention Approaches for Groups and Individuals with Dementia

Intervention	Purpose	Dementia Stage
Attention training (Sohlberg et al., 2001)	Provides stimulus drills to acting specific areas of attention.	All stages
Cognitive-semantic therapy (Chapey, 1977, 1986; Chapey & Lubinski, 1979; Chapey, Rigrodsky, & Morrison, 1977)	Stimulates all five mental operations to improve communication. Modifies patient responses through cuing, modeling, and reinforcement. Transfer knowledge to daily situations.	Mild

Table 4–9. *continued*

Intervention	Purpose	Dementia Stage
Errorless learning (Middleton & Schwartz, 2012)	Target information is presented to the patient for study or immediate reproduction without retrieval from long-term memory.	Mild-moderate
Graphic and written cues (Hoerster, Hickey, & Bourgeois, 2001)	Provides written information and/or familiar photographs to facilitate communication within a group or with an individual.	Mild-moderate
Low-tech AAC devices/software (Yasuda et al., 2009; Gentry et al., 2008; Bourgeois et al., 2010)	Provides external aids that use stimuli that reflect patient's daily life; provide practice.	All stages
Memory wallets (Bourgeois, 1992; Sohlberg & Mateer, 1986)	Provides patients in groups or individuals with pictures and sentences to trigger remote and recent memories.	All stages
Montessori-based Intervention (Orsulic-Jeras, Schneider, & Camp, 2000)	Creates structured, stimulating tasks appropriate for the group's or individual's cognitive abilities to facilitate social interaction.	Mild-moderate
Reality orientation (Folsom & Folsom, 1974)	Individual reality orientation to time, place, and person and through orienting patients to reality within a group setting.	All stages
Reminscence therapies (Harris, 2012; Harris & Norman, 2002)	Recall and guided reminiscences using props and a time period to stimulate discussion about remote memories.	Mild-moderate
Spaced retrieval training (Brush & Camp, 1998)	Person with dementia is given a piece of functional information or shown a behavior and asked to recall over time in response to a stimulus question.	Mild-moderate
Validation therapy (Toseland et al., 1997) (Feil, 1992)	Provides validation of what the patient with says regardless of accuracy through words or gestures without judgment.	All stages
Vanishing cues (Glisky, Schacter, & Tulving, 1986)	Systematic reduction of letter fragments to-be-learned words across trials to facilitate vocabulary learning or naming	Mild-moderate

minimized to lessen the amount of visual distractions for the person with dementia. Patients with dementia communicate best in face-to-face encounters in a quiet, orderly environment. Communication is more effective, also, if there is a combination of verbal, visual, and tactile stimuli for the topic of discussion. Environmental changes can also include arranging for communication partners in the home or in the long-term care environment to engage regularly with persons with dementia.

Another example of indirect therapy is the Breakfast Club (Pietro & Boczko, 1998), in which the group interacts around a life skill, specifically meal preparation. The Breakfast Club concept is a structured multimodality group communication intervention.

Indirect strategies also include training caregivers to work with their loved ones in the naturalistic setting. Most caregivers have developed effective strategies for helping the person with dementia at home, such as labeling the contents of frequently used rooms in the home, specifically the kitchen, bath, and bedroom. These workable strategies can be incorporated into an overall plan for facilitating communication. Other recommendations to caregivers can enhance their ability to communicate with a care recipient, including such techniques to enhance communication as: (1) avoiding open-ended question, (2) restating poorly understood information, (3) using eye contact when speaking to the patient, (4) using frequent gestures, (5) using literal and direct statement, (6) providing orientation information at the beginning of each conversation, (7) keeping topics familiar and observable, and (8) modifying statements in the patient's language (Shekim, 1990).

Ripich, Wykle, and Niles (1995), Ripich and Wykle (1996) and Ripich and Ziol (1999) designed a caregiver training program around seven specific communication strategies that can be used to alter communication interactions. The acronym FOCUSED organizes the seven strategies for easy recall: F is for functional and face-to-face; O is for orient to topic; C is for continuity of topic-concrete topics; U is for unstick any communication blocks; S is for structure with yes/no and choice questions; E is for exchange conversation/encourage interaction; D is for direct, short, simple sentences. The program's effectiveness has been demonstrated with family and professional caregivers, e.g., nursing assistants. Caregivers using the program report better communication between them and their care recipients when using this approach.

An additional program, designed by Ripich and Wykle (1996), is *The Alzheimer's Disease Communication Guide*, which is a structured program for caregivers. This guide offers six training modules that cover information about AD and dementia, techniques for interacting with persons with dementia and for maximizing their potential to use language, and realistic expectations. A summary of indirect approaches to therapy with persons with dementia may be found in Table 4–10.

Approaches to Caregiver Counseling

Caregivers are diverse in their cultural expectations and experiences, socioeconomic status, education, coping skills, and understanding of the patient's problems. Rather than anticipate the caregiver's level of understanding, the clinician should conduct an initial interview to determine what is needed (Clark, 1991). The answers can be a guide to planning

Table 4–10. Summary of Indirect Approaches Appropriate for Persons with Dementia

Approach	Description	Dementia Stage
Breakfast Club (Pietro & Boczko, 1998)	Clinician provides opportunity for persons with dementia to plan a meal and interact about meal preparations and dining. Considered a multimodality group intervention.	Mild-moderate
Caregiver education/ counseling (Ripich, Ziol, Fritsch, & Durand, 1999; Payne, 2009)	Clinician provides information about disorder, supports and counsels caregivers, and develops therapy protocols that caregivers can use in the patient's living environment.	All stages
Communication partners (Bourgeois, 1992)	Clinician structures opportunities for persons in the living situation to interact and share burden of conversation.	Mild-moderate
Environmental alterations (Brush, 2008)	Clinician modifies room ambience to maximize opportunities for personal interactions and to minimize environmental distractions.	All stages
Manipulating linguistic variables (Bayles & Kaszniak, 1987)	Clinician minimizes linguistic complexity used with patient; maximizes patient strengths in the areas of higher cognitive language functioning.	Mild-moderate
Using functionally relevant therapy stimuli (Bourgeois, 1992)	Clinician uses stimuli relevant to the patient's daily living environment by enhancing patient's ability to relate an object with daily activities, using scrapbooks, wallets, daily diaries, identification bracelets, and notebooks of directions for daily activities.	Mild-moderate

an appropriate program for counseling. Some suggested questions are:

1. What do you understand or what have you been told about the patient's disease?
2. How has the patient's disease affected you and other members of your family?
3. What changes in the patient's behavior, personality, and language have you observed? For how long?
4. How do you think the patient feels about the disease and the changes?
5. In your view, how does the speech-language pathologist work with patients with dementia?
6. What do you do to help the patient communicate better?
7. What are your most urgent concerns for the patient?
8. What feelings about dementia are held by your family and friends?

9. What alternative methods have you used to help the patient?
10. What are your feelings about caring for the patient at home? In the nursing home?

Answers to these questions will help to guide the clinician-caregiver encounter. An easily understood oral and written description should be provided with information about dementia and the effects on cognition, language, and personality during the course of the disease. This information should be individualized to the patient's dementia type. A description of the abilities that are preserved rather than those that are absent will provide a more positive approach to presenting information. However, caregivers should not be given a sense of optimism about the patient's progress or unrealistic recovery (Clark, 1991; Glista, 2006)).

Caregiver perceptions about the causes of dementia are important considerations. Culturally derived perceptions about dementia as shameful, as karma, or as an act of God can color perspectives about the need for speech-language therapy. Culturally different opinions about dementia should be listened to and respected; however, the emphasis should be on educating caregivers about the medical causes and the best treatment approaches. If the disease is inherited, caregivers should be given simplified information about the genetic basis of the disease.

Caregivers are the best resource for reinforcing what the patient is doing in therapy because they interact with the patient regularly. Several steps are necessary to ensure that caregivers will be able to work with persons with dementia with unnecessary frustration:

1. Specific techniques can be demonstrated during therapy sessions.

2. Therapy sessions can be videotaped for instructional purposes.
3. Caregivers should maintain a diary of their work and impressions of the patient's progress and behaviors.
4. Clinicians can arrange in-home observations periodically.
5. Progress can be monitored by the speech-language pathologist between therapy sessions in face-to-face conversations.

Cultural Considerations in Counseling Diverse Caregivers

There is a well-documented tendency for frail, elderly persons with dementia to remain in some communities well into the course of the disease. One major reason is a cultural expectation that adult children should provide a home for their parents. Another is a cultural preference for receiving care from familiar persons. Ripich (1991) noted that African American caregivers tend to assimilate communication strategies better than whites. These caregivers were more accepting, less judgmental, and able to handle grief with less anger (Goldberg, 1996).

Some of the cultural bias for remaining in the home with adult offspring also depends on whether the older person is native or foreign born. A large percentage of foreign-born Mexican Americans, for example, would prefer to live with their children in the event that they can no longer care for themselves. Foreign-born older Mexican Americans face more serious economic constraints than the native-born. Living with their children may be motivated in part by economic need (Angel, Angel, McClellan, & Markides, 1996).

Because of the increasing diversity of the patient population with dementia, therefore, Valle (1988–1989) has recommended that the educational and counseling materials available for patients with dementia and their families reflect the diversity in society. Brochures and other reading materials should be in English and in other languages and should contain pictures and situations that reflect the diverse community of patients.

Caring for the Caregiver

More than 7 out of 10 people with AD live at home, where family and friends provide almost 75% of their care (National Research Council, 2003). Caring for persons with dementia can be extremely challenging and frustrating. Caregivers can become so stressed that they too develop chronic illnesses and dementia (Rabin, 2012c). Relaxation training for patients and their caregivers is recommended (Murray, 2008) as a positive way to support patients and their families. For additional information on strategies for supporting caregivers, clinicians may refer to an article by Payne (2009) for suggestions for professionals who are working with caregivers.

The Alzheimer's Association has an interactive website for caregivers (http://www.alz.org). Clinicians should refer caregivers to this website and to AD support groups recommended by the Alzheimer's Association. Caregivers should also be referred to their local Social Security and Medicare offices to determine eligibility for and costs of health-related services. Caregivers may also need relief from home health workers. Clinicians can refer caregivers to their state or local administration on aging and to local offices of AARP for recommendations for home health agencies. Local administration offices on aging may also be helpful in identifying and recommending hospice care, long-term and respite care facilities, and caregiver support groups.

Universal Precautions

Clinicians caring for persons with dementia and other neurogenic disorders should use universal precautions during testing and treatment. This is particularly necessary to avoid exposure to hepatitis-B and HIV or AIDS. Frequent hand-washing and protective gloves are recommended.

Elder Abuse

Older persons with dementia, particularly older women, are particularly vulnerable to elder abuse. One 2009 study revealed that close to 50% of people with dementia experience some kind of abuse; a 2010 study found that 47% of participants with dementia had been mistreated by their caregivers (Cooper et al., 2009; Wiglesworth et al., 2010). Abuse of older persons is one of the most underrecognized and underreported social problems in the United States.

Elder abuse and neglect of older persons have become major public health issues. The National Center on Elder Abuse (2013) reports that elder abuse is most likely to occur in domestic and institutional settings and defines elder abuse in these settings as follows:

> *Domestic elder abuse* generally refers to any type of mistreatment committed by someone with whom the elder has a special relationship (e.g., a spouse, sibling, child, friend, caregiver).

> *Institutional abuse* generally refers to any type of mistreatment occurring in residential facilities (such as a nursing home, assisted living facility, group home, board and care facility, foster home, etc.) and is usually perpetrated by

someone with a legal or contractual obligation to provide some element of care or protection.

Elder abuse can affect people of all ethnic backgrounds and social status and can affect both men and women. Caregiver stress is frequently linked to domestic abuse. Abuse of another person may result when internal and external factors combine to impair the caregiver's judgment, including emotional problems, loss of employment, financial problems, lack of family or community support, and the severity of the mental or physical impairment of the person receiving care. Caregivers can be so debilitated by these issues that they react negatively when older family members need help. Older adults in poor health are more likely to be abused than those in good health.

Several types of abuse are commonly accepted as the major categories of elder mistreatment, such as:

◆ **Physical abuse.** Inflicting or threatening to inflict physical pain or injury on a vulnerable elder or depriving the elder of a basic need.
◆ **Emotional abuse.** Inflicting mental pain, anguish, or distress on an elder person through verbal or nonverbal acts.
◆ **Sexual abuse.** Nonconsensual sexual contact of any kind or coercing an elder to witness sexual behaviors.
◆ **Exploitation.** Illegal taking, misuse, or concealment of funds, property, or assets of a vulnerable elder.
◆ **Neglect.** Refusal or failure by those responsible to provide food, shelter, health care,

or protection for a vulnerable elder.
◆ **Abandonment.** The desertion of a vulnerable elder by anyone who has assumed the responsibility for care or custody of that person.

Although there are distinct types of abuse defined, it is not uncommon for an elder to experience more than one type of mistreatment at the same or different times. For example, a person financially exploiting an elder may also be neglecting to provide appropriate care, food, and medication.

Signs of Abuse and Professional Responsibilities

According to the National Center on Elder Abuse (2013), the following signs may indicate physical or emotional abuse, neglect, or exploitation:

◆ Bruises, pressure marks, broken bones, abrasions, and burns may be an indication of physical abuse, neglect, or mistreatment.
◆ Unexplained withdrawal from normal activities, a sudden change in alertness, and unusual depression may be indicators of emotional abuse.
◆ Sudden changes in financial situations may be the result of exploitation.
◆ Bedsores, unattended medical needs, poor hygiene, and unusual weight loss are indicators of possible neglect.
◆ Behavior such as belittling, threats, and other uses of power and control by spouses are indicators of verbal or emotional abuse.

◆ Strained or tense relationships, frequent arguments between the caregiver and elderly person are also signs.

A clinician who suspects elder abuse, neglect, or exploitation of a person in immediate danger should call 911 or the local police for help. Other resources are:

1. **Adult Protective Services** is the common name of the social services program that receives and looks into reported suspicions about abuse or neglect of people living in the community. If you suspect abuse or neglect of someone living in the community, contact the local Adult Protective Services in your area.

2. The **Long-Term Care Ombudsman** is the name of the social services program that receives and looks into reports of suspected abuse or neglect of someone living in long-term care (like a nursing home or assisted living facility).

Summary

Early intervention for dementia allows speech-language pathologists to plan and provide services to patients and their families. Although dementia is not curable, early intervention more often ensures a preferred quality of life for patients and provides mechanisms that enable patients to maintain cognitive and language functioning longer during the course of a dementia.

Dementia is an umbrella term that includes a number of diseases that compromise cognitive and language skills. A variety of tests for cognitive-language abilities are available that enable speech-language pathologists to develop profiles of strengths and deficits throughout the course of dementia, including comprehensive batteries, screening tools, and functional communication assessments that can be given at bedside or within a clinical setting. Informal testing complements standardized testing by providing more qualitative and descriptive information about a patient's functioning. Clinician observations also complement standardized testing and are useful in the planning of an appropriate program of intervention for patients and their caregivers within the naturalistic setting.

Caregiver counseling and education should be implemented to maximize patient compliance and caregiver reinforcement. Support groups and interactive websites are some of the resources that can be recommended to caregivers to help reduce the stress of caring for a person with dementia.

For personal safety, clinicians are urged to use universal precautions when assessing and treating patients. Clinicians are also advised to be observant about persons with dementia. Patients with dementia are particularly vulnerable to abuse, neglect, and exploitation both in the home and in institutional settings. Clinicians should be prepared to recognize and report suspected elder abuse to the appropriate authorities.

STUDY QUESTIONS

1. What defines dementia and what are dementia characteristics?

2. What are some causes of reversible dementia?

3. What are the risk factors for nonreversible dementia?

4. How is MCI defined? What role does MCI play in dementia?

5. What are some of the genetic mutations for Alzheimer's disease?

6. What are the differences in prevalence and clinical expression between AD, VaD, DLB, and FTD?

7. How do these dementias differ in the damage to cortical and subcortical structures and effects on cognition and language?

8. What is ApoE? What happens if it is abnormal?

9. How is VaD related to cardiovascular health?

10. What are the differences in etiology between PD and HD?

11. In what ways can HD and PD dementias affect cognition and language?

12. How does HIV cause auditory disorders?

13. What are the effects of the dementia associated with HIV on language and cognition?

14. How are alcohol abuse and thiamine deficiency tied to dementia?

15. Are all assessments for cognitive-language functioning appropriate at all stages of dementia? Which are most appropriate for patients in the mild to moderate stages?

16. What is the purpose of functional assessments? Name and describe at least three.

17. Why is it important for clinicians to observe patients with dementia in several different settings as they interact with others?

18. Name at least five neuropsychological assessments that may be used by a member on the interdisciplinary dementia team.

19. What are ways in which clinicians can provide direct intervention for cognitive-language disorders?

20. What is the difference between spaced retrieval and errorless naming strategies?

21. There are several methods of cueing patients to recall. What are they?

22. What is attention training?

23. Identify forms of indirect intervention for cognitive-language disorders.

24. In what ways can speech-language pathologists modify the patient's environment to maximize cognition?

25. Why are communication partners important for persons with dementia?

26. What are the benefits from low-tech augmentative and alternative communication devices for persons with a diagnosis of dementia? What is a disadvantage of digital voice for persons with a diagnosis of dementia?

27. What kinds of questions would be good to ask caregivers before planning a program of education and counseling for them?

28. Ripich and her colleagues designed two programs for caregivers. What are they?

29. What are universal precautions? Why are they important for clinicians to observe?

30. What the signs of elder abuse? How can the clinician report suspected elder abuse? To whom?

REFERENCES

Achiron, A., & Barak, Y. (2003). Cognitive impairment in probable multiple sclerosis. *Journal of Neurology, Neurosurgery, and Psychiatry, 74*, 443–446.

Adle-Biassette, H., Duyckaerts, C., Wasowicz, M., He, Y., Fornes, P. Foncin, J. P., . . . Hauw, J-J. (1996). βAP deposition and head trauma. *Neurobiology of Aging, 17*, 415–419.

Albert, M. (2012). Evaluating prevention therapies: Developing an Alzheimer's biomarker. *Alzheimer's Outlook 2012*. Johns Hopkins College of Medicine. Baltimore, MD: Author.

Alzheimer's Association. (2012). Alzheimer's disease facts and figures. *Alzheimer's and Dementia, 8*(2). Retrieved from http://www.alz.org/downloads/facts_figures_2012.pdf

Amato, M. P., Razzolini, L., Goretti, B., Stromillo, M. L., Rossi, F., Giorgio, A., . . . De Stefano, N. (2013). Cognitive reserve and cortical atrophy in multiple sclerosis. *Neurology, 80*, 1728–1733.

American Psychiatric Association. (2000a). *Diagnostic and statistical manual IV–Text Revision* (DSM-IV-TR). Retrieved from Behave-Net®Clinical Capsule™ website: http://www.behavenet.com/capsules/disorders/alzheimersTR.htm

American Psychiatric Association. (2000b). Delirium. In *Diagnostic and statistical manual of mental disorders DSM-IV-TR* (4th ed.). Arlington, VA: Author. Retrieved from http://www.psychiatryonline.com

American Speech-Language-Hearing Association. (2005a). *The roles of speech-language pathologists working with individuals with dementia-based communication disorders* [Technical report]. Retrieved from from http://www.asha.org/policy

American Speech-Language-Hearing Association. (2005b). *The roles of speech-language pathologists working with individuals with dementia-based communication disorders* [Position statement]. Retrieved from http://www.asha.org/policy.

Angel, J. L., Angel, R. L., McClellan, J. L., & Markides, K. S. (1996). Nativity, declining health, and preferences in living arrangements among elderly Mexican Americans: Implications for long-term care. *Gerontologist, 36*, 464–473.

Anstey, K. J., von Sanden, C., Salim, A., & O'Kearney, R. (2007). Smoking as a risk factor for dementia and cognitive decline: A meta-analysis of prospective studies. *American Journal of Epidemiology, 166*, 367–378.

Antinori, A., Arendt, G., Becker, J. T., Brew, B. J., Byrd, D. A., Cherner, M., . . . Wojna, V. E. (2007). Updated research nosology for HIV-associated neurocognitive disorders. *Neurology, 69*, 1789–1799.

Arber, S., & Ginn, J. (1991). *Gender and later life: A sociological analysis of resources and constraints*. London, UK: Sage.

Archibald, L. M. D., Orange, J. B., & Jamieson, D. J. (2009). Implementation of computer-based language therapy in aphasia. *Therapeutic Advances in Neurologic Disorders, 2*, 299–311.

Arkin, S. (1991). Memory training in early Alzheimer's disease: An optimistic look at the field. *American Journal of Alzheimer's Care and Related Disorders and Research, 7*, 17–25.

Ash, S., McMillan, C., Gross, R. G., Morgan, B., Boller, A., Dreyfuss, M., . . . Grossman, M. (2011). The organization of narrative discourse in Lewy body spectrum disorders. *Brain and Language, 119*, 30–41.

Azambuja, M. J., Radanovic, M., Haddad, M. S., Adda, C. C., Barbosa, E. R., & Mansur, L. L. (2012). Language impairment in Huntington's disease. *Arquivos de Neuro-psiquiatria. 6*, 410–415.

Barwood, C. H., & Murdoch, B. E. (2013). Language abilities of patients with primary progressive multiple sclerosis: A preliminary group and case investigation. *International Journal of Speech-Language Pathology, 15*, 234–244. doi:10.3109/17549507.2012.745605

Bayles, K. A. (1984). Language and dementia. In A. L. Holland (Ed.), *Language disorders in adults: Recent advances* (pp. 209–243). San Diego, CA: College-Hill Press.

Bayles, K. A. (1988). Dementia: The clinical perspective. In H. K. Ulatowska (Ed.), *Aging and communication. Seminars in Speech and Language, 9*, 149–166.

Bayles, K. A., & Kaszniak, A. W. (Eds.) (1987). *Communication and cognition in normal aging and dementia*. Boston, MA: College-Hill Press.

Bayles, K. A., & Tomoeda, C. K. (1993). *The Arizona Battery for Communication Disorders of Dementia*. Austin, TX: Pro-Ed.

Baylor, C., Yorkston, K., Barner, A., Britton, D., & Amtmann, D. (2010). Variables associated with communicative participation in people with multiple sclerosis: A regression analysis.

American Journal of Speech-Language Pathology, 19, 143–153.

Bear, M. F., Connors, B. W., & Paradiso , M. A. (2001). *Neuroscience: Exploring the brain* (2nd ed.). Philadelphia, PA: Lippincott Williams & Wilkins.

Bennett, D. A., Schneider, J. A., Buchman, A. S., Mendes, d. L. C., Bienias, J. L., & Wilson, R. S. (2005). The Rush memory and aging project: Study design and baseline characteristics of the study cohort. *Neuroepidemiology, 25*, 163–175.

Benton, A. (1975). Neuropsychological assessment. In T. N. Chase (Ed.), *The nervous system* (pp. 67–74). New York, NY: Raven.

Blessed, G. P., Tomlinson, B. E., & Roth, M. (1968). The association between quantitative measures of dementia and of senile change in the cerebral grey matter of elderly patients. *British Journal of Psychiatry, 114*, 797–811.

Bourgeois, M. S. (1991). Communication treatment for adults with dementia. *Journal of Speech and Hearing Research, 34*, 831–844.

Bourgeois, M. S. (1992). Evaluating memory wallets in conversation with persons with dementia. *Journal of Speech and Hearing Research, 35*, 1344–1357.

Bourgeois, M. S. (2013). Therapy techniques for mild cognitive impairment. *Perspectives on Neurophysiology and Neurogenic Speech and Language Disorders, 23*, 23–34.

Bourgeois, M., Fried-Oken, M., & Rowland, C. (2010, March 16). AAC strategies and tools for persons with dementia. *The ASHA Leader.*

Bouwman, F. H., Skolasky, R., Hes, D., Selnes, O. A., Glass, J. D., Nance-Sproson, T. E., . . . McArthur, J. C. (1998). Variable progression of HIV-associated dementia. *Neurology, 50*, 1814–1820.

Braak, H., & Braak, E. (1991). Neuropathological staging of Alzheimer-related changes. *Acta Neuropathologica (Berlin), 82*, 239–259.

Braak, H., & Braak, E. (1995). Staging of Alzheimer's disease related neurofibrillary changes. *Neurobiology of Aging, 16*, 271–278.

Brodt, H. R., Kamps, B. S., Gute, P., Knupp, B., Staszewski, S., & Helm E. B. (1997). Changing incidence of AIDS-defining illnesses in the era of antiretroviral combination therapy. *AIDS, 11*, 1731–1738.

Brush, J. A., (2008, June 17). *Environmental interventions and dementia: Enhancing meal-* *times in group dining rooms.* Retrieved from http://www.asha.org.Publications/leader/2008/080617/080617d.htm

Brush, J. A., & Camp, C. J. (1998). Using spaced retrieval as an intervention during speech-language therapy. *Clinical Gerontologist, 19*, 51–64.

Brush, J. A., & Camp, C. (1999, October, 9). Effective interventions for persons with dementia: Using spaced retrieval and Montessori techniques. *Perspectives on Neurophysiology and Neurogenic Speech and Language Disorders*, pp. 427–432.

Burns, M. S. (1997). *Burns Brief Inventory of Communication and Cognition.* Austin, TX: Pearson Assessment.

Burton, E. J., McKeith, I. G., Burn, D. J., Williams, E. D., & O'Brien, J. T. (2004). Cerebral atrophy in Parkinson's disease with and without dementia: A comparison with Alzheimer's disease, dementia with Lewy bodies and controls. *Brain, 127*, 791–800.

Carey, R. G., & Posavac, E. J. (1982). Rehabilitation program evaluation using a revised Level of Rehabilitation Scale (LORS-II). *Archives of Physical Medicine and Rehabilitation, 63*, 367–376.

Chandra, B., Kokmen, E., Schoenberg, B. S., & Beard, C. M. (1989). Head trauma with loss of consciousness as a risk factor for Alzheimer's disease. *Neurology, 39*, 1576–1578.

Chapey, R. (1977). A divergent semantic model of intervention in adult aphasia. In R. H. Brookshire (Ed.), *Clinical aphasiology: Conference proceedings* (pp. 257–264). Minneapolis, MN: BRK.

Chapey, R. (1986). Cognitive intervention: Stimulation of cognition, memory, convergent thinking, divergent thinking and evaluative thinking. In R. Chapey (Ed.), *Language intervention strategies in adult aphasia* (2nd ed., pp. 215–230). Baltimore, MD: Williams & Wilkins.

Chapey, R., & Lubinski, R. (1979). Semantic judgment ability in adult aphasia. *Cortex, 15*, 247–256.

Chapey, R., Rigrodsky, S., & Morrison, E. M. (1977). Aphasia: A divergent semantic interpretation. *Journal of Speech and Hearing Disorders, 42*, 287–295.

Chiaravalloti, N. D., & DeLuca, J. (2008). Cognitive impairment in multiple sclerosis. *Lancet Neurology, 7*, 1139–1151.

Cichowski, K. (1998). *Rehabilitation Institute of Chicago Functional Assessment Scale–V*. Chicago, IL: Rehabilitation Institute of Chicago.

Clark, L. W. (1991). Caregiver stress and communication management in Alzheimer's disease. In D. N. Ripich (Ed.), *Handbook of geriatric communication disorders* (pp. 127–141), Austin, TX: Pro-Ed.

Cohen, R. A., Boland, R., Paul, R., Tashima, K. T., Schoenbaum, E. E., Celentano, D. D., . . . Carpenter, C. C. (2001). Neurocognitive performance enhanced by highly active antiretroviral therapy in HIV-infected women. *AIDS, 15*, 341–345.

Coleman, L. M., Fowler, L. L., & Williams, M. E. (1995). Use of unproven therapies by people with Alzheimer's disease. *Journal of the American Geriatric Society, 43*, 747–750.

Cooper, J. A., Sagar, H. J., Jordan, J., Harvey, N. S., & Sullivan, E. V. (1991). Cognitive impairment in early, untreated Parkinson's disease and its relationship to motor disability. *Brain, 114*, 2095–2122.

Cooper, C., Selwood, A., Blanchard, M., Walker, Z., Blizard, R., & Livingston, G. (2009) Abuse of people with dementia by family carers: Representative cross-sectional survey. *British Medical Journal, 338*, b155.

Croisile, B. (1992). Progressive cognitive disorders due to focal cortical atrophy. *European Journal of Medicine, 1*, 177–182.

Cummings, J., & Benson, D. E. (1984). Subcortical dementia: Review of an emerging concept. *Archives of Neurology, 41*, 874–879.

Cummings, J., Darkins, A., Mendez, M., Hill, M. A., & Benson, D. F. (1988). Alzheimer's disease and Parkinson's disease: Comparison of speech and language alterations. *Neurology, 38*, 680–684.

Cummings, J., & Duchen, L. (1981). Klüver-Bucy syndrome in Pick's disease: Clinical and pathologic correlations. *Neurology, 31*, 1415–1422.

Damasio, A. R., Damasio, H., Rizzo, M., Varney, N., & Gersh, F. (1982). Aphasia with nonhemorrhagic lesions in the basal ganglia and internal capsule. *Archives of Neurology, 39*, 15–20.

Davies, P. (1991). Alz-50, A68 and the paired helical filaments of Alzheimer's disease. *Journal of NIH Research, 3*, 55–56.

DeJong, R. N., & Pope, A. (1975). Dementia. In T. N. Chase (Ed.), *The clinical neurosciences* (pp. 449–456). New York, NY: Raven.

Delis, D. C., Kaplan, E., & Kramer, J. H. (2001). *Delis–Kaplan Executive Function System™* (D–KEFS™). San Antonio, TX: Pearson Assessments.

Double, K. L., Halliday, G. M., Kril, J. J., Harasty, J. A., Cullen, K., Brooks, W. S., . . . Broes, G. A. (1996). Topography of brain atrophy during normal aging and Alzheimer's disease. *Neurobiology of Aging, 17*, 513–521.

Drozdick, L. W., Holdnack, J. A., & Hilsabeck, R. C. *Essentials of WMS–IV assessment (essentials of psychological assessment)*. Hoboken, NJ: John Wiley and Sons.

Dumas, E. M., van den Bogaard, S. J., Middelkoop, H. A., & Roos, R. A. (2013). A review of cognition in Huntington's disease. *Frontiers in Bioscience (Scholars Edition), 1*, 1–18.

Dungee-Anderson, D., & Beckett, J. O. (1992). Alzheimer's disease in African American and white families: A clinical analysis. *Smith College Studies in Social Work, 62*, 155–168.

Ebmeier, K. P., Calder, S. A., Crawford, J. R., Stewart, L., Cochrane, R. H. B., & Besson, J. A. (1991). Dementia in idiopathic Parkinson's disease: Prevalence and relationship with symptoms and signs of Parkinsonism. *Psychological Medicine, 21*, 69–76.

Edwards, E. D., & Egbert-Edwards, M. (1990). Family care and the Native American elderly. In M. S. Harper (Ed.), *Minority aging: Essential curricula content for selected health and allied health professions*. Health Resources and Services Administration, Department of Health and Human Services (DHHS Publication No. HRS [P-DV-90-4], pp. 145–164). Washington, DC: U.S. Government Printing Office.

Federico, A., Bianchi, S., & Dotti, M. T. (2005). The spectrum of mutations for CADASIL diagnosis. *Neurological Science, 26*, 117–124.

Feil, N. (1992). Validation therapy. *Geriatric Nursing, 13*, 129–133.

Ferrando, S., van Gorp, W., McElhiney, M., Goggin, K., Sewell, M., & Rabkin, J. (1998). Highly active antiretroviral treatment in HIV infection: Benefits for neuropsychological function. *AIDS, 12*, F65–F70.

Fink, R. B., Brecher, A., Sobel, P., & Schwartz M. F. (2005) Computer-assisted treatment of word retrieval deficits in aphasia. *Aphasiology, 19*, 943–954.

Fink, F., Eling, P., Rischkau, E., Beyer, N., Tomandi, B., Klein, J., & Hildebrandt, H. (2010). The association between California Verbal Learning Test performance and fibre impairment in multiple sclerosis: Evidence from diffusion tensor imaging. *Multiple Sclerosis Journal, 16,* 332–341. doi:10.1177/1352458509356367

Folsom, J. C., & Folsom, G. S. (1974). The real world. *Mental Health, 58,* 29–33. Arlington, VA: National Association for Mental Health.

Foster, N. L., Jagust, W. J., & Fox, N. C. (2013). A peek behind the curtain: amyloid imaging, referrals, and specialist memory evaluations. *Alzheimer's Disease and Associated Disorders, 27,* 1–3.

Frattali, C., & Lynch, C. (1989). Functional assessment: Current issues and future challenges. *ASHA, 31,* 70–74.

Frattali, C. M., Thompson, C. K., Holland, A. L., Wohl, C. B., & Ferketic, M. M. (1995). *Functional Assessment of Communication Skills for Adults (ASHA FACS).* Rockville, MD: American Speech-Language-Hearing Association.

Gatz, M., Reynolds, C., Finkel, D., Pederson, N. L., & Walters, E. (2010). Dementia in Swedish twins: Predicting incident cases. *Behavior and Genetics, 40,* 768–775. doi:10.1007/s10519-010-9407-4

Gentry, T., Wallace, J., Kvarfordt, C., & Lynch, K. (2008). Personal digital assistants as cognitive aids for individuals with severe traumatic brain injury: A community-based trial. *Brain Jury, 22,* 19–24.

Glisky, E. L., Schacter, D. L., & Tulving, E. (1986). Learning and retention of computer-related vocabulary in memory-impaired patients: method of vanishing cues. *Journal of Clinical and Experimental Psychology, 3,* 292–312.

Glista, S. (2006). Educating and supporting individuals with aphasia and their families. *Perspectives on Neurophysiology and Neurogenic Speech and Language Disorders, 16,* 425–431.

Goins, R. T., Spencer, S. M., McGuire, L. C., Goldberg, J, Wen, Y, & Henderson, J. A. (2011). Adult caregiving among American Indians: The role of cultural factors. *The Gerontologist, 51,* 310–320.

Goldberg, B. (1996). A very long goodbye. The ravishes of Alzheimer's disease. *ASHA, 38,* 24–31.

Gomez-Isla, T., Price, J. L., McKeel, D. W., Moms, J. C., Growdon, J. H., & Hyman, B. T. (1996). Profound loss of layer II entorhinal cortex neurons occurs in very mild Alzheimer's disease. *Journal of Neuroscience, 16,* 4491.

Gomez-Isla, T., Growdon, W. B., McNamara, M., Newell, K., Gomez-Tortosa, E., Hedley-Whyte, E. T., & Hyman, B. T. (1999). Clinico-

pathologic correlates in temporal cortex in dementia with Lewy bodies. *Neurology, 53,* 2003–2009.

Goodglass, H., & Kaplan, E. (1983). *The Boston Diagnostic Aphasia Examination.* Philadelphia, PA: Lea & Febiger.

Gordon, W. P., & Illes, J. (1987). Neurolinguistic characteristics of language production in Huntington's disease: A preliminary report. *Brain and Language, 31,* 1–10.

Gorelick, P. B., Scuteri, A., Black, S. E, Decarli, C., Greenberg, S. M., Iadecola, C., . . . Seshadri, S. (2011). *Vascular contributions to cognitive impairment and dementia. Statement for healthcare professionals from the American Heart Association/American Stroke Association.* Retrieved from http://stroke, ahaournals.org

Gotham, A. M., Brown, R. G., & Marsden, (1986). Depression in Parkinson's disease: A quantitative and qualitative analysis. *Journal of Neurology, Neurosurgery, and Psychiatry, 49,* 381–389.

Graff-Radford, N. R., Damasio, A. R., Hyman, B. T., Hart, M. N., Tranel, D., Damasio, H., . . . Rezai, K. (1990). Progressive aphasia in a patient with Pick's disease: A neuropsychological, radiologic and anatomic study. *Neurology, 40,* 620–626.

Groher, M. E. (1988). Modifications in speech-language assessment procedures for the older adult. In B. B. Shadden (Ed.), *Communication behavior and aging: A sourcebook for clinicians* (pp. 248–260). Baltimore, MD: Williams & Wilkins.

Gross, R. G., McMillan, C. T., Chandrasekaran, K., Dreyfuss, M., Ash, S., Avants, B., . . . Grossman, M. (2012). Sentence processing in lewy body spectrum disorder: The role of working memory. *Brain and Cognition, 78,* 85–93.

Gurland, B., Golden, K., & Challop, J. (1982). Unidimensional and multidimensional approaches to the differentiation of depression and dementia in the elderly. In S. Corkin, K. L. Davis, J. H. Growdon, & R. L. Wurtman (Eds.), *Alzheimer's disease: A report of progress* (Aging: Vol. 19, pp. 119–125). New York, NY: Raven.

Halabi, C., Halabi, A., Dean, D., Wang, P-N., Boxer, A. L., Trojanowski, J. Q., . . . Seely, W. W. (2013). Patterns of striatal degeneration in frontotemporal dementia. *Alzheimer's Disease & Associated Disorders, 27,* 74–83.

Hamos, J. E., DeGennaro, L. J., & Drachman, D. A. (1989). Synaptic loss in Alzheimer's disease and other dementias. *Neurology, 39,* 355–361.

Harris, J. L. (2012, October 30). SIGnatures: Speaking up about memories. *The ASHA Leader.*

Harris, J. L., & Norman, M. L. (2002). Reframing reminiscence as a cognitive-linguistic phenomenon. In J. D. Webster and B. Haight (Eds.), *Critical advances in reminiscence: From theory to application* (pp. 95–105). New York, NY: Springer.

Harezlak, J., Buchthal, S. Taylor, M., Schifitto, G., Zhong, J., Daar, E., . . . Navia, B. (2011). Persistence of HIV-associated cognitive impairment, inflammation, and neuronal injury in era of highly active antiretroviral treatment. *AIDS, 25,* 625–633. doi:10.1097/QAD.0b013e3283427da7

Harvey, R. F., & Jelleff, H. M. (1981). Functional performance assessment: Program approach. *Archives of Physical Medicine and Rehabilitation, 63,* 43–52.

Harvey, R. F., & Jellinek, H. M. (1979). *PECS: Patient evaluation and conference system.* Wheaton, IL: Marianjoy Rehabilitation Center.

Harvey, R. F., & Jellinek, H. M. (1981). Functional performance assessment: A program approach. *Archives of Physical Medicine and Rehabilitation, 62,* 456–460.

Haslam, C., Moss, Z., & Hodder, K. (2010). Are two methods better than one? Evaluating the effectiveness of combining errorless learning with vanishing cues. *Journal of Clinical and Experimental Neuropsychology, 9,* 973–985.

Hawes, C., Morris, J. N., Phillips, C. D., Mor, V., Fries, B. E., & Nonemaker, S. (1995). Reliability estimates for the Minimum Data Set for Nursing Home Resident Assessment and Care Screening (MDS). *Gerontologist, 35,* 172–178.

Hecht, S. W. (2008). Herbal contributions to the management of the multi-factorial cognitive disorders—Alzheimer's disease and vascular dementia. *Perspectives on Neurophysiology and Neurogenic Speech and Language Disorders, 18,* 114–123.

Helm-Estabrooks, N. (2001). *Cognitive Linguistic Quick Test.* San Antonio, TX: Pearson.

Henry, M. (2010). Treatment for progressive impairment of language. *Perspectives on Neurophysiology and Neurogenic Speech and Language Disorders, 20,* 13–20. doi:10.1044/nnsld20.1.13

Heyman, A., Wilkinson, W. E., Stafford, J. A., Helms, M. J., Sigmon, A. H., & Weinberg, T. (1984). Alzheimer's disease: A study of epidemiologic aspect. *Annals of Neurology, 15,* 335–341.

Hinckley, J. (2009). Clinical decision-making for stroke and aphasia in the older adult. *Perspectives on Gerontology, 14,* 4–11. doi:10.1044/gero14.1.4

Hodges, J. R. (2003). A study of stereotypic behaviours in Alzheimer's disease and frontal and temporal variant frontotemporal dementia. *Journal of Neurology, Neurosurgery and Psychiatry, 74,* 1398–1402.

Hodges, J. R., Salmon, D. P., & Butters, N. (1991). The nature of the naming deficit in Alzheimer's and Huntington's disease. *Brain, 114,* 1547–1558.

Hoerster, L., Hickey, E. M., & Bourgeois, M. S. (2001). Effects of memory aids on conversations between nursing home residents with dementia and nursing assistants. *Neuropsychological Rehabilitation, 11,* 399–427.

Holland, A. L., Frattali, C., & Fromm, D. (1999). *Communication Abilities in Daily Living* (2nd ed.). Austin, TX: Pro-Ed.

Holland, A. L., McBurney, D. H., Moossy, J., & Reinmuth, O. M. (1985). The dissolution of language in Pick's disease with neurofibrillary tangles: A case study. *Brain and Language, 243,* 36–58.

Hopper, T. (2005, November 8). *Assessment and treatment of cognitive-communication disorders in individuals with dementia.* Retrieved from http://asha.org/Publications/leader/2005/0511108/051108d.htm

Hopper, T., Bourgeois, M., Pimenthal, J., Qualls, C. D., Hickey, E., Frymark, T., & Schooling, T. (2013). An evidence-based systematic review on cognitive intervention for individuals with dementia. *American Journal of Speech-Language Pathology, 22,* 126–145.

Hsaio, K., Chapman, P., Nilsen, S., Eckman, C., Harigaya, Y., Younkin, S., . . . Cole, G. (1996). Correlative memory deficits, Aβ elevation, and amyloid plaques in transgenic mice. *Science, 274,* 99–102.

Hughes, C. P., Berg, L., Danzinger, W. L., Coben, L. A., & Martin, R. L. (1982). A new clinical scale for staging of dementia. *British Journal of Psychiatry, 140,* 566–572.

Illes, J. (1989). Neurolinguistic features of spontaneous language production dissociate three forms of neurodegenerative disease: Alzheimer's, Huntington's and Parkinson's. *Brain and Language 37,* 628–642.

Indiana University School of Medicine. (1995). *Facts about finding the HD gene: DNA banking and genetic testing for Huntington's disease.* Indianapolis, IN: Author.

Jokel, R., Cupit, J., Rochon, E., & Leonard, C. (2009). Relearning lost vocabulary in nonfluent progressive aphasia with MossTalk Words®. *Aphasiology, 23,* 175–191.

Jongen, P. J., Ter Horst, A. T., & Brands, A. M. (2012). Cognitive impairment in multiple sclerosis. *Minerva Medica, 103,* 73–96.

Kalimo, H., Ruchoux, M. M., Viitanen, M., & Kalaria, R. N. (2002). CADASIL: A common form of hereditary arteriopathy causing brain infarcts and dementia. *Brain Pathology, 12,* 371–384.

Kalimo, H., Viitanen, M., Amberla, K., Juvonen, V., Marttila, R., Pöyhönen, M., . . . Winblad, B. (1999). CADASIL: Hereditary disease of arteries causing brain infarcts and dementia. *Neuropathology and Applied Neurobiology, 25,* 257–265.

Kallail, K. J., Downs, D. W., & Scherz, J. W. (2008). Communication disorders in individuals with HIV/AIDS. *Kansas Journal of Medicine, 1,* 62–69.

Katz R. C., & Wertz, R. T. (1997) The efficacy of computer-provided reading treatment for chronic aphasic adults. *Journal of Speech- Language- Hearing Research, 40,* 493–507.

Katzman, R., Brown, T., Fuld, P., Peck, A., Schechter, R., & Schimmel, H. (1983). Validation of a short orientation-memory-concentration test of cognitive impairment. *American Journal of Psychiatry, 140,* 734–739.

Katzman, R., Galasko, D. R., Saitoh, T., Chen, X., Pay, M. M., Booth, A., & Thomas, R. G. (1996). Apolipoprotein-epsilon 4 and head trauma: Synergistic or additive risks? *Neurology, 46,* 889–891.

Kean, J., & Locke, D. E.C. (2008). Neuropsychological consequences of cancer and cancer treatment. *Perspectives on Neurophysiology and Neurogenic Speech and Language Disorders, 18,* 114–151.

Keilman, L. I. (2003). *Functional Communication Profile Revised.* East Moline, IL: Linguisystems.

Kertesz, A., Hudson, L., Mackenzie, I. R. A., & Munoz, D. G. (1994). The pathology and nosology of primary progressive aphasia. *Neurology, 44,* 2065–2072.

Kesler, A., Artzy, T., Yaretzky, A., & Kott, E. (1995). Slowly progressive aphasia, a left temporal variant of probably Pick's disease: 15 years follow-up. *Israel Journal of Medical Science, 31,* 626–628.

Khoza-Shangase, K. (2011) An analysis of auditory manifestations in a group of adults prior to antiretroviral therapy. *African Journal of Infectious Diseases, 6,* 11–22.

Kitamoto, T., Tateishi, J., Tashima, T., Takeshita, I., Barry, R. A., DeArmond, S. J., & Prusiner, S. B. (1986). Amyloid plaques in Creutzfeldt–Jakob disease stain with prion protein antibodies. *Annals of Neurology, 20,* 204–208.

Knibb, J. A., & Hodges, J. R. (2005). Semantic dementia and primary progressive aphasia: A problem of categorization? *Alzheimer's Disease and Associated Disorders, 19*(Suppl. 1), S7–S14.

Kobayashi, K., Kurachi, M., Gyoubu, T., Fukutani, Y., Inao, G., Nakamura, I., & Yamaguchi, J. (1990). Progressive dsphasic dementia with localized cerebral atrophy: Report of an autopsy. *Clinical Neuropathology, 9,* 254–261.

Kokmen, E. (1984). Dementia-Alzheimer's type. *Mayo Clinic Proceedings, 59,* 35–42.

Kokmen, E., Naessens, J. M., & Offord, K. P. (1987). A short test of mental status: Description and preliminary results. *Mayo Clinical Proceedings, 62,* 281–288.

Kramer, A. F., & Erickson, K. I. (2007). Capitalizing on cortical plasticity: Influence of physical activity on cognition and brain function. *Trends in Cognitive Sciences, 8,* 342–348.

Kramer, A. F., Hahn S., Cohen, N. J., Banich, M.T., McAuley, E., Harrison, C. R., . . . Colcombe, A. (1999). Ageing, fitness and neurocognitive function. *Nature. 400,* 418–419.

LaPoint, S. F., Patel, U., & Rubio, A. (2000). Cerebral autosomal dominant arteriopathy with subcortical infarcts and leukoencephalopathy (CADASIL). *Advances in Anatomic Pathology, 7,* 307–321.

Laures-Gore, J., & Marshall, R. S. (2008). Acupuncture as a treatment technique for aphasia and cognitive impairments. *Perspectives on Neurophysiology and Neurogenic Speech and Language Disorders, 18,* 107–113.

Lewy Body Dementia Association. (2013). *What is LBD?* Retrieved from http://www.lbda.org

Lieberman, P., Friedman, J., & Feldman, L. S. (1990). Syntax comprehension deficits in Parkinson's disease. *The Journal of Nervous and Mental Health, 178,* 360–365.

Liu, W. (2004). Behavioral disorders in the frontal and temporal variants of frontotemporal dementia. *Journal of Neurology, 5,* 742–748.

Lorenzen, B., & Murray, L. L. (2008). Benefits of physical fitness training in healthy aging and neurogenic patient populations. *Perspectives on Neurophysiology and Neurogenic Speech and Language Disorders, 18*, 99–106.

Lye, T. C., & Shores, E. A. (2000). Traumatic brain injury as a risk factor for Alzheimer's disease: A review. *Neuropsychology Review, 2000*, 115–129.

Lyketos, C. G. (2012). Deep brain stimulation for Alzheimer's disease. *Alzheimer's Outlook 2012.* Johns Hopkins College of Medicine. Baltimore, MD: Author.

MacDonald, S. (2005). *Functional Assessment of Verbal Reasoning and Executive Strategies* (FAVRES). CCD Publishing (http://www.iccd publishing.com).

Mahendra, N., & Hopper, T. (2013). Dementia and related cognitive disorders. In I. Papathanasiou, P. Coppens, & C. Potagas (Eds.), *Aphasia and related neurogenic communication disorders* (pp. 397–425). Burlington, MA: Jones & Bartlett Learning.

Marshall, R. S., & Laures-Gore, J. (2008). CE Introduction: What is complementary and alternative medicine? *Perspectives on Neurophysiology and Neurogenic Speech and Language Disorders, 18*, 86–89.

Mason-Baughman, M. B., & Lander, A. (2012). Communication strategy training for caregivers of individuals with dementia. *Perspectives on Gerontology, 17*, 78–83. doi:10.1044/gero17.3.78

Mattioli, F., Stampatori, C., Bellomi, F., Capra, R., Rocca, M., & Filippi, M. (2010). Neuropsychological rehabilitation in adult multiple sclerosis. *Neurological Sciences* (Suppl. 2), S271–S274.

Mattis, S. (2001). *Dementia Rating Scale–2™ (DRS–2™)* Lutz, FL: PAR.

Mayer, J. F., Bishop, L. A., & Murray, L. L. (2012). The feasibility of a structured cognitive training protocol to address progressive cognitive decline in individuals with vascular dementia. *American Journal of Speech-Language Pathology, 21*, 167–179.

Mayeux, R., Stern, Y., Herman, A., Greenbaum, L., & Fahn, S. (1986). Correlates of early disability in Huntington's disease. *Annals of Neurology, 20*, 727–731.

McArthur, J. C., Haughey, N., Gartner, S., Conant, K., Pardo, C., Nath, A., & Sacktor, N. (2003). Human immunodeficiency virus-associated dementia: An evolving disease. *Journal of Neurovirology, 9*, 205–221.

Mehta, V., Pei, W., Yang, G., Li, S., Swamy, E., Boster, A., . . . Pi, D. (2013) Iron is a sensitive biomarker for inflammation in multiple sclerosis lesions. *PLoS ONE 8*(3): e57573. doi:10.1371/journal.pone.0057573

Merrilees, J., Dowling, G. A., Hubbard, E., Mastick, J., Ketelle, R., & Miller, B. L. (January-March, 2013). Characterization of apathy in persons with frontotemporal dementia and the impact on family caregivers. *Alzheimer's Disease & Associated Disorders, 27*, 62–67.

Mesulam, M. M. (2001). Primary progressive aphasia. *Annals of Neurology, 49*, 425–432.

Mesulam, M. M., Mufson, E. J., Wainer, B. H., & Levey, A. I. (1983). Central cholinergic pathways in the rat: An overview based on an alternative nomenclature (Ch1–Ch6). *Neuroscience, 10*, 1185–1201.

Middleton, E. L., & Schwartz, M. F. (2012). Errorless learning in cognitive rehabilitation: A critical review. *Neuropsychological Rehabilitation, 22*, 138–168.

Mortimer, J. A. (1983). Alzheimer's disease and senile dementia: Prevalence and incidence. In B. Reisberg (Ed.), *Alzheimer's disease* (pp. 141–148). New York, NY: Free Press.

Mungas, D., Marshall, S. C., Weldon, M., Haan, M., & Reed, B. R. (1996). Age and education correction of Mini-Mental State Examination for English and Spanish-speaking elderly. *Neurology, 46*, 700–706.

Murdoch, B. (2010). *Acquired speech and language disorders* (pp. 110–150). Chichester, UK: John Wiley and Sons.

Murray, L. L. (2008). The application of relaxation training approaches to patients with neurogenic disorders and their caregivers. *Perspectives on Neurophysiology and Neurogenic Speech and Language Disorders, 18*, 90–98.

Nasreddine, Z. S., Phillips, N. A., Bedirian, V., Charbonneau, S., Whitehead, V., Collin, L., Cummings, J. L., & Chertkow, H. (2005). The Montreal cognitive assessment, MoCA: A brief screening tool for mild cognitive assessment. *Journal of the American Geriatrics Society, 53*, 695-699.

National Center on Elder Abuse. (2013). Administration on Aging. Department of Health and Human Services. Retrieved from http://www.ncea.aoa.gov/resources/index.aspx

National Center on Elder Abuse (Administration on Aging). *Statistics/Data.* Accessible from http://www.ncea.aoa.gov/Library/Data/index.aspx

National Center for Health Statistics. (2013). CDC. *ICD-9-CM guidelines, conversion table, and addenda.* Classification of Diseases, Functioning, and Disability. Retrieved from http://www.cdc.gov/nchs/icd9cm_addenda_guidelines.htm

National Institute of Neurological Disorders and Stroke (NINDS). (2012a). Infarction page. Retrieved from http://www.ninds.nih.gov/disorders/cadasil

National Institute of Neurological Disorders and Stroke (NINDS). (2012b). *Dementia with Lewy bodies information page.* Retrieved from http://www.ninds.nih.gov/disorders/dementiawithlewybodies/dementiawithlewybodies.htm

National Institute of Neurological Disorders and Stroke (NINDS). (2012c). *Frontotemporal dementia information page.* Retrieved from http://www.ninds.nih.gov/disorders/picks/picks.htm

National Institute of Neurological Disorders and Stroke (NINDS). (2013a). *Cruetzfeld-Jakob fact sheet.* Retrieved from http://www.ninds.nih.gov/disorders/cjd/detail_cjd.htm

National Institute of Neurological Disorders and Stroke (NINDS). (2013b). *Huntington's disease.* Retrieved from http://www.nlm.nih,gov/medline plus/huntingtonsdisease/html

National Multiple Sclerosis Society. (n.d.). *What we know about MS.* Retrieved on May 23, 2013 from http://www.nationalmssociety.org/about-multiple-sclerosis/what-we-know-about-ms/what-causes-ms/index.aspx

National Research Council. (2003). *Elder mistreatment: Abuse, neglect and exploitation in an aging America.* Washington, DC: National Academies Press.

Navia, B. A., Jordan, B. D., & Price, R. W. (1986). The AIDS dementia complex: I. Clinical features. *Annuals of Neurology, 19,* 517–524.

Noe, E., Marder, K., Bell, K. L., Jacobs, D. M., Manly, J. J., & Stern, Y. (2004). Comparison of dementia with Lewy bodies to Alzheimer's disease and Parkinson's disease with dementia. *Movement Disorders, 19,* 60–67.

O'Halloran, R. T., Worrall, L. E., Toffolo, D., Code, C., & Hickson, L. M. H. (2004). IFCI: Inpatient functional communication interview. Oxon, UK: Speechmark.

Orsulic-Jeras, S., Schneider, N. M., & Camp, C. J. (2000). Special feature: Montessori-based activities for longterm care residents with dementia. *Topics in Geriatric Rehabilitation, 16,* 78–91.

Overman, C. A., & Geoffrey, V. C. (1987). Alzheimer's disease and other dementias. In H. G. Mueller & V. C. Geoffrey (Eds.), *Communication disorders in aging: Assessment and management* (pp. 271–297). Washington, DC: Gallaudet University Press.

Parkside Associates, Inc. (1986). Level of Rehabilitation Scale III. Park Ridge, IL: Author.

Payne, J. C. (2009, April). Supporting family caregivers: The role of speech-language pathology and audiology. *The ASHA Leader.*

Payne, J. C. (2011, November). Cultural competence in treatment of adults with cognitive and language disorders. *The ASHA Leader.*

Pendlebury, S. T., & Rothwell, P. M. (2009). Prevalence, incidence, and factors associated with pre-stroke and post-stroke dementia: A systematic review and meta analysis. *Lancet Neurology, 8,* 1006–1018.

Pérez-Ruiz, C., & Prado-Alcalá (1989). Retrograde amnesia induced by lidocaine injection into the striatum: Protective effect of the negative reinforcer. *Brain Research Bulletin, 22,* 599–603.

Perry, E. K., & Perry, R. H. (1985). A review of neuropathological and neurochemical correlates of Alzheimer's disease. *Danish Medical Bulletin, 32*(Suppl. 1), 27–34.

Petersen, R. C. (2004). Mild cognitive impairment as a diagnostic entity. *Journal of Internal Medicine, 256,* 183–194.

Pfeffer, R. I., Kuroski, T. T., Harrah, C. H., Chance, J. M., & Filos, S. (1982). Measurement of functional activities in older adults in the community. *Journal of Gerontology, 37,* 323–329.

Pietro, M. J. S., & Boczko, F. (1998). The Breakfast Club: Results of a study examining the effectiveness of a multi-modality group communication treatment. *American Journal of Alzheimer's Disease and Other Dementias, 13,* 146–158.

Pillon, B., Duboic, B., Ploska, A., & Agid, Y. (1991). Severity and specificity of cognitive impairment in Alzheimer's, Huntington's and Parkinson's diseases and progressive supranuclear palsy. *Neurology, 41,* 634–643.

Plassman, B. L., Havlik, R., Steffens, D. C., Helms, M. J., Newman, T. N., Drosdick, D., . . . Breitner, J. C. (2000). Documented head injury in early adulthood and risk of Alzheimer's disease and other dementias. *Neurology, 55,* 1158–1166.

Plassman, B., Langa, K. M., Fisher, G. G., Heeringa, S. G., Weir, D. R., Ofstedal, M. B., . . . Wallace, R. B. (2007). Prevalence of dementia in the United States: The aging, demographics, and memory study. *Neuroepidemiology, 29*(1–2), 125–132. doi:10.1159/000109998

Power, C., & Johnson, R. T. (1995). HIV-1 associated dementia: Clinical features and pathogenesis. *Canadian Journal of Neurological Sciences, 22*, 92–100.

Prado-Alcalá, R. A. (1989). The striatum as temporary memory store. In A. Ardila & F. Ostrosky-Solis (Eds.), *Brain organization of language and cognitive processes* (pp. 219–224). New York, NY: Plenum Press.

Prestia, A., Drago, V., Rasser, P. E., Bonetti, M., Thompson, P. M., & Frisoni, G. (2010). Cortical changes in incipient Alzheimer's disease. *Journal of Alzheimer's Disease, 22*, 1339–1349.

Provenzano, F. A., Muraskin, J., Tosto, G., Narkhede, A., Wasserman, B. T., Griffith, E. Y., . . . Brickman, A. M., for the Alzheimer's Disease Neuroimaging Initiative. (2013). White matter hyperintensities and cerebral amyloidosis: Necessary and sufficient for clinical expression of Alzheimer's disease. *Journal of the American Medical Association, 4*, 455–461. doi:10.1001/jamaneurol.2013.1321

Rabin, P. V. (2012a). Novel drug therapies for Alzheimer's disease. *Alzheimer's Outlook 2012.* Johns Hopkins College of Medicine. Baltimore, MD: Author.

Rabin, P. V. (2012b). The latest thinking about MCI. *Alzheimer's Outlook 2012.* Johns Hopkins College of Medicine. Baltimore, MD: Author.

Rabin, P. V. (2012c). Alzheimer's caregivers at risk for dementia. *Alzheimer's Outlook 2012.* Johns Hopkins College of Medicine. Baltimore, MD: Author.

Rao, S. M., Leo, G.J., Bernardin, L., & Unverzagt, F. (1991). Cognitive dysfunction in multiple sclerosis. *Neurology, 41*, 685–691. doi:10.1212/WNL.41.5.685

Randolph, C. (2012). *Repeatable battery for the assessment of neuropsychological status update.* San Antonio, TX: Pearson Assessments.

Reisburg, B., Feris, S. H., deLeon, M. J., & Cook, T. (1982). The global deterioration scale for assessment of primary degenerative dementia. *American Journal of Psychiatry, 139*, 1136–1139.

Ripich, D. N. (1991). Language and communication in dementia. In D. N. Ripich (Ed.), *Handbook of geriatric communication disorders* (pp. 255–283). Austin, TX: Pro-Ed.

Ripich, D. N., & Horner, J. (2004, April 27). The neurogenerative dementias: Diagnosis and interventions. *The ASHA Leader.*

Ripich, D. N., & Terrell, B. Y. (1988). Patterns of discourse cohesion and coherence in Alzheimer's disease. *Journal of Speech and Hearing Disorders, 53*, 8–15.

Ripich, D. N., & Wykle, M. L. (1996). *Alzheimer's disease communication guide.* Tucson, AZ: Communication Skills Builders.

Ripich, D. N., Wykle, M., & Niles, S. (1995). Alzheimer's disease caregivers: The FOCUSED program: A communication skills training program helps nursing assistants to give better care to patients with Alzheimer's disease. *Geriatric Nursing, 16*, 15–19.

Ripich, D. N., Ziol, E., Fritsch, T., & Durand, E. J. (1999). Training Alzheimer's disease caregivers for successful communication. *Clinical Gerontologist, 21*, 37–56.

Roberts, G. W., Allsop, D., & Bruton, C. (1990). The occult aftermath of boxing. *Journal of Neurology, Neurosurgery & Psychiatry, 53*, 373–378.

Rogers, M. A., & Alarcon, N. B. (1998a). Dissolution of spoken language in primary progressive aphasia. *Aphasiology,12*, 635–650.

Rogers, R. L., Meyer, J. S., Mortel, K. F., Mahurin, R. K., & Judd, B. W. (1986). Decreased cerebral blood flow precedes multi-infarct dementia, but follows senile dementia of Alzheimer's type. *Neurology, 36*, 1–6.

Ross-Swain, D. (1996). *Ross information processing test, Second edition* (RIPA-2). Austin, TX: Pro-Ed.

Ross-Swain, D. G., & Fogle, P. (1996). *Ross information processing test , geriatric* (RIPA-G). Austin, TX: Pro-Ed.

Roundtree, S. D., Waring, S. C., Chan, W. C., Lupo, P. J., Darby, E. J., & Doody, R. S. (2007). Importance of subtle amnestic and non-amnestic deficits in mild cognitive impairment: Prognosis and conversion to dementia. *Dementia and Geriatric Cognitive Disorders, 24*, 476–492.

Ruchoux, M. M., & Maurage, C. A. (1997). CADASIL: Cerebral autosomal dominant arteriopathy with subcortical infarcts and leukoencephalopathy. *Journal of Neuropathology and Experimental Neurology, 56*, 947–964.

Rudelli, R., Strom, J. O., & Ambler, M. W. (1982). Posttraumatic premature Alzheimer's disease. *Archives of Neurology, 39*, 570–575.

Ruet, A., Deloire, M., Charré-Morin, J., Hamel, D., & Brochet, B. (2013). Cognitive impairment differs between primary progressive and relapsing-remitting MS. *Neurology. 80*, 1501–1508.

Rusanen, M., Kivipelto, M., Quesenberry, C. P., Zhou, J., & Whitmer, R. A. (2010). Heavy smoking in midlife and long-term risk of Alzheimer's disease and vascular dementia. *Archives of Internal Medicine, 171*, 333–339.

Sacktor, N., McDermott, M. P., Marder, K., Giovanni, S., Solnes, O. A., McArthur, J. C., . . . Epstein, L. (2002). HIV-associated cognitive impairment before and after the advent of combination therapy. *Journal of NeuroVirology, 8*, 136–142. doi:10.1080/13550280290049615

Santacruz, K. S., & Swagerty, D. (2001). Early diagnosis of dementia. *American Family Physician, 63*, 703–714.

Saxton, J., McGonigle, K. L., Swihart, A. A., & Boller, F. (1993). *Severe Impairment Battery*. Bury St. Edmunds, UK: Thames Valley Text Company.

Scheltens, P., Hazenberg, G. J., Lindeboom, J., Valk, J., & Wolters, E. C. (1990). A case of progressive aphasia without dementia: Temporal Pick's disease? *Journal of Neurology, Neurosurgery, and Psychiatry, 53*, 79–80.

Scheltens, P., Ravid, R., & Kamphorst, W. (1994). Pathologic findings in a case of primary progressive aphasia. *Neurology, 44*, 279–282.

Shadden, B. B. (1988). Education, counseling, and support for significant others. In B. B. Shadden (Ed.), *Communication behavior and aging: A sourcebook for clinicians* (pp. 309–328). Baltimore, MD: Williams & Wilkins.

Shadden, B. B. (1990). Degenerative neurological disorders. In E. Cherow (Ed.), *Proceedings of the research symposium in communication sciences and disorders and aging. ASHA Report 19* (pp. 99–113). Rockville, MD: American Speech-Language-Hearing Association.

Shekim, L. O. (1990). Dementia. In L. L. LaPointe (Ed.), *Aphasia and related neurogenic language disorders* (pp. 210–220). New York, NY: Thieme Medical.

Smith, M. M., Mills, J. A., Epping, E. A., Westervelt, H. J., & Paulsen, J. S. (2012). Depressive symptom severity is related to poorer cognitive performance in prodromal Huntington's disease. *Neuropsychology, 26*, 664–669. doi:10. 1037/a0029218

Snowdon, D. A., Kemper, S. J., Mortimer, J., Greiner, L. H., Wekstein, D. R., & Markesbery, W. R. (1996). Linguistic ability in early life and cognitive function and Alzheimer's disease in late life: Findings from the Nun Study. *Journal of the American Medical Association, 275*, 528–532.

Sobel, B. P. (2001). Bingo vs. physical intervention in stimulating short-term cognition in Alzheimer's disease patients. *American Journal of Alzheimer's Disease and Other Dementias, 16*, 115–120.

Sohlberg, M. M., Johnson, L., Paule, L., Raskin, S. A., & Mateer, C. A. (2001). *Attention Process Training–II: A program to address attentional deficits for persons with mild cognitive dysfunction* (2nd ed.). Wake Forest, NC: Lash & Associates.

Sohlberg, M. M., & Mateer, C. A. (1986). *Attention Process Training (APT)*. Puyallup, WA: Association for Neuropsychological Research and Development.

Speedie, L. J., Brake, N., Folstein, S. E., Bowers, D., & Heilman, K. M. (1990). Comprehension of prosody in Huntington's disease. *Journal of Neurology, Neurosurgery, and Psychiatry, 53*, 607–610.

Staff, N. P., Lucchinetti, C. F., & Keegan, B. M., (2009). Multiple sclerosis with predominant, severe cognitive impairment. *Archives of Neurology, 66*, 1139.

State University of New York at Buffalo. (1993). *Guide for use of the Uniform Data Set for Medical Rehabilitation: Functional Independence Measures*. Buffalo, NY: Author.

Stipe, J., White, D., & Van Arsdale, E. (1979). Huntington's disease. *American Journal of Nursing, 79*, 1428–1435.

Tang, M. X., Maestre, G., Tsai, W. Y., Liu, X. H., Feng, L., Chung, W. Y., . . . Mayeux R. (1996). Effect of age, ethnicity, and head injury on the association between ApoE genotypes and Alzheimer's disease. *Annals of the New York Academy of Sciences, 802*, 6–15.

Tárraga, L., Boada, M., Modinos, G., Espinosa, A., Diego, S., Morera, A., . . . Becker, J. T. (2006). A randomised pilot study to assess the efficacy of an interactive, multimedia tool of cognitive stimulation in Alzheimer's disease. *Journal of Neurology, Neurosurgery, and Psychiatry, 77*, 1116–1121.

Taylor, C., Kingma, R. M., Croot, K., & Nickels, L. (2009). Speech pathology services for primary progressive aphasia: Exploring an emerging area of practice. *Aphasiology, 23*(2), 161–174.

Tonkovich, J. L. (1988). Communication disorders in the elderly. In B. B. Shadden (Ed.), *Communication behavior and aging: A sourcebook for clinicians.* Baltimore, MD: Williams & Wilkins.

Toseland, R. W., Diehl, M., Freeman, K., Manzanares, T., Naleppa, M., & McCallion, P. (1997). The impact of validation group therapy on nursing home residents with dementia. *Journal of Applied Gerontology, 16,* 31–50.

Tozzi, V., Balestra, P., Galgani, S., Narciso, P., Ferri, F., Sebastiani, G., & Benedetto, A. (1999). Positive and sustained effects of highly active antiretroviral therapy on HIV-1-associated neurocognitive impairment. *AIDS, 13,* 1889–1897.

Turner, M. A., Moran, N. F., & Kopelman, M. D. (2002). Subcortical dementias. *British Journal of Psychiatry, 180,* 148–15.1 doi:10.1192/bjp.180.2.148

Ulatowska, H. K., & Olness, G. S. (2001a) Dialectal variants of verbs in narratives of African Americans with aphasia: Some methodological considerations. *Journal of Neurolinguistics, 14,* 93–110.

Ulatowska, H. K., Olness, G. S., Wertz, R. T., Thompson, J. L., Keebler, M. W., Hill, C. L., & Auther, L. L. (2001b). Comparison of language impairment, functional communication, and discourse measures in African-American aphasic and normal adults. *Aphasiology, 15,* 1007–1016.

Ulatowska, H. K., Wertz, R., Chapman, S., Hill, C., Thompson, J., Keebler, M., . . . Auther, L. (2001c). Interpretation of fables and proverbs by African-Americans with and without aphasia. *American Journal of Speech-Language Pathology, 10,* 40–50.

UCSF Memory and Aging Center. (2012). *Vascular dementia.* Retrieved from http://memory.ucsf.edu/education/diseases/vascular

UNAIDS. (2000). *AIDS Epidemic: Update, December 2000.* Geneva, Switzerland: Joint United Nations Programme on HIV/AIDS.

U.S. Department of Health and Human Services. (n.d.). *The Privacy Act.* Retrieved from http://www.hhs.gov/foia/privacy/index.html

Valcour, V., Paul, R., Neuhaus, J., & Shikuma, C. (2011). The effects of age and HIV on neuropsychological performance. *Journal of the International Psychological Society, 17,* 190–195. doi:10.1017/S1355617710001438

Valle, R. (1988–1989, Winter). Outreach to ethnic minorities with Alzheimer's disease: The challenge to the community. *Health Matrix, 6,* 13–27.

Velozo, C. A., Magalhaes, L. C., Pan, A-Y., & Leiter, M. (1995). Functional scale discrimination at admission and discharge: Rasch analysis of the level of rehabilitation scale III. *Archives of Physical Medicine and Rehabilitation, 76,* 705–712. Retrieved from http://dx.doi.org/10.1016/S0003-9993(95)80523-0

Vetrivel, K. S., Zhang, Y-W., Xu, H., & Thinakaran, G. (2006). Pathological and physiological functions of presenilins. *Molecular Neurodegeneration, 1,* 4.

Vickrey, B. G., Mittman, B. S., Connor, K. I., Pearson, M. L., Della Penna, R. D., Ganiats, T. G., . . . Lee, M. (2006). The effect of a disease management intervention on quality and outcomes of dementia care: A randomized, controlled trial. *Annals of Internal Medicine, 145,* 713–726.

Voyzey, (2009). Intervention strategies for the staged individual with dementia. *Perspectives on Gerontology, 14,* 19–27.

Wallesch, C. W., & Fehrenbach, R. A. (1988). On the neurolinguistic nature of language abnormalities in Huntington's disease. *Journal of Neurology, Neurosurgery, and Psychiatry, 51,* 367–373.

Wallesch, C. W., & Hundsalz, A. (1994). Language function in delirium: A comparison of single word processing in acute confusional states and probable Alzheimer's disease. *Brain and Language, 46,* 592–606.

Waters, C. (1995). Management of the complicated patient. *Parkinson's Report, 16,* 6–8.

Webb, M., & Trzepacz, P. T. (1987). Huntington's disease: Correlations of mental status with chorea. *Biological Psychiatry, 22,* 751–761.

Whitehouse, P. J., Price, D. L., Clark, A. W., Coyle, J. T., & DeLong, M. R. (1981). Alzheimer's disease: Evidence for selective loss of cholinergic neurons in the nucleus basalis. *Annals of Neurology, 10,* 122–126.

Whitmer, R. A., Gustafson, D. R., Barrett-Connor, E., Haan, M. N., Gunderson, E. P., & Yaffe, K. (2008). Central obesity and increased risk of dementia more than three decades later. *Neurology, 71,* 1057–1064.

Whitwell, J. L., Weigand, S. D., Shiung, M. M., Boeve, B. F., Ferman, T. J., Smith, G. E., . . . Jack, C. R. (2007). Focal atrophy in dementia with Lewy bodies on MRI: A distinct pattern from Alzheimer's disease. *Brain, 130,* 708–719.

Wiglesworth, A., Mosqueda, L., Mulnard, R., Liao, S., Gibbs, L., & Fitzgerald, W. (2010). Screening for abuse and neglect of people with dementia. *Journal of the American Geriatrics Society, 58,* 493–500.

Wiig, E. H., Nielsen, N. P., Minthon, L., & Warkentin, S. (2002). *Alzheimer's Quick Test (AQT) Assessment of Temporal-Parietal Function.* New York, NY: Harcourt Assessment.

Williamson, R., Rossor, M., Owen, M., & Hardy, J. (1991). Segregation of a missence mutation in the amyloid precursor protein gene with familial Alzheimer's disease. *Nature, 349,* 704–706.

Wilson, B. A., Greenfield, E., Clare, L., Baddeley, A., Cockburn, J., Watson, P., . . . Nannery, R. (2008). *Rivermead Behavioural Memory Test–3rd edition.* San Antonio, TX: Pearson Assessments.

Witter, M. (2011). Entorhinal cortex. *Scholarpedia, 6,* 4380.

World Health Organization. (2001). *International classification of functioning disability and health.* Geneva, Switzerland: Author.

Yaffe, K., Lindquist, K., Schwartz, A. V., Vitartas, C., Vittinghoff, E., Satterfield, S., Simonsick, E. M., & Harris, T. (2011). Advanced glycation end product level, diabetes, and accelerated cognitive aging. *Neurology, 77,* 1351–1356.

Yasuda, K., Kuwabara, K., Kuwahara, N., Abe, S., & Tetsutani, N. (2009). Effectiveness of personalized reminiscence photo videos for individuals with dementia. *Neuropsychological Rehabilitation, 19,* 603–619.

Yates, C. M., Simpson, J., Maloney, A. F. J., Gordon, A., & Reid, A. H. (1980). Alzheimer's-like cholinergic deficiency in Down's syndrome. *Lancet, 2,* 979.

Yorkston, K. M., Miller, R. M., & Strand, E. A. (1995). *Management of speech and swallowing in degenerative diseases.* Tucson, AZ: Communication Skills Builders.

Zetusky, W. J., Jakovic, J. L., & Pirozzolo, R. J. (1985). The heterogeneity of Parkinson's disease: Clinical and prognostic implications. *Neurology, 35,* 522–526.

CHAPTER 5

Traumatic Brain Injury

Joan C. Payne, Wilhelmina Wright-Harp, and Alaina Davis

Intense media attention has focused on traumatic brain injuries (TBIs) in light of former congresswoman Gifford's remarkable recovery from a penetrating head injury, because of concerns for athletes who sustain closed head injuries during football, boxing, and soccer competitions, and out of concern for the thousands of returning armed services personnel who have sustained multiblast head and multisystem injuries during their tours of duty in the Middle East. Speech-language pathologists are members of the interdisciplinary teams for TBI assessment and treatment and are in the unique position to provide the best practices in assessing and managing cognitive and communication disorders in patients with TBI and in offering hope and encouragement to their families.

TBI DEFINITION

TBI is defined as an alteration in brain function, or other evidence of brain pathology, caused by an external force (Menon, Schwab, Wright, & Maas, 2010). It is a brain injury from externally inflicted trauma that may result in significant impairment of an individual's physical, cognitive, and psychosocial functioning. Specifically, TBI is a nondegenerative, noncongenital insult to the brain that can lead to permanent or temporary impairment of cognitive, physical, and psychosocial functions. TBI may result in diminished or altered brain functioning due to an external mechanical force that may disrupt the individual's normal state of consciousness (Dawodu & Campagnolo, 2010). It is important to note then that TBI does not include brain damage resulting from cerebrovascular accidents, tumors, and progressive neurological disorders. Moreover, not all blows or jolts to the head will result in a TBI.

There are three major types of TBIs to be covered in this chapter. One is nonpenetrating or closed head injury, usually caused by the impact of an external force, usually blunt force, which causes rapid acceleration, deceleration, and rotation of the brain within the cranial vault (skull). The injury does not produce a disruption in the continuity of the skull or dura but may alter an individual's consciousness. The second type is penetrating head injury, which is a visible injury and may be the result of an accident, gunshot wound, or a variety of external factors. The injury is usually located at a focal point in the brain where a penetrating object, such as a shattered piece of skull or a bullet, has entered and disrupted the skull and the underlying meninges. The third type is a missile blast injury during which blasts from detonated explosives apply pressure to the brain and produce a supersonic overpressurization shock wave (Brain Injury Association, 1995; Groher, 1977; LaPointe, Murdoch, & Stierwalt, 2010; Wallace, 2006).

Closed and penetrating head injuries can happen to individuals of any age. Sports injuries and missile blast injuries that cause TBI are generally observed in younger rather than older adults; however, some older adults are also affected. Falls are the major category of TBIs in older adults. For the purposes of this chapter, therefore, discussions about TBI focus on the prevalence and sequela of TBI in younger and older adults. As many mature adults also have chronic conditions that can worsen TBI outcome, a considerable discussion is given to effects of TBI on an aging neurological system.

EPIDEMIOLOGY

TBI is one of the major causes of mortality and disability in the United States with approximately 1.7 million injuries occurring annually affecting individuals of all ages, races/ethnicities, and incomes (Centers for Disease Control and Prevention [hereafter CDC], 2010a; Timmons & Menaker, 2010). Of the 1.7 million, 80.7%

are treated in emergency rooms, 16.3% are hospitalized, and 3.0% result in death (CDC, 2010b). Recent estimates indicate that TBI is a contributing factor to a third (30.5%) of all injury-related deaths in the United States, and those who survive often suffer from permanent disabilities affecting motor, cognitive, language, and swallowing function along a continuum ranging from mild to severe impairment. The financial cost for hospital care continues to rise as nearly 5.3 million people are living with TBI-related disabilities today, resulting in an estimated cost of $76.5 billion, including direct and indirect medical expenses such as lost productivity, each year (Finkelstein, Corso, & Miller, 2006; Langlois, Rutland-Brown, & Wald, 2006; Thompson et al., 2012).

Among the elderly, defined as persons age 65 years and older, trauma is the seventh leading cause of mortality, and TBI is responsible for over 80,000 emergency department visits annually (Langlois et al., 2006; Rutland-Brown, Langlois, & Thomas, 2006). As individuals born during the baby boom generation age, the number of people over the age of 65 will reach 71 million by 2030 and represent 20% of the U.S. population (Timmons & Menaker, 2010). During the period from 2005 to 2050, the elderly population in the United States is projected to more than double. In the same period, the number of those over the age of 85 is expected to grow to greater than 20 million (Timmons & Menaker, 2010). Consequently, with the increased number of elderly, the incidence of age-related TBIs is also expected to rise (DiRusso et al., 2002).

Currently, nearly 5.3 million people are living with TBI-related disabilities. In 2006, over $2.8 billion was spent on treating TBI in individuals older than age 65 years (National Healthcare Quality and

Disparities Reports, 2010). Thus, with the projected increase in head injury among the elderly, it is anticipated that there will be a corresponding increase in expenses required for hospitalization and long-term care among this population.

Persons who are elderly are at great risk for head injuries (Payne & Ommaya, 1997; Timmons, & Menaker, 2010). More common with advancing age are the progressive accumulation of disease processes, age-related deterioration of vision and hearing, and changes in coordination, balance, motor strength, and postural stability, which reduce the ability to react quickly and avoid environmental hazards. Other conditions, such as dementia, age-related cognitive impairments, congestive heart disease, postural hypotension, and arthritis, further exacerbate these limitations, increasing the risk for head injuries (Santora, Schinco, & Trooskin, 1994; DiRusso et al., 2002).

Recent advances in the treatment of chronic conditions such as cardiovascular diseases, diabetes, and arthritis have increased life longevity and improved the health of older persons during their later years. A direct outcome is that older adults are more physically active and mobile than in previous generations. However, the consequences of advanced age and increased longevity and activity expose older adults to more opportunities for head injuries resulting from falls and motor vehicle and pedestrian-related vehicular accidents (Payne & Ommaya, 1997).

In order of prevalence, causes of head injuries among older persons are falls (51%), automobile accidents (20%), pedestrian-struck accidents (19%), and a combination of causes, for example, assaults, abuse, and alcohol consumption/intoxication (10%) (Rutland-Brown et al., 2006; Thompson, McCormick, & Kagan, 2006). Figure 5–1 shows the causes of TBI among older adults.

PATHOPHYSIOLOGY OF TBI

Recovery for any patient who sustains a head injury is determined by several

Major Causes of TBI in the Elderly

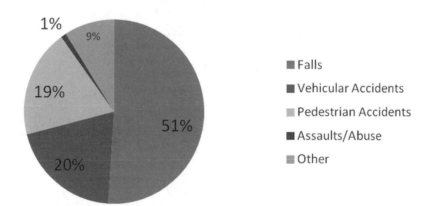

Figure 5–1. Major causes of TBI in the elderly (Rutland-Brown, Langlois, & Thomas, 2006; Thompson, H. J., McCormick, W. C., & Kagan, S. H., 2006).

factors. The patient's age determines the resiliency of the central nervous system, the overall health of the individual, and the extent to which chronic diseases are already present. The pre-injury status of the brain is an important prognostic indicator for recovery. Previous strokes, dementia, chronic alcohol use, drug abuse, or repeated head injuries are cumulative with the existing TBI and complicate the patient's clinical presentation and prognosis for recovery of function. If the head injury is severe, the total amount of immediate damage has implications for the degree of loss of consciousness (duration of coma) and other focal signs (National Institute of Neurological Diseases and Stroke, 2013, hereafter NINDS). Finally, the additive effects of secondary and intracranial insults can worsen an already compromised neural system in an older adult, in a returning veteran who may have been exposed to repeated blast injuries, or in an athlete who has sustained previous head injuries (Payne & Ommaya, 1997, p. 190).

Penetrating Versus Nonpenetrating Injuries

The primary damage associated with TBI is classified into two broad categories: penetrating and nonpenetrating injuries. In a nonpenetrating or closed head injury, the underlying dura mater remains intact even if the skull is fractured. In contrast, a penetrating or open head injury occurs when the skull fracture penetrates the underlying dura mater and/or the brain is penetrated by an object, such as in a gunshot to the head or other missile injury.

Penetrating TBI

The penetrating type of injury occurs when a foreign object pierces the skull,

damages the underlying dura mater, and extends into the cerebral tissue. The most frequent causes of penetrating brain injuries are either high velocity missiles, as a bullet from a gun, or low velocity impacts (e.g., a stab wound or blows to the head). Penetrating insults produce focal injuries with substantial damage to areas surrounding the direct site of trauma (Payne & Ommaya, 1997) and can also damage major blood vessels in the cerebrum, causing a hemorrhage or bleeding within the skull or within brain tissue. The resulting neurological damage is similar to focal hemorrhage or infarction caused by a cerebrovascular accident.

Motor vehicle accidents are a possible cause of penetrating head injuries when the brain is injured from a skull fracture, which results when the bone of the skull cracks or breaks (National Highway Traffic Safety Administration, 2012). Skull fractures can cause infection to the wound itself as well as to the brain. There are two types of fractures: depressed and penetrating. A depressed skull fracture occurs when pieces of the broken skull press into the tissue of the brain. A penetrating skull fracture occurs when something pierces the skull, such as a bullet, leaving a distinct and localized injury to brain tissue (NINDS, 2012).

Nonpenetrating or Closed Head Injury

A closed head injury presents with a diffuse, bilateral pathology unless there is co-occurrence with brain injury resulting from focal damage (Payne & Ommaya, 1997). Although the cranium and underlying tissue may not be damaged in a closed head injury, it is not always less severe than open head injuries. Primary damage resulting in a closed head injury is the result of mechanical forces involving direct impact and inertia (Ivancevic, 2009). Nonpenetrating (closed) head injuries may be of two types: acceleration-deceleration, in which the brain is thrown around in the cranial vault, and nonacceleration, which is caused when extraordinary weight is placed on the skull and underlying brain tissue. Of the two, acceleration-deceleration injuries are more serious (Roseberry-McKibben & Hegde, 2006).

Acceleration/Deceleration Injury. During acceleration and deceleration, the head is set into motion by external physical forces. When the head begins to move, the brain is still stationary but soon begins to move. When the head movement stops, the brain continues moving inside the

skull forcefully, in what Ommaya and Gennarelli (1974) described as both rotational and forward and backward movements, or rotational acceleration (Gutierrez et al., 2001). As the brain moves within the rigid structure of the cranium, delicate brain tissue is damaged. The exact point of impact causes a coup injury, while the area the brain strikes opposite the initial site of impact creates a contrecoup injury (Figures 5–2 and 5–3). In addition, the bony projections on the base of the skull cause the moving brain to be lacerated or torn.

As the brain moves around the rough and somewhat sharp and jagged inner surfaces of the skull (primarily located on the temporal bone), bruising and contusions can occur, including multifocal

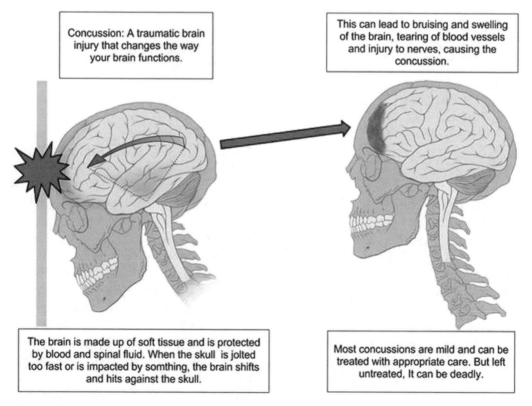

Concussion: A traumatic brain injury that changes the way your brain functions.

This can lead to bruising and swelling of the brain, tearing of blood vessels and injury to nerves, causing the concussion.

The brain is made up of soft tissue and is protected by blood and spinal fluid. When the skull is jolted too fast or is impacted by somthing, the brain shifts and hits against the skull.

Most concussions are mild and can be treated with appropriate care. But left untreated, It can be deadly.

Figure 5–2. Concussion mechanics (Max Andrews / Wikimedia Commons / CC-A-SA-3.0 Unported).

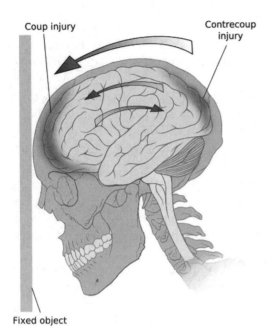

Figure 5–3. Coup–contrecoup damage in TBI (Patrick J. Lynch, Medical Illustrator, http://patricklynch.net; and C. Carl Jaffe, MD, Cardiologist / Wikimedia Commons / CC-A-SA-3.0 Generic).

contusions in the temporal and anterior frontal lobes (Grieve & Zink, 2009). The acceleration-deceleration movement can cause diffuse axonal injury (DAI), a result of shearing of the axons in the white matter in the parasagittal area and brainstem from angular acceleration, such as when a car crash victim's head fully extends, then fully hyperextends in rapid succession (Timmons & Maneker, 2010). The rapid acceleration-deceleration motion also causes stretching (or shearing) of white fiber tracts in the brain and damages individual neurons and their connections, causing a breakdown of overall communication among neurons in the brain.

Nonacceleration Injuries. Nonacceleration injuries occur when a restrained head is hit by a moving object. Although the cranium remains at rest following the impact, the brain continues moving until it bounces against the skull. An example is when an object squashes the head. At the time of impact, a tremendous amount of force may be exerted on the head. In the extreme case, the impact can crush the head, resulting in death. In the majority of cases, however, non-acceleration injuries may fracture the skull, resulting in less serious damage to the brain (Roseberry-McKibben & Hegde, 2006).

Concussion

The least severe and the most common type of TBI associated with a closed head injury is a concussion, which is classified as mild TBI (mTBI). A concussion is a short loss of consciousness due to temporary loss of brain function in response to a head injury. Concussion results from diffuse versus focal brain injury, and is considered to be a milder form of diffuse axonal injury because the stretching of axons is less extensive. A concussion causes a variety of often subtle physical, cognitive, and emotional symptoms, which may go undetected.

The symptoms of concussion usually fall into four categories, including thinking/remembering, physical, emotional/mood, and sleep (CDC, 2010b). Some of these symptoms may appear immediately, while others may not be noticed for days or months following the injury or in some cases not until more demands are placed upon the individual as he/she resumes everyday life activities. However, in most cases (80–90%), concussions resolve within 7 to 10 days. Table 5–1 shows the signs and symptoms of concussion.

Ommaya and his associates, (Ommaya, 1979, 1995, 1997; Ommaya & Gennarelli, 1974; Ommaya, Goldsmith & Thibault, 2002) hypothesized that in

Table 5–1. Symptoms of Concussion

⚙ Thinking/ Remembering	Ɏ Physical	⚡ Emotional/ Mood	👁 Sleep
Difficulty thinking clearly	Headache Fuzzy or blurry vision	Irritability	Sleeping more than usual
Feeling slowed down	Nausea or vomiting (early on) Dizziness	Sadness	Sleep less than usual
Difficulty concentrating	Sensitivity to noise or light Balance problems	More emotional	Trouble falling asleep
Difficulty remembering new information	Feeling tired, having no energy	Nervousness or anxiety	

Source: Centers for Disease Control and Prevention. (2010a). Concussion: What are the sign and symptoms of concussion? Retrieved from http://www.cdc.gov/concussion/signs_symptoms.html

cerebral concussion, blunt force trauma produces a mechanically induced strain on the brain in a centripetal sequence of disruptive effects on function and structure. According to this hypothesis, the injury sequence begins at the cortical surface in mild cases and extends inward to affect the diencephalic-mesencephalic core at the most severe levels of trauma. The centripetal force on the brain is a swirling movement of the fragile cerebral structures within the cranial vault. As the brain moves, axons within their myelin sheath are twisted and sheared. The brain is accelerated or decelerated and arrested as the frontal and temporal poles impact against the wall of the anterior and middle cranial fossae (Miller, 1983). The damage is bilateral, cumulative, and diffuse. When the amount of strain is great enough to affect the rostral brainstem, the effect upon consciousness is severe enough to cause paralytic coma of traumatic unconsciousness.

Ommaya (1995) also observed that the "talk and die or deteriorate" (TADD) syndrome begins at grade I (no loss of conscious) to grade II (brief loss of consciousness) injury cases, during which there is a measurable period of lucidity that allows the patient to engage in coherent speech. The patient appears to be normal but then proceeds to coma and death or survival with disabilities of severe head injury within a short period of time. This is called the second impact syndrome. Autopsy data on persons with TADD reveal either no evidence of DAI or a very low incidence for axonal lesions. Ommaya (1995) proposed that there are two types of TBI according to type of onset of traumatic coma:

Type I Immediate onset of coma after head injury with production of DAI lesions

Type II Delayed onset of coma after head injury with a variable period of lucidness with no initial coma and with insignificant DAI lesions (TADD)

TBI SYMPTOMS

The symptoms associated with TBI vary depending on the site and extent of neurological damage. TBI symptoms generally fall into one or more of the following categories:

- Physical: headache, nausea, vomiting, dizziness, altered consciousness (stupor, coma), blurred vision, sleep disturbance, weakness, paresis/plegia, sensory loss (smell, taste), spasticity, insomnia, balance disorders, disorders of coordination, or seizure disorder
- Behavioral/emotional: depression, poor emotional control, social withdrawal, hallucinations, delusions, confabulations, anxiety, agitation, irritability, impulsivity, or aggression
- Cognitive: poor concentration; memory loss; decreased speed of processing new learning; problems with attention, planning, reasoning, judgment, executive control, self-awareness, language, or abstract thinking
- Communication: mutism, confused language, aphasia, dysphagia, dysarthria, apraxia, anomia, preservation, reduced verbal fluency, difficulty initiating conversation, difficulty with turn taking in conversation, problems with topic initiation and maintenance, impaired narrative cohesion, impaired prosody, imprecise language, difficulty with abstract language, problems with reading and writing, auditory comprehension deficits, and impaired pragmatics (Dennis, 2009; Roseberry-McKibben & Hegde, 2006).

Patients typically present with one or more of these symptoms, which are interdependent and usually present with subtle, complex, and overlapping manifestations (Dennis, 2009). Physical symptoms are easily identified; however, some symptoms are not visible, making them harder to diagnose, as in the following:

- Mild TBI (concussion)
- Auditory manifestations (peripheral and central auditory disorders, tinnitus)
- Cognitive and memory impairments and executive function disorders
- Visual manifestations (vision loss and visual disturbances)
- Emotional/behavioral disturbances
- Posttraumatic stress disorder (PTSD)
- Pain
- Fatigue
- Memory impairments
- Musculoskeletal disorders
- Small embedded fragments

PRIMARY AND SECONDARY BRAIN INJURY

Trauma to the head may result from mechanical forces that cause damage to the nerve cells of the brain. Outcome from head injury is determined by two substantively different stages, which are primary and secondary injuries. Depending upon the extent of brain injury, the TBI is described as primary injury, secondary injury, or a combination of the two (Hammeke & Gennarelli, 2003; Porth, 2007). Table 5–2 summarizes the effects of primary and secondary brain injuries in TBI.

Primary Injury

The primary damage, known also as primary insult or mechanical damage, occurs at the moment of impact and can range from large to microscopic brain lesions. Primary damage includes contusion, skull fracture, damage to blood vessels, and axonal shearing (when the axons of neurons are stretched and torn). In instances of contusion, laceration, and intracranial hemorrhage, the damage is classified as focal due to the mechanism of the contact injury. However, the primary insult may also lead to diffuse brain damage in acceleration-deceleration injury types in which there is DAI or brain swelling (Werner & Engelhard, 2007).

Contusions

A contusion is a distinct area of swollen brain tissue, mixed with blood released from broken blood vessels. A contusion can occur in the absence of skull fracture in response to shaking of the brain back and forth within the confines of the skull (coup–contrecoup). Contusions are typically found on the inferior frontal lobes and poles of the frontal lobes, the lateral and inferior aspects of the temporal lobes, and the cortex above and below the operculum of the left, right, or both sylvian fissures (Ribbers, 2013).

Skull Fracture

A fracture of the skull can occur as a result of a severe impact or blow to the head (i.e., falls, automobile accidents, physical assault, and sports injuries). There are four types:

Simple fracture—a break in the bone without damage to the skin

Linear skull fracture—a break in a cranial bone resembling a thin line, without splintering, depression, or distortion of bone

Depressed skull fracture—a break in a cranial bone (or "crushed" portion of skull) with depression of the bone in toward the brain

Compound fracture—involves a break in or loss of skin and splintering of the bone

In some cases, a fracture may not cause severe consequences to the underlying brain tissue (Klatzo, 1979). However, when damage does occur, it can disrupt the functions of the hippocampus and other medial temporal lobe limbic structures and cause posttraumatic amnesia (PTA) memory disorders (Levin, Grossman, & Kelly, 1976). Studies on the severity of the injury have shown that there is a greater loss of consciousness in patients admitted with a principal diagnosis of intracranial injury rather than a diagnosis of skull fracture (Ommaya et al., 1996). Skull fractures are primary head injuries that may lead to secondary injuries such as contusion or bruising of brain tissue. In a contusion, edema (swelling) develops in a specific area of brain tissue and is mixed with blood released from broken blood vessels (NINDS, 2005, 2013)

Table 5–2. Primary and Secondary Brain Damage

Primary Damage	Secondary Damage
Skull fracture: a break in the skull. There are four types: simple, linear, depressed, and compound fractures.	Cerebral atrophy and ventricular enlargement: brain shrinkage with corresponding enlargement of the ventricular system.
Damage to blood vessels resulting in hemorrhage. Four types include: intracerebral, subdural, subarachnoid, and epidural	Arterial hypoxemia: reduction of oxygen to the most severely injured parts of the brain
Intracerebral hemorrhage, a subcategory of intracranial hemorrhage in which blood flows directly into cerebral tissue	Intracranial hematoma: blood clot in the brain
Subdural hemorrhage	Subdural hematoma: blood clot between the inner surface of the dura mater and the brain
Subarachnoid hemorrhage	Arterial hypotension: low arterial blood pressure
Epidural hemorrhage: bleeding between the dura mater and the skull	Hypercapnia: excessive carbon dioxide levels in the blood
Cerebral contusion: bruising of cerebral tissue	Cerebral edema: diffuse posttraumatic brain swelling
Cerebral laceration: a cut or tear of cerebral tissue observed following a skull fracture or stab wound to the head in penetrating brain injury.	Ischemia: insufficient blood flow to cerebral tissue
Axonal shearing: axon fibers are stretched and torn during an acceleration-deceleration head injury	Increased intracranial pressure: increased pressure within the skull due to the buildup of fluids from edema, hematomas, contusions, which in severe cases may lead to brain herniation
Diffuse axonal injury (DAI) is a result of shearing of the axons in the white matter and brain stem from angular acceleration.	Brain herniation: parts of the brain are squeezed and exit past structures in the skull
	Meningitis: inflammation of the meninges.
	Brain abscess: a collection of pus, immune cells, and other material in the brain

Source: Hammeke, T. A., & Gennarelli, T. A. (2003). Traumatic brain injury. In R. B. Schiffer, S. M. Rao, & B. S. Fogel (Eds.), *Neuropsychiatry.* Hagerstown, MD: Lippincott Williams & Wilkins, p. 1150.

Primary damage related to falls produces a different clinical manifestation. At the point of impact (coup), the vertex of the head is struck forcefully. The decelerated forces of the skull cause an upward displacement of the brain and corpus callosum (Payne & Ommaya, 1997). The corpus callosum is forcefully impacted against the inferior, sickle-shaped edge of the falx cerebri, which usually hangs above the cingulate gyrus. Consequently, the degree of displacement is substantial (Vogel, 1979).

Secondary Injury

Also known as secondary insult or delayed nonmechanical damage, secondary injury represents a series of pathological processes initiated at the moment of injury as a direct consequence of the primary damage with subsequent clinical features. Secondary damage worsens the primary injury and is correlated with severity of overall injury, poorer prognosis for recovery, and residual cognitive impairments (Youse, Le, Cannizzaro, & Coelho, 2002). The neurophysiological and anatomical changes associated with secondary damage occur minutes to days later and are for the most part preventable and treatable. Examples include anoxia (oxygen deprivation), edema (brain swelling), infection, hematoma, and increased intracranial pressure (Aschkenasy & Rothenhaus, 2006; Balestreri, Cozosnya, & Hutchinson, 2006; Porth, 2007; Youse. Lee, Cannizzaro, & Coelho, 2002).

Damage from anoxia occurs more selectively in the hippocampal regions and produces significant memory deficits. Edema has been linked to severe memory impairment (Uzzell, Obrest, Dolinkas, & Langfitt, 1986). Cerebral atrophy and ventricular enlargement have been related to various deficits of higher cognitive functioning, such as impaired judgment, memory, intellect, and language (Cullum & Bigler, 1986; Levin, Benton, & Grossman, 1982).

Increased Intracranial Pressure

Another condition associated with secondary brain injury is increased intracranial pressure (ICP), the result of the buildup of fluids from edema, hematomas, and contusions, for example. ICP occurs when there is no more space in the cranium to accommodate the extra volume of the mass, blood, or fluid produced from the TBI. Various treatments exist to prevent increases in ICP after trauma. These include shunting of the cerebrospinal fluid to the spinal subarachnoid space, increasing cerebrospinal fluid absorption, and shunting venous blood out of the skull (Balestreri et al., 2006; Brain Injury Association of America, 2013). If these compensations fail, the ICP rises. Elevated ICPs are a marker for poor outcome. A mean ICP greater than 20 mm Hg increases the possibility of patient mortality.

Intracranial Hemorrhages

Intracranial hemorrhages fall into four categories: epidural, subdural, subarachnoid, and intraparenchymal (intracerebral). If the accumulating blood is not evacuated, a hematoma (a semisolid mass of blood within or surrounding the brain) will occur, creating pressure on the surrounding brain tissue.

The resulting symptomatology is related in large part to the location of the hematoma. For example, an epidural hematoma is located between the skull and the dura (the outermost meninges/membrane covering the brain). In a subdural hematoma, bleeding is confined to the area between the dura and the surface of the brain (Biros & Heegaard, 2009). Subdural hematomas are classified as either acute or chronic. The acute form is a very severe brain injury with a sudden onset that typically causes unconsciousness and is fatal in about 50% of cases. A subdural hematoma is more common in the elderly because of age-related brain atrophy (shrinkage). This atrophy weakens the veins and causes them to stretch, making them more likely to tear, even after a minor head injury (Biros & Heegaard, 2009). Common causes of subdural hematomas are assault, car accidents, falls, and medications (i.e., blood thinners like Coumadin). Acute subdural hematomas are often caused by whiplash, which occurs when a sudden stop while driving causes the head to move violently forward and back.

A chronic subdural hematoma occurs when blood leaks from the veins slowly over time or a fast hemorrhage is left to clear up on its own. In this chronic type, the hematoma can accumulate in several small, separate episodes of bleeding (Biros & Heegaard, 2009). A chronic subdural hematoma typically follows a fairly minor head injury in a person who is elderly or is taking blood-thinning medications or whose brain has shrunk as a result of alcohol abuse or dementia. Symptoms develop gradually over 1 to 6 weeks. The most common symptoms are drowsiness, inattentiveness or confusion, headaches, changes in personality, seizures, and mild paralysis (Biros & Heegaard, 2009).

A third type is called intracerebral hemorrhage, caused by bleeding within the brain parenchyma. The resulting intra-cerebral hematoma compresses the surrounding brain tissue, affecting function (Czosnyka et al., 2007). Possible cause is either a direct impact to the brain (i.e., coup injury) or an indirect (or contrecoup) injury in which the force of an impact on one side of the brain causes a second area of damage on the side of the brain opposite the original impact.

Older patients who sustain minor head trauma with no loss of consciousness and who are neurologically intact on arrival to the emergency room may develop an intracerebral hematoma. Although small, this incidence is increased if the patient is taking warfarin and perhaps other anticoagulants or antiplatelet agents (Li, Brown, & Levine, 2001).

TBI SEVERITY

The severity of a TBI may range from mild (a brief change in mental status or consciousness) to severe (an extended period of unconsciousness or amnesia after the injury). The majority of TBIs (about 75%) that occur each year are concussions or other forms of mTBI (CDC, 2010b). However, advanced age is well recognized as an independent predictor of worse outcome after TBI, even with relatively minor head injuries (Czosnyka et al., 2005; Susman et al., 2002).

Normal consciousness, according to Ommaya (1995) is the state of awareness that allows the individual to integrate and utilize incoming sensory information and respond appropriately. Conversely, a coma, also called persistent vegetative state, is a profound state of unconsciousness in which an individual has lost awareness of the surroundings and the ability to think (NINDS, 2013). A coma state reflects significant damage to or depression of the function of the central nervous system and is a life-threatening complication of serious CNS involvement. Ommaya (1995) and Ommaya and Gennarelli (1974) argued that prolonged coma after TBI represented damage to the brain stem because of severe injury to the overlying cortical and subcortical structures.

Therefore, a major determination of TBI severity is duration and loss of consciousness based upon results from the Glasgow Coma Scale (GCS; Teasdale & Jennett, 1974). However, more recently the determination of TBI severity has been based on length and severity of amnesia from the Galveston Orientation and Amnesia Test (GOAT; Levin, O'Donnell,

& Grossman, 1979). Table 5–3 gives a summary of TBI severity. Criteria for the GCS and GOAT are shown in Tables 5–4 and 5–5, respectively.

The majority (75%) of TBIs are classified as mild in severity. According to Youse et al. (2002), mTBI (Table 5–6) is associated with closed head injuries (concussion) resulting in a trauma-induced physiological disruption of brain function, as evidenced by at least one of the following:

- loss of consciousness for not greater than 30 minutes
- a GCS score of at least 13 within 30 minutes post-injury

Table 5–3. Classification of Mild TBI (Concussion)

Grade	Cantu (1992)	Colorado	AAN
1	No LOC; PTA < 5 minutes	No LOC; confusion without amnesia	Transient confusion; no LOC. Concussive symptoms resolve < 15 minutes
2	LOC < 5 minutes; PTA > 30 minutes	No LOC; confusion with amnesia	Transient confusion; no LOC. Concussive symptoms last > 15 minutes
3	LOC > 5 minutes; PTA > 24 hours	Any LOC	Any LOC either brief (seconds) or prolonged (minutes)

Source: Colorado = Workers Compensation Board, State of Colorado; AAN = American Academy of Neurology; see "Practice Parameter" (1997).

Table 5–4. Measurement of TBI Severity

Classification	GCS Score	Duration of Coma	Length of PTA
Severe	3–8	Over 6 hours	Over 24 hours
Moderate	9–12	Less than 6 hours	1–24 hours
Mild	13–15	20 minutes or less	60 minutes or less

Source: Sohlberg & Mateer, 2001; Lezak, 1995

Table 5–5. Glasgow Coma Scale

Parameter	Test	Patient Response	Score
Eye Opening	Verbal command	Spontaneous with blinking at baseline	4 points
	Verbal command	To verbal command—opens eyes when asked in a loud voice	3 points
	Pain	only opens eyes when pinched (not applied to face)	2 points
	Pain	No response—does not open eyes	1 point
Verbal Response	Speech	Carries on a conversation correctly and is oriented to person, place and time	5 points
	Speech	Confused conversation, but able to answer questions	4 points
	Speech	Inappropriate words	3 points
		Incomprehensible speech, produces sounds that examiner cannot understand	2 points
	Speech	No response	1 point
Motor Response	Commands	Obeys simple commands for movement	6 points
	Pain	Purposeful movement pulls examiner's hands away when pinched	5 points
	Pain	Withdraws in response to pain, pulls a part of the body away when pinched	4 points
	Pain	Flexion in response to pain (decorticate posturing)	3 points
	Pain	Extension response in response to pain (decerebrate posturing)	2 points
	Pain	No motor response to pain	1 point

GCS Categorization of Coma: No eye opening, no ability to follow commands, no word verbalizations (GCS score 3–8)

Head Injury Classification: Severe Head Injury—GCS score of 8 or less, Moderate Head Injury—GCS score of 9 to 12, Mild Head Injury—GCS score of 13 to 15.

Sources: CDC, 2003; Teasdale & Jennett, 1974.

- PTA, a loss of memory for events before or after injury lasting less than 24 hours
- any alteration in mental state
- focal neurological damage that may or may not be transient.

When standard radiological studies (e.g., CT scan, MRI) are done, they must be interpreted as normal.

Although symptoms of mTBI are mild, it is possible for an individual with mTBI to have significant damage to the

Table 5–6. Galveston Orientation and Amnesia Test (GOAT)

Question	Error Score	Notes
What is your name?	−2 _____	Must give both first name and surname.
When were you born?	−4 _____	Must give day, month, and year.
Where do you live?	−4 _____	Town is sufficient.
Where are you now:		
(a) City	−5 _____	Must give actual town.
(b) Building	−5 _____	Usually in hospital or rehab center. Actual name necessary.
When were you admitted to this hospital?	−5 _____	Date.
How did you get here?	−5 _____	Mode of transport.
What is the first event you can remember after the injury?	−5 _____	Any plausible event is sufficient (record answer)
Can you give some detail?	−5 _____	Must give relevant detail.
Can you describe the last event you can recall before the accident?	−5 _____	Any plausible event is sufficient (record answer)
What time is it now?	−5 _____	−1 for each half-hour error.
What day of the week is it?	−3 _____	−1 for each day error.
What day of the month is it? (i.e., the date)	−5 _____	−1 for each day error.
What is the month?	−15 _____	−5 for each month error.
What is the year?	−30 _____	−10 for each year error.
Total Error:		
Total Actual Score = (100 − total error) = 100 − _____ =		Can be a negative number.

76–100 = Normal

66–75 = Borderline

<66 = Impaired

Source: Levin, H. S., O'Donnell, V. M., & Grossman, R.G. (1979). The Galveston Orientation and Amnesia Test. A practical scale to assess cognition after head injury. *Journal of Nervous and Mental Diseases,167*, 675–684. Reprinted with permission.

brain or its surrounding structures. This is especially true for older persons who are taking blood thinners (e.g., Coumodin, Plavix) and in cases where there is a history of heavy alcohol use.

In the classification of TBI, there has been a long-standing debate about the nature, diagnosis, pathophysiology, history, and terminology of mTBI. Although the terms *concussion* and *mild TBI* are often used interchangeably, the designation of mTBI may be inappropriately used to describe unresolved brain injury, and *concussion* may be the more appropriate term.

Concussion is a form of TBI, although it is clinically and diagnostically distinct from more severe forms of TBI. In some circumstances, the term *concussion* may be preferred, particularly when talking with patients about their condition to indicate the mild, transient nature of the injury and to stress the prospect of recovery.

TBI PREVALENCE

Three groups have emerged with distinct profiles of TBI. Among adolescents and young adults (ages 15–29), the highest risk group comprises those age 15 to 19, with a prevalence of 400 to 700 per 100,000 individuals. Another high risk group are persons who are 75 years and older, among whom the incidence is higher than in the general population: about 300 per 100,000 persons (CDC, 2010b; Human Service Transportation Delivery, 2010; Langlois et al., 2006; Roseberry-McKibbin & Hegde, 2006). A third group are the very young (children aged 0 to 4 years), who have been found to have the highest rate of head injuries, resulting typically from falls (839 per 100,000) (CDC, 2010b). With regard to gender, males are more prone to suffer a TBI, with more than twice as many having suffered a head injury than women (Frost,

Farrer, Primosch, & Hedges, 2012). Males age 0 to 4 years have the highest rates of TBI-related emergency department visits, hospitalizations, and deaths combined (CDC, 2010b). Another high risk group are the incarcerated, because the prevalence of TBI is higher than among the general population (Farrer & Hedges, 2011; Hagelson, 2010).

In addition to those mentioned as high-risk, there are reports of persistent racial disparities in emergency room visits for TBI in persons with mTBI and in outcomes for those who have sustained moderate to severe TBI (Bazarian, Pope, McClung, Cheng, & Flesher, 2003; Bowman, Martin, Sharar, & Zimmerman, 2007; Shafi et al., 2007). These disparities can decrease the accuracy of reporting annual prevalence and recovery of TBI among diverse cultural and ethnic groups in the United States and possibly lead to an underestimation of the numbers of persons from diverse communities who sustain head trauma.

TBI CAUSES

Motor vehicle accidents are the leading cause of head injuries among the general population, accounting for approximately 50% of all TBIs, and are the major cause of mortality, with rates highest for young adults age 20 to 24. In contrast, falls are reported as the major cause of TBIs among older persons, historically at 51% of head injuries (Rutland-Brown et al., 2006), and continue to rise in incidence among this population, with recent rates as high as 60.7% (CDC, 2010b).

Falls

The most common cause of a head injury among adults is fall for those adults aged

65 years and older (CDC, 2010b) Thompson et al., 2006). Falls are also the most common cause of nonfatal injuries and hospital admissions for trauma, with 20% to 30% of elderly patients injured suffering a moderate to severe head injury. In 2010, 2.3 million nonfatal fall injuries among older adults were treated in emergency departments, and more than 662,000 of these patients were hospitalized (CDC, 2010b).

Falls occur for a variety of reasons. Some are due to safety hazards in the home or the community environment. Others are due to debilitating health or medical conditions. The rate of falls requiring hospitalization increased from 339 per 100,000 in people age 65 to 69 to 3,637 per 100,000 in those age 85 and older (Faul, Xu, Wald, & Coronado, 2010).

Although falls may occur anywhere, most falls among the elderly occur at or around the home at ground level. In the home, falls are often due to inadequate or lack of proper safety measures, such as poor lighting, slick floors, loose area rugs, and absence of handicap bars in the bathtub or railings on stairs (NIH Senior Health, 2011). For elderly in the nursing home environment, there is also a risk of falls due to improper transfer (e.g., from bed to wheelchair) and poor balance while using a walker or cane (Aschkenasy & Rothenhaus, 2006; Stevens, 2006).

There are a number of risk factors that have been associated as possible causes of falls. Three major factors are medical problems, medication side effect, and fear of falling. The major medical problems that contribute to falls are arthritis, osteoporosis, hypotension, hip fractures, muscle paresis or paralysis following a cerebrovascular accident, poor vision due to cataracts or glaucoma, impaired hearing, and muscle weakness of the extremities, leading to poor balance and gait (NIH Senior Health, 2011).

Medication side effects present other risks for falls. Huang and associates (2012) found that pharmacological factors that place the elderly at greater risk for drug-related side effects include changes in body composition, serum albumin, total body water, and hepatic and renal functioning. Psychotropic medications (antidepressants, neuroleptics, and sedatives) and antihypertensives (beta-blockers, calcium blockers, and diuretics) have been identified as major risk factors in falls because they can cause dizziness and problems with balance. Less commonly associated medications are antiepileptic and glaucoma agents. The risk is even greater among those who take multiple medications, also known as polypharmacy. Polypharmacy, the use of usually four or more medications, is common among individuals as they age and can lead to negative health outcomes and greater risks for a fall than the taking of fewer medications (Haijar, Cafiero, & Hanlon, 2007; NIH Senior Health, 2011).

A third risk factor is fear of falling, which can affect motivation to engage in physical activity. Inactivity results in diminished muscle strength, flexibility, and endurance, which can cause an older person to be unsteady and fall (NIH Senior Health, 2011; Santora et al., 1994).

Vehicular and Pedestrian Accidents

After falls, motor vehicle and pedestrian accidents are the second leading cause of head injuries among older adults (Langlois et al., 2006; Faul et al., 2010; Thompson et al., 2006). Persons over age 65 are also the fastest growing segment of the driving population, due in large part to increased longevity (Payne & Ommaya, 1997; Yee, Cameron, & Bailey, 2006). Studies on this population have shown a higher incidence of motor vehicle accidents (MVAs) among older persons (National Highway Traffic Safety Administration, 2012; Sjogren & Bjornstig, 1991), particularly those 70 years or older because of decreased visual acuity, diminished cognitive function in the areas of reasoning and memory, and physical changes such as slower reaction time. Moreover, following an MVA, elderly trauma patients tend to have poorer outcomes (Malik, Dal, & Talpur, 2012; Sklar, Demarest, & McFeeley, 1989). In light of these factors, the rising incidence of TBIs related to MVAs among the elderly is a major concern.

Elderly persons living in urban areas are particularly susceptible to traffic accidents. Older Americans have the highest accident rate for numbers of miles driven of any age group and the most severe injuries from vehicular and pedestrian accidents (Payne & Ommaya, 1997; Yee et al., 2006). Statistics also show that older drivers are more likely than younger ones to be involved in multivehicle crashes, particularly at intersections (National Highway Traffic Safety Administration, 2012). It is thought that three factors account for the higher rate of multivehicle accidents among older adults specifically: poor judgment in making left-hand turns, drifting out of the traffic lane, and decreased ability to modify behavior in response to an unexpected or rapidly changing situation.

Older persons are also at increased risk for pedestrian-related vehicular accidents and make up a significant percentage of pedestrians who have suffered head injuries from being struck by a motor vehicle (McCoy, Johnstone, & Duthie, 1989; National Center for Health Statistics, 2012; Sklar et al., 1989). Slower ambulation, impaired reflexes, misjudgment, disturbed gait, and visual/auditory impairments appear to be the primary risk factors, as elderly persons are frequently struck within marked crosswalks or walk directly into the path of an oncoming vehicle.

Studies examining the incidence of injuries among elderly pedestrians struck by a motor vehicle report an increased fatality rate (Sklar et al., 1989; Subramanian, 2012). Fatal injuries typically result from severe head injury or major vascular damage, with the majority of deaths occurring at the accident scene or in the emergency department (Sklar et al., 1989). Recent data reveal that age plays a tremendous role in type and severity of injury in pedestrian-related MVAs. Injuries to the brain as well as to other areas—including the spine, thorax, and skeleton—increase dramatically with age (Demetriades et al., 2004). Depending on the extent of injury, elderly survivors present with language, cognitive, motor speech, and pragmatic deficits that affect their communication in activities of daily living as well as in their social interactions.

Assaults and Abuse

Although approximately 20% of TBIs among the general population result from violent assaults, the incidence among the elderly accounts for only 1% of all TBIs (Thompson et al., 2006). However, ethnicity, income level, and area of residence (urban or rural) make some elders more susceptible to injurious assaults. These factors also affect the prevalence of TBIs with assaults accounting for the majority of head injuries in some inner-city urban settings (Barber & Webster, 1974; McCrary, 1992; Payne & Ommaya, 1997).

Elder abuse, another cause of TBIs, is a growing problem in this nation.

Like all forms of abuse and neglect, it is insidious, and underreported. According to the National Elder Abuse Incidence Study (National Center on Elder Abuse, 1998), nearly 450,000 persons over age 60 have experienced some form of domestic abuse, although only 16% of these cases are reported. Recent data from the World Health Organization (2011) indicate that approximately 4% to 6% of older adults have experienced some form of abuse at home. Elder maltreatment can lead to serious physical injuries, including head trauma, resulting in long-term consequences. Elder abuse is often undetected because victims are often afraid to report cases of maltreatment to family, friends, or the authorities.

Elder abuse also occurs in senior residential facilities. A survey of nursing-home staff in the United States indicates that rates of elder abuse in long-term care institutions may be high. Approximately 10% of paid caregivers reportedly committed at least one act of physical abuse toward an elderly patient annually; and even more alarming, 36% of staff respondents witnessed at least one incident of physical abuse of an elderly patient in the previous year (World Health Organization, 2011).

Frail, elderly, cognitively compromised women over the age of 80 are particularly at risk for elder abuse. The abuse takes many forms and may lead to head injuries. Further descriptions of types of elder abuse and resources for reporting elder abuse may be found in Chapter 4.

Alcohol-Related TBIs

Alcohol abuse and alcoholism are frequent causes of TBI. Alcohol abuse is a common but often undiagnosed problem among older adults. Surveys indicate that 6% to 11% of older patients admitted to hospitals and 14% of elderly patients in emergency rooms exhibit symptoms of alcoholism (Council on Scientific Affairs, 1996). The prevalence of problem drinking in nursing homes is as high as 49% in some studies, depending in part on survey methods (Joseph, 1997). Late-onset alcohol problems also occur in some retirement communities, where drinking at social gatherings is often the norm (Atkinson, Tolson, & Turner, 1990).

Alcohol use is a major predisposing cause of head injuries among older adults and is associated with vehicular accidents (U.S. Department of Transportation, 2010) and frequent falls (Aschkenasy & Rothenhaus, 2006; Nordell, Jarnlo, Jetsen, Nordstrom, & Thorngren, 2000), as well as assaults and elder abuse (CDC, 2012; National Center on Elder Abuse, 1998; Payne & Ommaya, 1997). One-third of older adults who are alcohol abusers develop a more severe problem with alcohol in later life, while the other two-thirds exhibit the medical and psychosocial consequences of early-onset alcoholism as they age.

Alcohol-involved traffic accidents are a major cause of trauma among older adults, who are the fastest growing segment of the driving population. A person's crash risk per mile increases starting at age 55, exceeding that of a young beginning driver by age 80 (National Institute on Alcohol Abuse and Alcoholism, 2011). In addition, older drivers tend to be more seriously injured than those who are younger in crashes of equivalent magnitude (Waller, 1996). The combination of older age and alcoholism can also dramatically increase driving risk. After consuming the same amount of alcohol, an elderly driver with a history of alcoholism is more impaired and more susceptible to a vehicular accident than an elderly driver without a history of chronic alcohol use (Waller, 1998).

Some surveys yield data that compare young and older adults on their drinking habits. Compared to younger adults, some results suggest that the elderly consume less alcohol and have fewer alcohol-related problems. However, longitudinal surveys indicate that a person's drinking pattern remains relatively stable with age, perhaps reflecting societal norms that prevailed when the person began drinking (National Institute on Alcohol Abuse and Alcoholism, 1988). Some living environments are implicated in the drinking habits of older adults. Within long-term settings, survey results document an increasing prevalence of alcoholism among the older population, which places them at greater risk for falls and repeat head injuries.

Sports Injuries

Although sports injuries are more prevalent in children and adolescents, accounting for 20% to 30% of head injuries, they are becoming a growing cause of TBIs among older adults. With an increased longevity and the emphasis on staying healthy through exercise (National Institute of Neurological Disorders and Stroke, 2012), older adults are now more active and engaged in sports activities. Consequently, sports-related injuries result from problems in balance, sensory deficits (vision and hearing), and muscle weakness, affecting flexibility, strength, and endurance. Horse riding is the single most dangerous sport in the context of head injury. In golf, blunt force injuries may be likely to occur. Individuals who

have experienced a prior head injury are at greater risk for sports-related injuries due to the serious impact a TBI can have on balance (Disabled World News, 2011).

Research data clearly indicate that blunt force injuries incurred in sports have long-lasting consequences. Repeated mTBIs occurring over an extended period of time may cause cumulative neurological and cognitive deficits. Retired American professional football players with a history of three or more TBIs were five times more likely to have mild cognitive impairment (Guskiewicz et al., 2005). Professional boxers are well known to have a risk of significant cognitive decline and alterations in brain function (Jordan et al., 1997). However, there is increasing concern that cumulative effects may also be occurring in athletes who sustain more routine injuries as a function of playing a contact sport such as football or ice hockey (Collins et al., 1999; Matser, Kessels, Lezak, Jordan, & Troost, 1999). Long-term effects of repeated concussions include chronic motor and neuropsychological deficits.

Guskiewicz and associates (2005) noted a greater than average incidence of earlier onset of Alzheimer's disease among retired football players than in the general American male population. Their findings suggest that the onset of dementia-related syndromes may be initiated by repetitive cerebral concussions in professional football players. Potential catastrophic outcome as a result of a repeated concussion injury during recovery from an initial injury may occur because cellular, metabolic, axonal, and vascular disturbances are amplified, and profound cerebral edema develops, producing coma and severe neurological disability, or death.

Multisystem Missile Blast Injuries

Blast injury is considered to be the "signature injury" of the war (Elder & Cristian, 2009; Hoge et al., 2008; Jett, 2010). Since 2001, 2.4 million servicemen and women served in Operation Iraqi Freedom (OIF), Operation Enduring Freedom (OEF), and Operation New Dawn (OND) (Spelman, Hunt, Seal, & Burgo-Black, 2012). New and sophisticated missile warfare during the Global War on Terror has exposed U.S. military troops to strong air-pressure blasts that cause multilevel/multisystem injuries (Wallace, 2006). Advanced head and body protective gear such as Kelvar helmets are keeping service members alive by reducing penetrating injuries; however, because the brain is shaken within the skull, military personnel are sustaining closed head brain injuries/concussions that result in mTBI (Okie, 2005; Wallace, 2006).

Incidence and Prevalence

TBI is the major cause of mortality and morbidity from the war. Blast injury is the most common cause (Elder & Cristian, 2009). Seventy-nine percent of service members have sustained TBI with loss of consciousness (LOC) (Elder & Cristian, 2009; Hoge et al., 2008). Within that percentage, 15% to 20% meet the criteria for mTBI (Elder & Cristian, 2009; Hoge et al., 2008; MacGregor, Dougherty, Morrison, Quinn, & Galarneau, 2011).

In a survey by Hoge et al. (2008), 124 out of 2,525 U.S. Army infantry soldiers reported an injury with LOC and 260 reported an injury with altered mental status without LOC. Injuries without LOC or altered mental status from other events such as falls or handling heavy equipment were reported in 435 soldiers. In addition, soldiers who reported mTBI were significantly younger, junior in rank, and male (Hoge et al., 2008). Elder and Cristian (2009) report that 20% of the first 1.6 million who served in the Global War on Terror sustained a TBI; of those injured, about 60% were not assessed by health care workers, and a large number were not recognized prior to discharge. Of those seen by health care professionals at Walter Reed Army Medical Center, 59% of blast injuries sustained a TBI (Okie, 2005).

The alarming rate of head injuries in returning service members has become a new focus of research for the Veterans Affairs and the Department of Defense (VA/DOD) and within the field of speech-language pathology. Forty-seven percent of returning veterans are between the ages of 17 and 31 (Spelman et al., 2012). These are young adults who will want to either return to active duty or reenter civilian life. Some will want to obtain a college degree, return to their families, start a family, or find a job. Re-entry after mTBI can be challenging, particularly when comorbid symptoms such as physical, cognitive, emotional, and social impairments are present. Figures 5–4, 5–5, and 5–6 show DOD numbers for TBI, incidence of TBI by severity, and TBI incidence by military branch, respectively.

Explosives

Explosives to which service personnel are frequently exposed are categorized as high order and low order. High-order explosives are made up of chemicals with a high rate of reaction, such as nitroglycerin, C-4, and dynamite. These types of explosives create shattering effects from the blast waves, whereas low-order explo-

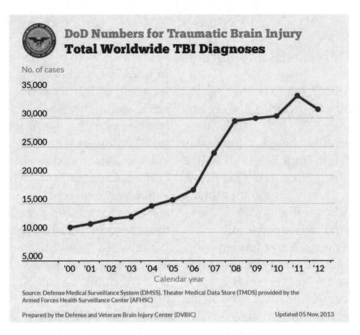

Figure 5–4. Total worldwide TBI diagnosis. Total worldwide TBI diagnosis from 2000–2012. (From Armed Forces Health Surveillance Center, Defense and Veterans Brain Injury Center, 2013. *Department of Defense numbers for traumatic brain injury*. Retrieved from http://www.dvbic.org/dod-worldwide-numbers-tbi.). Accurate as of January 2014.

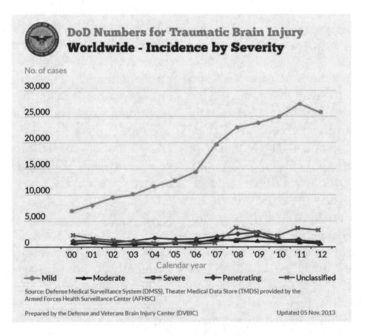

Figure 5–5. TBI incidence by severity. TBI incidence by severity from 2000–2012. (From Armed Forces Health Surveillance Center, Defense and Veterans Brain Injury Center, 2013. *Department of Defense numbers for traumatic brain injury*. Retrieved from http://www.dvbic.org/dod-worldwide-numbers-tbi.). Accurate as of January 2014.

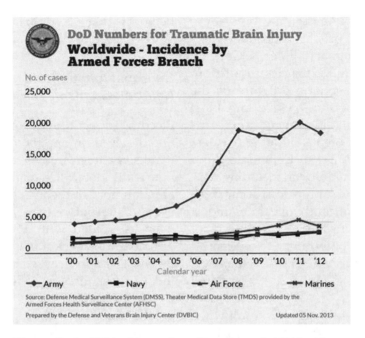

Figure 5–6. TBI incidence by military branch. TBI incidence by military branch from 2000–2012. (From Armed Forces Health Surveillance Center, Defense and Veterans Brain Injury Center, 2013. *Department of Defense numbers for traumatic brain injury.* Retrieved from http://www.dvbic.org/ dod-worldwide-numbers-tbi.). Accurate as of January 2014.

sives produce a blast wind that has a pushing effect (Wallace, 2006). Low-order explosives are designed to burn and gradually release at a slow rate. These include improvised explosive devices, which are considered to be the source of the explosion (Moore & Jaffe, 2010). The energy that is released can be in the forms of electrical, thermal, and kinetic energy (Moore & Jaffe, 2010).

Blast injuries, also referred to as blast-induced neurotrauma (Cernak, 2007; Jett, 2010) and combat-acquired brain injury (Parrish, Roth, Roberts, & Davie, 2009), are the result of blasts from detonated explosives that apply pressure to the brain, low-order explosives, and explosives that produce a supersonic over-pressurization shock wave (Elder & Cristian, 2009; Wallace, 2006). Explosions in

the atmosphere are characterized by the release of energy in a short period of time in a small volume, which results in a non-linear shock and pressure wave of finite amplitude that spreads from the major cause of blasts. Rocket-propelled grenades are another form of low-order explosives and include pipe bombs, gunpowder, and Molotov cocktails (Elder & Cristian, 2009; Wallace, 2006).

Types of Multiblast Injuries

Polytrauma refers to the multiorgan/multisystem injuries that affect more than one physical region and organ system, resulting in cognitive, physical, psychological, or psychosocial impairments and functional disability (Scott, Belanger, Vanderploeg, Massengale, & Scholten, 2006;

Wallace, 2006). Polytrauma injuries are categorized as primary, secondary, tertiary, and quaternary (Elder & Cristian, 2009). Primary blast injuries result from increased atmospheric pressure or the combination of shock wave and blast wind that results in damage to the air- and fluid-filled organs (Elder & Cristian; Moore & Jaffe, 2010). Concussion and damage to the middle ear, including tympanic membrane rupture, can occur (Wallace, 2006). Scott and colleagues report that within their sample ($n = 50$), 66% of patients with polytrauma experienced concussion, 31% had soft-tissue damage, 28% had hearing loss, and 20% suffered lung injury.

Secondary blast injuries result when the individual is struck by objects, such as shrapnel and bullets put in motion by a blast (Elder & Cristian, 2009; Moore & Jaffe, 2010). Secondary injuries are similar to penetrating injuries. Small pieces of shrapnel lodged within the brain can be dangerous because as the body recognizes that it is a foreign object, it can then begin to shift in order to remove itself. This movement may eventually damage vital structures of the brain, causing hemorrhaging.

Tertiary blast injuries result when an individual is set into motion forcefully by a blast and collides with a solid object (Elder & Cristian, 2009; Moore & Jaffee, 2010). Service personnel can be thrown from vehicles during roadside bombings or jolted onto the ground into an object when a bomb detonates. The movement of the brain is reminiscent of the acceleration-deceleration movement seen in motor vehicle accidents that cause coup/contrecoup injuries. Quaternary blast injuries include burns, crush injuries, and significant blood loss, which can lead to

hemorrhaging (Moore & Jaffe; Roth, 2007; Wallace, 2006).

Neuropathologies and Neuromechanisms of Blast Injuries

Bleeding, direct tissue damage, and DAI are the best understood mechanisms, thanks in part to studies on civilian head injuries (Elder & Cristian, 2009). There are a number of theories that attempt to explain the pathophysiological mechanism associated with TBI. One theory describes the effect of blasts on the brain by ghost shrapnel caused by shock waves that cause an increase in air pressure that is approximately one thousand times greater than normal air pressure. This increase forms small bubbles throughout the brain that eventually pop and leave holes (Lawhorne & Philpott, 2010). It is possible that pieces of shrapnel are broken down into millions of tiny fragments that kill cells and then appear as tiny holes; however, to date, there is no research to validate the theory of ghost shrapnel.

A second theory relates to blast-induced vascular changes (Elder & Cristian, 2009). This theory suggests that oscillating high-pressure waves are transmitted through the systematic circulation to the vasculature of the brain, causing damage to structures close to cerebral vessels, including axonal fibers and cells. However, there is no direct support for this theory. Validation of the peripheral mechanism theory might be useful and would support the development of new types of body armor and helmets that would absorb or deflect blast waves in order to protect against central nervous system injuries (Elder & Cristian, 2009).

Research on the effects of repeated blast injuries comes from data on athletes who sustain multiple incidences of TBI. Chronic traumatic encephalopathy (CTE) was discovered by Dr. Bennet Omalu in 2002 through an autopsy on a National Football League player who sustained multiple concussions during his career. CTE is defined by Omalu, Hamilton, Kamboh, DeKosky, and Bailes (2010) as a progressive neurodegenerative syndrome caused by repetitive blunt force impacts to the head and transfer of acceleration-deceleration forces to the brain. An identifier of CTE is the tau protein. Tau protein is implicated in traumatic axonal injury and forms tangles that are characteristic of Alzheimer's and frontotemporal dementia.

Tau protein is a highly soluble microtubule-associated protein, mostly found in neuronal rather than non-neuronal cells in humans. The protein is found in neurofibrillary tangles, which are involved in the pathogenesis of Alzheimer's disease and other tau pathology (Yeh, Oakes, & Riedy, 2012). Neurofibrillary tangles are most commonly seen associated with repetitive mTBI. Recent studies have revealed that traumatic axonal injury is an active progressive deterioration of white and gray matter (Yeh et al., 2012).

There is a growing body of research that is utilizing postmortem brain research and animal models to study the effects of single and repetitive blasts on the brain. Analysis of deep brain tissue reveals multifocal loci of diffuse tauopathy (the primary proteinopathy) and possible accompaniment of low-grade and multifocal white matter rarefraction, microgial activation, and parenchymal histiocytes (Omalu et al., 2011a). A single case study by Omalu and colleagues (2011b) examined the brain of an Iraqi War veteran who was exposed to repetitive TBIs and played football and hockey for leisure. He suffered from PTSD and committed suicide by hanging. Postmortem analysis identified tauopathy as the primary proteinopathy in the form of multifocal sparse to frequent topographic neurofibillary tangles and neuritic threads throughout the lobes of the brain, but primarily in the frontal lobe. In addition, the apolipoprotein E genotype was identified. This allele is high risk for Alzheimer's disease and adverse effects of TBI.

It is important to understand that most service members are returned to full duty shortly after the injury-causing event (MacGregor et al., 2011). Civilian studies, particularly in athletes (football, soccer, boxing, among others), have found detrimental physiological, cognitive, and emotional health effects from sustaining multiple concussions (McKee, Cantu, & Nowinski, 2009; Neselius et al., 2012; Omalu et al., 2011a). MacGregor and colleagues (2011) conducted one of the first studies to report on repeated concussion among military personnel in a combat-deployed setting. Their study included 113 service members with two or more diagnosed concussions during OIF from March 2004 to April 2008. Over 90% of first and second injury events were combat-related and the result of blast mechanisms. At least 19% of repeated concussions occurred within 2 weeks of the first event and 87% occurred within 3 months of the first event. Results of the study suggested that although the time between events was not associated with an increase in clinical utilization, severity of the events was significantly associated with deterioration of mental health status. Those with a repeat concussion less than 3 months after the first event trended toward higher odds of needing mental health and neurology services (MacGregor et al., 2011).

The reasons for this persistent deterioration of mental status may be the cumulative effects of repeated concussions. Ultrasound brain studies of blast injury in rats show expanded perineural spaces, the appearance of cytoplasmic vacuoles, myelin deformation, and axoplasmic shrinkage, which is reminiscent of DAI. Imaging studies have also shown disrupted axonal transport and transient alterations in the disruption of neurofilament proteins in cortical regions after blasts to the head (Cernak, 2007; Cernak Wang, Jiang, Bian, & Savic,, 2001).

Summary

The epidemiology of TBI varies according to age, racial/ethnic group, geographical region (urban versus rural), and predisposing conditions, such as medication use and history of alcoholism. Falls account for the largest number of head injuries in older adults and have been linked to accidents in the home or long-term care facility as well as to medication side effects and polypharmacy. Other etiologies of head injury include motor vehicle incidents, pedestrian-related accidents, assaults, elder abuse, sports injuries, and missile blast injuries during wartime. Assaults are the leading cause of head injury in some urban settings among certain older racial/ethnic groups (i.e., African and Hispanic Americans), unlike the general population. These differences in the incidence and causes of head trauma are linked to living in high-impact urban areas where older adults may be more vulnerable to head injuries as a result of interpersonal violence. Therefore, among some racial/ethnic groups, the rank order of causes for head injuries is falls, assaults, and vehicular accidents.

There is a disparity in the availability of quality health care provided individuals from diverse racial/ethnic groups, particularly African Americans and Hispanics. African Americans and Hispanics with a history of alcohol and/or drug abuse have limited access to care or experienced greater delays in care compared with non-Hispanic whites.

Alcohol abuse is a factor in the high prevalence of head injury among older adults and is associated with all causes of TBI, including vehicular accidents, falls, and assaults. Alcohol-involved traffic accidents are a major cause of trauma among the elderly, but older drivers tend to be more seriously injured than younger drivers regardless of the cause or seriousness of the crash.

Elder abuse, another cause of TBIs, is a growing but often underreported problem in the United States. Older individuals are more susceptible to abuse because they are more physically frail, may suffer from visual and hearing problems, or have cognitive impairments that make them extremely vulnerable. Older, frail, and cognitively impaired women are most at risk. Abuse can occur in the elder's home, usually from family caregivers, or can occur in residential facilities where older adults experience abuse from paid caregivers. Most often, incidences of physical abuse, neglect, or exploitation are imposed on older adults by persons in the support network who are directly responsible for their care and who are under considerable stress. Elder abuse takes many forms, however. TBI can be caused by blunt force trauma or by overmedicating the individual. A complete description of the forms of elder abuse and the actions professionals should take to report elder abuse are found in Chapter 4.

Different challenges are presented by the population of returning armed services personnel from Middle East conflicts compared with older, civilian adults. Many service personnel have been repeatedly exposed to blast injuries and experience CTE, which progressively worsens. The nature of these brain injuries also increases the possibility that individuals will have a diagnosis of mental health crises. Alzheimer's disease may also be a sequela of blast injuries because of the pathology associated with neurofibrillary tangles and tauopathy.

POSTTRAUMATIC STRESS DISORDER

Definition and Epidemiology

In addition to complications from TBIs, many returning servicemen and women experience Posttraumatic Stress Disorder (PTSD), an anxiety disorder that develops after an individual experiences a terrifying or traumatic event that either caused or threatened physical harm (Schneider, Haack, Owens, Herrington, & Zelek, 2009). Individuals who are at risk for PTSD include civilians who have experienced traumas such as motor vehicle accidents or sexual assault (Gibson, 2012) and military service members who have been exposed to blasts and traumatic combat situations. Military service members with mTBI are particularly at high risk for developing PTSD after surviving explosions, witnessing wounds or fatalities among other survivors, or being hospitalized with serious medical problems secondary to explosions (Capeheart & Bass, 2012).

Mental illness is highly prevalent within the military population with PTSD, and depression is the most commonly diagnosed and treated disorder (Nayback, 2008; Schneider et al., 2009). At least half of those who served multiple deployments are estimated to have PTSD and it is anticipated that the incidence of this disorder will continue to increase as more service members are identified (Gibson, 2012). According to Huckens and colleagues (2010) and Capeheart and Bass (2012), the prevalence of PTSD in OIF/OEF veterans who sought treatment at a VA health care facility was 13% to 21% and 49% in OIF/OEF veterans who reported combat-related LOC.

PTSD is not a new phenomenon, nor is it specific to the troops returning from Afghanistan and Iraq. The symptoms of PTSD were recognized in troops after World War I (1914–1918) when the high explosive trinitrotoluene was utilized in artillery shells. The symptoms were designated as NYDN (Not Yet Diagnosed, Neurologic), neurasthenia, or shell shock. By World War II and the Korean War, the condition was known as combat or battle fatigue. After the Vietnam War, troops suffered from psychological problems that were referred to as Vietnam syndrome, a condition related to exposure to Agent Orange, a pesticide and herbicide spray. By 1980, the symptoms were collectively termed posttraumatic stress disorder by the third edition (1980) of the *Diagnostic and Statistical Manual of Mental Disorders* (Shively & Perl, 2012).

Almost 19% of Vietnam War veterans developed war-related PTSD during their lifetimes and 9.1% (between 2% and 17%) continued to experience PTSD approximately 11 to 12 years after the war (Gibson, 2012). This fairly large percentage of residual PTSD in Vietnam veterans and a high percentage of PTSD in recently returning OIF/OEF/OND veterans suggests that speech-language pathologists and other health care professionals should participate in assessing and treating persons over age 50 with PTSD.

Hoge et al. (2008) provide evidence that PTSD is strongly associated with mTBI. Soldiers in the study who reported mTBI, particularly with LOC, were at high risk for physical and mental health problems. It was also found that blast injuries associated with altered mental status (compared with other injuries) and combat intensity were significantly associated with PTSD. Forty percent of soldiers with injuries associated with loss of consciousness met the criteria for PTSD, which is representative of a substantial percentage reported by Huckens and colleagues (2010). A logistic-regression model indicated that only LOC and combat intensity were significantly associated with PTSD. The analyses also suggested that the high rates of physical health problems reported by soldiers with mTBI 3 to 4 months after deployment are mediated largely by PTSD or depression (Hoge et al., 2008).

Clark, Scholten, Walker, and Gironda (2009) concluded that traumatic injuries associated with emotional problems such as PTSD can aggravate pain and complicate treatment. PTSD was significantly more frequent among those in the combat group, a similar but nonsignificant trend for major depression. PTSD diagnoses were four times more common in polytrauma patients injured by blasts than those with combat injuries incurred by other means, and almost 20 times more common than among those injured in noncombat settings (i.e., convoys with supplies).

The military consists of demographics that are representative of the United States; however, it is also a cultural subgroup with its own values and beliefs. In addition to being competent in cultural and linguistic diversity, clinicians must become knowledgeable of the culture of the military to provide best practices (U.S. Department of Veterans Affairs, 2010). Nayback's (2008) review on health disparities in veterans reported that although there are more men in the military that are exposed to combat, PTSD is more likely to occur in women. However, women are also more likely to seek help. In terms of race, Hispanic and Asian Americans have greater dispositions toward developing PTSD. Among African Americans, there was a lower percentage of service-related disability ratings for PTSD than for other veterans. African American veterans also had higher rates of homelessness and increased dependence on welfare, poorer quality of life outcomes, and lower annual incomes than those who received disability benefits regardless of types of combat-related injuries.

Spoont, Hodges, Murdoch, and Nugent (2009) investigated race and ethnicity in mental health services among veterans with PTSD and found that minorities were less likely to receive mental health treatment in the 6 months following PTSD diagnosis than non-Hispanic whites. The study suggested that ethnic identity continues to play a role in some aspects of the use of mental health services. African Americans and Hawaiian/Pacific Islanders were more likely than non-Hispanic whites to receive medications but were less likely to receive at least four 1-month supplies. African Americans and Hawaiian/Pacific Islanders were also more likely to participate in counseling. Differences were found in that African Americans were more likely than non-Hispanic whites to receive at least eight counseling sessions. Overall, Native Americans were as likely as other groups to receive treatment but less likely to receive psychotropics. It was suggested that the difference may be due to treatment preferences among groups.

PTSD Symptoms

The symptoms of PTSD include re-experiencing, avoidance, and hypervigilance or increased arousal (Lawhorne & Philpott, 2010; Slone & Friedman, 2008). Re-experiencing includes flashbacks, bad dreams, and frightening thoughts. These experiences can be triggered by words, objects, and situations that are reminiscent of events during active duty (Jones, Young, & Leppma, 2010). Avoidance or numbing is a symptom that complicates social adjustment. Persons may become isolated by staying away from places, events, and objects that remind them of traumatic experiences. In addition, persons suffering from PTSD tend to show little interest in activities that they previously enjoyed.

Service members and veterans with PTSD also are easily startled, report feelings of being tense or on edge, and may have angry outbursts. Events and places with large crowds are often not attended because the noise can trigger a flashback and cause great anxiety. PTSD can interfere with initiating sleep through hyperarousal and with maintaining sleep through nightmares (Capeheart & Bass, 2012). Some will stay up late at night to walk the parameters of their homes and may be armed.

From the literature, social behaviors seen in patients with PTSD can include:

- drug/alcohol abuse
- high-risk behaviors such as criminal violence
- feelings that something is wrong with them
- dangerous or suicidal thoughts

- inability to function at home, work, or in interpersonal relationships
- problems interacting with friends, families, coworkers, and public authorities
- further injury
- becoming homeless (Jett , 2010; Schneider et al., 2009).

The patient may also:

- lack inhibitions that result in difficulty adhering to social rules
- present with an inability to perceive interpersonal cues
- show aggression
- be violent against themselves or others
- have adverse reactions to stressful or demanding situations
- have limited awareness of changes in his/her behavior
- show intensification of preexisting problem behaviors
- experience strong guilt or depression (Harman & Kelly, 2012).

There are a number of cognitive, physical, and social-emotional symptoms of mTBI that overlap with symptoms of PTSD and make assessment and diagnosis difficult (Schneider et al., 2009).

TBI/PTSD Symptoms

There is considerable overlap between the symptoms associated with TBI and the symptoms found for PTSD. Among these are cognitive, social-emotional, and physical problems.

Overlapping TBI and PTSD cognitive symptoms include difficulty organizing and completing tasks, difficulty in recall of information from short- and long-term memory, maintaining attention to tasks, and reasoning/problem solving. When given an assignment, a person with a diagnosis of PTSD is likely to have difficulty organizing information to complete the task. Executive functioning skills are often impaired, which results in decreased flexibility in problem solving and goal setting (Schneider et al., 2009).

In addition to cognitive impairments, these individuals also exhibit changes in their social-emotional behaviors, including impulsivity, aggression, social inappropriateness, and denial of deficits (Canteen, 2011; Harman & Kelly, 2012). Social cues, content of conversations, and social interactions become difficult to evaluate. Initiating and sustaining peer and family relationships are challenging.

Complaints of pain are commonly reported in patients who have PTSD, regardless of traumatic experience such as military combat, MVA, burns, or even musculoskeletal injury (Gibson, 2012). The physical symptoms associated with mTBI and PTSD include headaches, dizziness, and fatigue, changes in sleep patterns, and impaired coordination and balance (Schneider et al., 2009). Exposure to shrapnel can cause visual disturbances, and the effects of blasts also cause sensitivity to noise and light (Schneider et al., 2009). The most common single injury associated with blast is noise-induced hearing injury caused by blast overpressure (Godunsky & Reiter, 2005; Helfer et al., 2011).

PTSD and Substance Abuse

PTSD is associated with a high rate of drug addiction and problems with the law, as well as the contemplation of suicide (Lawhorne & Philpott, 2010). Substance use can aggravate mood, anxiety, or cognition either as a direct substance effect or indirectly by interfering with sleep (Capeheart & Bass, 2012). Substance use disorders associated with TBI—for example, alcohol, cannabis, and stimulants, which includes cocaine and similar stimulants—were studied in 2008 (Graham & Cardon, 2008). Study findings suggest a general decrease in alcohol use after TBI; however, problematic alcohol use after TBI represents a subgroup of patients who need special attention and are likely to have a more difficult clinical course. This subgroup may include individuals with mTBI who also have a diagnosis of PTSD. The National Comorbidity Survey revealed a higher rate of cannabis use among persons with either a current or lifetime diagnosis of PTSD (Kessler, Sonnega, Bromet, Hughes, & Nelson, 1995).

Capeheart and Bass (2012) also found that alcohol and/or drug use disorders were highly associated with PTSD in OIF/OEF veterans. Sixty-three percent of veterans with either alcohol or drug use disorders were diagnosed with PTSD and 76% of veterans with both alcohol and drug use disorder were found to have PTSD (Capeheart & Bass, 2012). A review of the data from the 1991 Gulf War revealed that an alcohol use disorder was 2.7 times more likely to occur among veterans with PTSD than among veterans with no diagnosis of PTSD. In addition, alcohol or drug use disorder prevalence rates were found to be between 39% and 84% among Vietnam veterans (Capeheart & Bass, 2012).

Suicide is also a major concern with TBI/PTSD. PTSD is associated with increased risk for suicidal thoughts and behaviors, which may be further enabled by psychiatric comorbidity (Capeheart & Bass, 2012; Lawhorne & Philpott, 2010). In 2012, the number of suicides in the U.S. military surpassed the number of deaths in combat in Afghanistan (Chapel, 2013).

COMMUNICATION DISORDERS

Communication impairments are a well-established consequence of TBI, particularly for moderate to severe head injuries. Deficits range from motor speech impairments of dysarthria and apraxia of speech (Goozée, Murdoch, Theodoros, & Stokes, 2000; Jaeger, Hertrich, Stattrop, Schönle, & Ackerman, 2000) to impaired language skills such as word finding (Bittner & Crowe, 2005; Hoofien, Gilboa, Vakil, & Donovick, 2001; Kerr, 1995; Olver, Ponsford, & Curran, 1996) and problems in pragmatic ability (Channon & Watts, 2003; Douglas, 2010; McDonald, 1993, 1998, 2007; Snow, Douglas, & Ponsford, 1997, 1998; Turkstra, McDonald, & Kaufmann, 1995). Adults who have experienced a TBI frequently exhibit communication disorders that result from impairments in these areas.

Disorders of Pragmatics and Social Interaction

In the area of pragmatics, or language use, McDonald (1993) evaluated the pragmatic language skills of two adults with closed head injuries by asking the subjects to explain how to play a game. Trained judges found that verbal productions of the experimental group were judged to be significantly inferior to that of the controls. Verbal output was found to be overly repetitive or too sketchy in detail. Errors in sequencing and inclusion of irrelevant propositions contributed to the disorganized and confusing nature of the language used by subjects with head injuries to give game instructions. Frontal lobe deficits in monitoring and regulation of performance were implicated. Pragmatics were also investigated by Milton, Prutting, and Binder (1984), who found that patients with head injuries most often engaged in pragmatic behaviors that interfered with conversation, such as inappropriate prosody, affect, topic selection, topic maintenance, turn-taking, and conciseness.

Major problems may be seen in social interaction skills and conversation, especially because of impaired pragmatic abilities, discourse cohesion, word fluency, and higher cognitive dysfunctions in storage and retrieval. Significant disorders of language that affect social interaction include impairments of nonverbal communication. Nonverbal communication deficits are the result of the inability to apply previously learned rules for vocal changes in intensity, pitch, rate, intonation, and quality in congruence with the culture of the individual and the communication context (Kennedy & DeRuyter, 1991).

COGNITIVE IMPAIRMENTS

Cognitive impairments are the most common consequences of TBI and include impairments of attention, memory, and executive functioning (thinking, planning, organization, reasoning, problem solving) at all levels of severity (Arciniegas, Held, & Wagner, 2002). The patient may present with impairment in one or any combination of areas. Disturbances of attention and prospective memory when present are especially problematic, because disruption of these relatively basic cognitive functions may cause or worsen additional disturbances in executive function, communication, and other relatively more complex cognitive skills (Arciniegas et al., 2002; Groot, Wilson, Evans, & Watson, 2002; Squire, 2004).

Injury severity has been correlated with severity of cognitive deficits, as patients with mTBI tend to have less cognitive deficits than those with moderate to severe TBI. Military service members and veterans have been exposed to multiple injury events (e.g., multiblast injuries). The additive effect of these multiple mTBI events may result in cognitive deficits equal to more severe degrees of injury (Dennis, 2009). In all cases, whether civilian or military, cognitive impairments have a significant impact on quality of life, community reintegration, and return to work.

Attention and Concentration

Attention is a complex system consisting of several component skills, each of which may be affected by a TBI. Lesions to the frontal lobe and widespread DAI are associated causes in attention deficits (Adamovich, Henderson, & Auerbach, 1985). Attention relates to a group of processes including alertness, selective attention, attention span, speed of processing, divided attention, alternating attention, and sustained attention (Beukelman & Yorkston, 1991; Stierwalt & Murray, 2002). As a group, these processes form the basis for other cognitive activity. Attention processes are also affected by abnormalities in other cognitive processes and the familiarity of the stimulus to the individual (Beukelman & Yorkston, 1991).

Attention is the ability to focus on a specific stimulus without being distracted (Honsinger & Yorkston, 1991). The inability to attend to a stimulus compromises memory because the stimuli cannot be held in storage long enough for processing. Disorders of attention have been found to cause other problems, such a preserveration, impulsivity, distractibility, slowed processing, and impersistence (Auerbach, 1986).

Impaired selective attention is often present in patients with TBI. When present, impaired attention decreases the patient's ability to attend to one element out of an array of incoming sensory stimuli (Honsinger & Yorkston, 1991; Olson & Henig, 1983). In defining selective attention, Beukelman and Yorkston (1991) said: "[T]o focus on one element out of a large array [it] is necessary for us to inhibit or disregard all or most of the other stimuli impinging on our sense and thoughts" (p. 106). The disruption of the selection process causes: (1) an inability to pick out the important things to attend to and (2) erratic jumping from one thought to another and topic to topic without purposeful sequence. The term *perseveration* or *mental inertia* is used to describe the patient who literally gets stuck on one thought or activity and is unable to switch to another effectively.

The inability to sustain attention (or impaired vigilance) is one of the most frequently reported problems associated with TBI. Patients are unable to focus intentionally on a thought, task, or stimulus for a sustained period of time (Beukelman & Yorkston, 1991).

Memory

Memory is the ability to encode, store, and recall information. The three main processes involved in human memory are therefore encoding, storage, and recall. Memory impairment after TBI includes a high frequency of forgetting, interference, reduced recall for text, and an inability to use compensatory strategies (Blachstein, Vakil, & Hoofien, 1993; Crosson, Novak, Trenerry, & Craig, 1988; Haut & Shutty, 1992; Millis & Ricker, 1994; Shum, Valentine, & Cutmore, 1999). Not only do survivors of TBI demonstrate memory impairment, they may also have difficulty predicting what they will or will not remember (Kennedy & Nawrocki, 2003; Kennedy & Yorkston, 2000; Shum et al., 1999).

Payne and Ommaya (1997) argue that clinical and experimental studies support the position that there are two memory systems. The most convincing evidence is the clinical picture of patients with bilateral lesions in the hippocampus region and related structures. Patients with these lesions can register information but are unable to retain it. The two memory systems include a short-term memory registration phase and transition into a retention phase. The registration phase lasts only a few seconds. This is based on the shortest period of memory loss prior to an uncomplicated cerebral concussion. The short-term memory registration phase, which lasts approximately 10 seconds, is the time that information may influence behavior but not necessarily enter into a permanent memory phase. The second phase (retention) is the consolidation and laying of these memories into permanent storage. During the second phase, a repeated neural process is set into motion and eventually results in retention (Joynt, 1975).

Disorders of memory are common and persistent sequelae of diffuse TBI (Kennedy & Nawrocki, 2003; Levin, 1985; Levin, Benton, & Grossman, 1982). Deficits in memory occur from focal lesions when there is damage to specific structures of the brain or when there is diffuse cerebral damage (Auerbach, 1986). The most common sites of lesion include the fornix, hippocampus, mammillary bodies of the diencephalon, and the thalamus. Lesions in the frontal limbic system, specifically in the diencephalon, can also produce a disturbance to memory.

The functional consequences of memory impairments may be devastating and can affect the patient on a number of levels. Some include the ability to retrieve information and to recall personal life events, the ability to learn new information, and the ability to complete a schedule of activities (Beukelman & Yorkston, 1991).

Posttraumatic Amnesia

Memory status following a TBI has been described as a time continuum (Beukelman & Yorkston, 1991). Immediately following the onset of severe brain injury, patients may experience a period of coma that is produced by severe depression of central nervous system function. A comatose patient is not able to be roused and is unaware of internal or external stimuli. As the patient emerges from coma and becomes slightly more responsive, a period of disorientation and confusion often occurs. Posttraumatic amnesia has been defined as "the time from the moment of injury to the time of resumption of normal continuous memory" (Lishman, 1978, p. 201). Length of coma and PTA depend on the severity of injury, and both have been correlated with the degree of recovery.

PTA may be short term or can last longer (often over a month), but it is hardly ever permanent. The duration of PTA serves as a prognostic indicator for recovery. After PTA, the patient may recover cognitive function completely; however, some patients who experience a short period of PTA also experience persistent memory problems. After a prolonged period of PTA lasting more than a week, memory disorders may be more severe and persistent (Brooks, 1983).

The time period preceding the injury that the patient is unable to remember is known as retrograde amnesia. Patients with retrograde amnesia experience the loss of memories that were formed shortly before the injury, particularly where there is damage to the frontal or anterior temporal regions. In severe cases of TBI, individuals may present with retrograde amnesia, a loss of memory for events preceding the accident. In some cases the impairment may also affect recall of the events in the remote past. However, these individuals with retrograde amnesia may be able to encode and memorize new things that occurred after the onset of the amnesia. Retrograde amnesias of more than a few minutes are rarely seen with PTA of less than a few days or a week. During recovery, as the retrograde amnesia decreases, remote memories are recovered first and recent memories are recovered last (Joynt, 1975).

In contrast, those with anterograde amnesia (AGA) have problems with creating new memories after the injury has taken place. In some cases, AGA may not develop until several hours after the injury. When continuous memory returns, the person can usually function normally. Those with retrograde amnesia may partially regain memory later, but memories are never regained with AGA because of impaired encoding. New information is processed normally but almost immediately forgotten, never making it into the regions of the brain where long-term memories are stored (Squire, Stark, & Clark, 2004). Individuals with AGA may repeat comments or questions several times, or fail to recognize people they met just minutes before.

AGA may occur following an acute event such as a concussion. It also has been linked to damage to the hippocampus, an area of the brain responsible for long-term memory, or the medial aspects of the temporal lobe, which plays a role in the memory for both visual and auditory events and has been identified as the site of lesion in individuals with retrograde amnesia (Payne & Ommaya, 1997).

Behavioral and Personality Sequelae

Another consequence of TBI is that patients present with many emotional/behavioral problems, including anger, depression, apathy, anxiety, irritability, paranoia, confusion, agitation, frustration, sleep problems, and mood swings. Dennis (2009) reports that behavioral sequelae may include aggression and violence, impulsivity, acting out, noncompliance, social inappropriateness, emotional outbursts, childish behavior, impaired self-control, impaired self-awareness, inability to take responsibility or accept criticism, and alcohol or drug abuse/addiction. In some cases, a patient's personality problems may be so severe that the patient is diagnosed with a personality disorder. Symptoms associated with PTSD may overlap with symptoms of mTBI. Differential diagnosis of brain injury and PTSD is required for correct diagnosis and treatment.

Impaired Executive Functioning

Executive functioning is the cognitive process that regulates an individual's ability to organize thoughts and activities, prioritize tasks, manage time efficiently, and make decisions. This functioning is ascribed to the frontal lobes, and Chapter 6 describes right-hemisphere damage and its role in executive disorders.

Frontal lobe damage from TBI impairs executive functioning as well as working memory and attention. Constantinidou and Kennedy (2013) note that the preponderance of symptoms associated with frontal lobe damage distinguishes TBI from other types of brain injury and conjecture that the lost interconnectedness between the frontal lobes and other, more posterior structures is a hallmark of TBI.

Brooks, Fos, Greve, and Hammond (1999), for example, reported that mTBI patients did not perform as well as controls on tests of auditory serial association and controlled word association. Peach (2013) found, from analyses of sentence patterns of persons with TBI, that microlinguistic impairments of individuals with TBI are associated with variations in the organization and monitoring of language representations in working memory. According to Peach (2013), organization and monitoring of language are key operations of the executive system that facilitates language processing and inhibition of extraneous language representations. Furthermore, an association with pragmatics was explored by Douglas (2010), who reported a significant association between executive impairment and pragmatic disorders.

Rehabilitation of executive functioning, is, therefore, a process of remediation and compensation for functions previously subsumed by more posterior structures. According to Constaninidou and Kennedy (2013), treatment in these areas should form the bases for cognitive rehabilitation.

GENERAL ASSESSMENT— INITIAL STAGES OF RECOVERY

Following a head injury, the individual will go through a recovery period that can vary depending on severity of the initial injury. Initial assessment is initially brief depending upon the medical condition of the patient. During this period, if the patient is regaining consciousness, responses may be inconsistent, disoriented, and disorganized. Behavioral characteristics may include restlessness, irritation, and distractibility (Cavanna, 2010). The initial assessment is typically performed at bedside. As shown in Table 5–7, several commonly used assessment tools during this stage and throughout subsequent stages of recovery are the *Glascow Coma Scale* (GCS: Teasdale & Jennett, 1974) and its related scales, the *Glascow Outcome Scale* (GOS: Jennett & Bond, 1975; Teasdale, Pettigrew, Wilson, Murray, & Jennett, 1998) and the *Glascow Outcome Scale Extended* (GOSE: Wilson et al., 2007; Wilson, Pettigrew, & Teasdale, 1997); the *Galveston Orientation and Amnesia Test* (GOAT: Levin, O'Donnell, & Grossman, 1979); the *Age and Education Corrected Mini-Mental State Examination* (MMSadj; Folstein, Folstein, & McHugh, 1975; Mungas, Marshall, Weldon, Haan, & Reed, 1996); and the *Comprehensive Level of Consciousness Scale* (CLOCS; Stanczak et al., 1984).

Table 5–7. Suggested Tests for Initial Assessment

Assessment	Age	Description	Skills Tested
Age and Education Corrected Mini-Mental State Examination (MMadj)	18–100	Screens for cognitive impairment and/or dementia. Documents changes in intellectual ability over time.	Orientation, registration, attention and calculation, recall, and language. Assesses potential therapy techniques on cognitive function.
Comprehensive Level of Consciousness Scale (CLOCS)	Adult	Assesses the patient's initial status. Includes brainstem indicators and assesses a variety of responses.	Posture, resting eye position, spontaneous eye opening, ocular movements, pupillary reflexes, motor functioning, responsiveness, and communicative effort.
Galveston Orientation and Amnesia Test (GOAT)	All age groups	Designed to assess the extent and duration of confusion and posttraumatic amnesia (PTA).	Measures orientation for person, place, and time.
Glasgow Coma Scale (GCS)	All age groups	Describes all posttraumatic states of unconsciousness.	Eye opening, motor response, and verbal response.

Age and Educated Corrected Mini-Mental Status (MMSadj)

This is a widely used screening test of cognitive function among the elderly and individuals with TBI ranging from 18 to 100 years. Normed on persons from different education levels and ethnicities, the MMSadj is a preferable measure of cognitive impairment for a multicultural, multiethnic population with varying levels of education. Several areas are evaluated, including orientation, attention, calculation, memory (immediate and short-term), language, and visuospatial skills. The test is based on a total of 30 points, with severity ratings ranging from normal (23–30), to borderline (19–23), to impaired (<19). The test can be used to establish a baseline and track recovery following a head injury.

Comprehensive Level of Consciousness Scale (CLOCS)

The CLOCS is used to assess the patient's initial consciousness. Several areas are rated, including posture, resting eye position, spontaneous eye opening, ocular movements, pupillary reflexes, motor functioning, responsiveness, and communicative effort (Roseberry-McKibben & Hegde, 2006).

Galveston Orientation and Amnesia Test (GOAT)

An important indicator of TBI severity is PTA, a period during which memories are not stored following a TBI that prevents new learning. PTA includes the period of coma and extends until the patient's memory for ongoing events becomes accurate, reliable, and consistent (Sohlberg & Mateer, 2001, p. 33). Assessment of memory problems includes evaluation of PTA, which includes three components: disorientation, AGA, and retrograde amnesia (Roseberry-McKibben & Hegde, 2006).

The GOAT is commonly used to determine the relationship between length of PTA and severity of injury. The length of PTA is considered the best predictor of permanent impairment (Sohlberg & Mateer, 2001). It is a brief questionnaire developed to evaluate the progression of cognitive function during the subacute stage of recovery. Three major areas are evaluated, including amnesia, orientation, and memory. The GOAT can be administered daily to obtain self-reported information about orientation to person, place, and time as well as retrograde amnesia (Payne & Ommaya, 1997; Sohlberg & Mateer, 2001). Severity can be rated at one of three levels: normal (76–100), borderline (66–75), and impaired (<66). A score of 78 or more on three consecutive administrations is considered to indicate that the patient no longer is experiencing PTA.

Glasgow Coma Scale (GCS). Glasgow Outcome Scale (GOS), Glasgow Outcome Scale Extended (GOSE)

The severity of injury in trauma patients is correlated with the duration of coma. TBI patients may initially be in a comatose state,

an extended period of unconsciousness. In most cases the greater the injury severity, the longer the duration of coma. The GCS, developed by Teasdale and Jennett (1974), is administered during the initial period of hospitalization as well as throughout recovery to monitor patient improvement.

The GCS provides an objective and reliable measurement of the initial conscious state of the head trauma patient based upon three parameters: eye opening, motor response, and verbal response. A commonly used instrument, it is administered to all trauma patients in first aid, emergency rooms, and intensive care units. Later in subacute care hospitals, it is administered to monitor recovery in chronic patients. Each parameter is rated with the resulting points reported as a composite score (e.g., E4V4M5 = GCS13). Level of brain injury severity is classified as either severe = GCS <9, moderate = GCS 9–12, or minor = GCS ≥13 (CDC, 2003; Teasdale & Jennett, 1974).

The *Glascow Outcome Scale* (GOS: Jennett & Bond, 1975; Teasdale, Pettigrew, Wilson, Murray, & Jennett, 1998) and the *Extended Glascow Outcome Scale* (GOSE: Wilson, Pettigrew, & Teasdale, 1997; Wilson et al., 2007) expand the categories available to clinicians. The GOS has five categories: Dead, Vegetative State, Severe Disability, Moderate Disability, and Good Recovery. The GOSE provides more detail with 8 categories ranging from Death to Upper Good Recovery. The GOSE is accessible at http://www.tbi_impact.org.cde/mod_templates/12_F_01_GOSE. pdf

ASSESSMENT DURING RECOVERY

As soon as the patient is alert and conscious, it will be necessary to assess the patient's recovery. Among the measurements that are appropriate to use are the *Disability Rating Scale* (DRS; Rappoport, Hall, Hopkins, Belleza, & Cope, 1982; Wright, 2000), the *Functional Independence Measure* (FIM; Keith, Granger, Hamilton, & Sherwin, 1987), the *Rancho Los Amigos Scales of Cognitive Levels* (LOCF; Malkamus & Stenderup, 1974), the *Montreal Cognitive Assessment* (MoCA; Nasreddine et al., 2005), and the *JFK Coma Recovery Scale–Revised* (CRS-R; Giacino, Kalmar, & Whyte, 2000).

Disability Rating Scale (DRS)

The DRS is used to evaluate changes in head injury patients during recovery. The DRS was developed specifically for TBI patients and measures level of disability as the patient transitions from coma to community. The total score ranges from 0 to 30. The lower the score, the better the outcome. Eight dimensions of behavior are assessed, including eye opening, verbal responses, motor responses, feeding, toileting/grooming, independence, and employability.

Functional Independence Measure (FIM)

The FIM provides reliable and quantifiable methods for evaluating physical and cognitive recovery in adults with head injury. The FIM has two major components: motor and cognitive. The FIM measures degree of independence in activities of self-care, sphincter control, transfers, locomotion, communication, and cognition. The FIM scores range from 1 (total or >75% assistance) to 7 (complete independence). Total scores range between 18 and 126. Subscores are available for motor and cognitive items. Scores may be used raw or converted to interval scores. The FIM is most useful as a measure of progress during inpatient rehabilitation. It has extensive normative data and excellent psychometric properties. It is most appropriate for severe and moderate disability levels of the *Glasgow Outcome Scale Extended*; ceiling effects limit utility in good recovery. The FIM is not sufficiently sensitive for mTBI.

Areas evaluated in the motor component include feeding, grooming, bathing, dressing, toileting, bladder/bowel management, transfers, and ambulation. The cognitive component includes items to evaluate comprehension, expression, social interaction, problem solving, and memory.

JFK Coma Recovery Scale–Revised (CRS-R)

The CRS-R is a standardized behavioral assessment designed to measure neurobehavioral function in patients with disorders of consciousness. It comprises six subscales designed to assess auditory, visual, motor, oromotor/verbal, communication, and arousal functions. The CRS-R is the only standardized assessment measure that directly incorporates the diagnostic criteria for coma, vegetative state, minimally conscious state, and emerging from a minimally conscious state. The scale is intended for use by medical and allied health professionals. The CRS-R has strong diagnostic sensitivity and specificity, correlates well with functional outcome, is useful for monitoring treatment effectiveness, and is available in nine languages.

Montreal Cognitive Assessment (MoCA)

The MoCA was validated on individuals with mild cognitive impairment. A complete description of this test may be found in Chapter 4. The MoCA is freely accessible to clinicians at http://www.mocatest.com

Ranchos Los Amigos Levels of Cognitive Functioning (LOCF)

The LOCF is a commonly used instrument to assess cognition and behavior of patients as they emerge from coma and to monitor patient recovery (Hagen, 1984). Two versions exist comprising ten levels: no response, generalized response, localized response, confused/agitated, confused/nonagitated, confused/appropriate, automatic/appropriate, and purposeful/appropriate at three levels of independence. The original scale was developed by Hagen, Malkamus, and Durham (1972; 1979) and Hagen (1998) at Ranchos Los Amigos Hospital. A revised comprehensive version (Malkamus & Stenderup, 1974) can be accessed at http://www.northeastcenter.com/ranchos_los_amigos_revised.htm and the third edition by Chris Hagen, Rancho Levels of Cognitive Function-Revised (1998), is available at http://rancho.org/research/cognitive_levels.pdf

OTHER RECOVERY SCALES

Another scale developed to measure the severity of injury is based upon a combination of three factors: GCS score, coma duration, and length of PTA (Sohlberg &

Mateer, 2001). PTA severity ranges from mild (duration <60 minutes) to extremely severe (persisting for >24 hours). PTA extending beyond 7 days indicates the presence of a very severe brain injury.

Monitoring the patient's status is essential during the initial stage of recovery. Sohlberg and Mateer (2001) have proposed the following guide for use during the early recovery period:

1. **Coma:** unresponsive; eyes closed
2. **Vegetative state:** no cognitive responses; gross wakefulness; sleep-wake cycles
3. **Minimally conscious state:** purposeful wakefulness; responds to some commands
4. **Confusional state:** recovered speech; amnesic (PTA); severe attentional deficits; agitated; hypoaroused; possible labile behavior
5. **Postconfusional, evolving independence:** resolution of PTA; cognitive improvement; achieving independence in daily self-care; improving social interaction; developing independence at home
6. **Social competence, community re-entry:** recovering cognitive abilities; goal-directed behaviors; social skills; personality; developing independence in the community; returning to academic or vocational pursuits

PROGNOSTIC INDICATORS

Prognosis is dependent on the nature and extent of the brain injury. Recovery is determined by several factors such as age, history of previous injuries, and overall health. The age of the patient determines the resiliency of the central nervous system.

For example, older age has been well recognized as an independent predictor of worse outcome after TBI, even with relatively minor head injuries (CDC, 2012). The pre-injury status of the brain and extent of other chronic disease entities (e.g., stroke, degenerative disease, chronic alcohol use, presence of cerebral damage from previous head injuries) are important factors to consider in determining the patient's prognosis for recovery. Damage from repeated head injuries is cumulative and can complicate the patient's clinical presentation and recovery of function. If the head injury is severe, the total amount of immediate damage has implications for the degree of loss of consciousness and other focal signs (Payne & Ommaya, 1997, p. 190). Moreover, the additive effects of secondary and intracranial insults to the already damaged brain greatly exacerbate the already compromised nervous system.

The prognostic outlook is based on the severity of the injury. Morris and Marshall (2000) proposed the following guidelines:

- **Mild head injuries:** Usually the prognosis is very good. Although some people experience PTA, this typically goes away after about 3 months. Although improvement may be gradual, in most cases, there is no long-term damage.
- **Moderate head injuries:** The greatest improvement usually occurs within the first 1 to 6 weeks—after which there may be some residual problems in the areas of memory or attention; however, they may not be permanent.
- **Severe head injuries:** Approximately half (50%) of severe head injuries are fatal.

Among the survivors, about 20% suffer severe disabilities.

Prognosis is typically good with treatment; however, a persistent mutism following the initial recovery period may suggest a relatively poor prognosis. The duration of PTA is another factor that influences prognosis. The longer the period of PTA, the poorer the individual's prognosis for a complete recovery.

ASSESSMENT OF COMMUNICATIVE-COGNITIVE FUNCTIONING

Assessment of individuals following a head injury requires careful consideration of information gathered from a variety of sources. Each patient must be examined carefully to determine the specific diagnosis and extent of cognitive and language impairments that need to be targeted in further testing and rehabilitation. Comprehensive assessment of the TBI patient includes several components: case history, patient observation, and family interview, as well as assessment with standardized and/or nonstandardized client-specific measures. Information gathered from these sources is used to determine the patient's prognosis (i.e., potential for recovery with treatment and the most efficacious treatment approach utilizing evidence-based treatment). Another important component is patient monitoring to determine treatment effectiveness (American Speech-Language-Hearing Association, 2004; Turkstra et al., 2005).

Case History

The purpose of the case history is to begin the data collection process. The case history must be comprehensive and serve to organize the interviews of the patient and family and other caregivers. Some of the information obtained during this process is the patient's medical status, education, vocation, and socioeconomic, cultural, and linguistic backgrounds (Hegde, 2008). Case history intake is discussed in detail in Chapters 4 and 6.

Patient Observation

Critical information about the level of functioning is ascertained during preliminary observations of the patient (e.g., level of alertness and responsiveness), including, if bilingual, whether there are differential language skills in the two languages. Other initial observations should include the presence of hemiplegia or paresis, sensory impairments (visual and hearing), and ability to follow simple commands.

Family Interview

The family interview provides critical information and can be particularly helpful to a clinician who is working with an adult from a diverse cultural or linguistic community. It is important to assess the family's language and communication patterns (e.g., language preference, communication style, availability of communication partners). When unsure of the language or cognitive features observed, the speech-language pathologist should consult with members of the patient's community (see Chapter 2 for the Culturally and Linguistically Appropriate Services Standards). It is also important to request information during the family interview about the patient's pre-injury status, including education, literacy skills,

occupation, hobbies, and interests. If the patient is seen in the home environment, other observations can be made, including identification of possible safety hazards, like unsecured rugs, the adequacy of lighting to ensure optimum communication and possible distractors that limit the patient's communication and cognitive functioning. This information will be useful in planning treatment.

Neuroimaging Reports

Neuroimaging techniques continue to advance as technology is improved within the medical field. Research in the area of neurogenic communication disorders is making strides to keep up with the latest advances in TBI research. Functional magnetic resonance imaging (fMRI) provides helpful information on the structural changes of the brain after injury. However, Yeh, Oakes, and Riedy (2012) pointed out that fMRI and other imaging techniques, such as computed tomography, have not been able to identify structural changes that occur with mTBI. Neuroimaging of moderate and severe TBI is typically illustrated by petechial hemorrhage and small speckled lesions from traumatic microbleeds of shearing capillaries as well as clinical signs of LOC. This damage is representative of axonal injury, i.e., DAI, secondary to trauma. There is currently no standardized way of assessing the severity of DAI in TBI patients, and conventional neuroimaging findings have not been able to fully assess its severity, functional deficits, or long-term outcomes (Yeh et al., 2012).

In more recent years, a new type of diffused fMRI has been developed, called diffusion tensor imaging (DTI). Aoki, Inokuchi, Gunshin, Yahagi, and

Suwa (2012) consider DTI to be a potential biomarker in mTBI patients because of its ability to detect white matter microstructure changes. One form of measurement used in DTI is fractional anisotropy (FA), which quantifies the orientation and integrity of white matter tracts. Decreased FA may indicate axonal degradation and discontinuities with excess water between tracts or in perivascular spaces, which also occurs in mTBI. Aoki and colleagues (2012) reviewed studies that focused on the corpus callosum, the largest white matter structure in the brain. The corpus callosum is identified as an area that consistently experiences deformation and decreased FA and can be identified in DTI studies. Whole-brain analysis is useful to investigate overall white matter changes rather than analyzing specific tracts or areas. The researchers concluded that reduced FA indicates differences in cellular membrane integrity, fiber myelination, fiber diameter, and directionality in the corpus callosum after TBI. The meta-analysis revealed that there are age-related changes with FA. These changes appear to increase during childhood and adolescence, peak around age 30, and then gradually decrease after age 30. External trauma such as TBI may accelerate loss of FA in adults. The studies reviewed by Aoki and colleagues (2012) did not include those with mental health disorders, which is a population that should be included in future DTI studies considering the large number of service members with concurrent mTBI and PTSD.

Niogi and associates (2008) inquired whether impairments that result from mTBI are categorized or if the severity of cognitive deficits is dependent on the extent of white matter damage. It was hypothesized that damage to the white matter pathways predicts dysfunction in the corresponding cognitive domains. The regions of the frontal lobe that were examined include the uncinate fasciculus (UF), the superior longitudinal fasciculus, and the genu of the corpus callosum. The right UF was found to be statistically correlated with memory. While the left UF did not have statistical significance, there was a trend for memory, therefore the UF has bilateral association with memory performance. The findings of this study were attributed to the UF's predisposition to rotational shear injury. Findings such as these assist in validating DTI in its ability to diagnose cognitive impairment in mTBI (Niogi et al., 2008).

The most recent technological advance in neuroimaging for brain injury is called susceptibility weighted imaging (SWI). SWI picks up on damage to axons and small blood vessels in the form of cerebral microbleeding. This can present as bleeding, severe reductions in deoxyhemoglobin, impaired neural vascular tone, or reduced blood flow and blood volume. SWI can identify hemorrhaging, thrombosis, and loss of local oxygen saturation in the medullary and pial veins in the brain. This type of venous damage may be seen in mTBI and may explain why patients whose brains appear unaffected on other types of imaging demonstrate neurocognitive problems (Haacke, 2013).

COGNITIVE ASSESSMENT MEASURES

Cognitive assessment is often shared by the speech-language pathologist and the neuropsychologist. The following is a list of assessment measures useful for evaluation of cognitive disorders in individuals with TBI. These assessment measures are shown in Table 5–8.

Table 5–8. Suggested Tests of Cognitive Abilities

Assessment	Age	Description	Skills Tested
Behavior Rating Inventory of Executive Function	18–90	Assess executive functioning. Useful for evaluating and planning treatment strategies.	Behavioral regulation, metacognition, global executive functions.
Behavioural Assessment of the Dysexecutive Syndrome	16–87	Assesses everyday life skills.	Temporal judgment, thought flexibility, problem solving, strategy formation, and planning.
Brief Symptom Inventory	18 and older	Provides a brief self-report measure of psychological distress.	Depression, anxiety, and somatization.
Comprehensive Assessment of Prospective Memory	Young and Older Adults	Designed to measure specific, everyday prospective memory lapses. A self-rating scale.	Perceived frequency of failure related to basic ADLs and IADLs, concerns about failures, reasons associated with successes/failures.
Craig Handicap Assess & Rep Tech	Adults	Objectively measures the degree to which impairments and disabilities impact participation.	Physical independence, cognitive independence, mobility, occupation, social integration, and economic self-sufficiency.
Delis-Kaplan Executive Function System	8–89	Standardized set of tests to evaluate higher level cognitive functions in children and adults.	Comprehensively assesses the components of executive functions mediated primarily by the frontal lobe.
Doors and People	5:1–Adult	A test of long-term explicit memory.	Visual recognition, visual recall, verbal recognition, and verbal recall.
Dysexecutive Questionnaire		Designed to sample everyday problems commonly associated with frontal system dysfunction.	Emotion, motivation, behavior, and cognition. Can be used to validate the BADS.
The Montreal Cognitive Assessment	Adults	A rapid screening instrument for mild cognitive dysfunction.	Attention and concentration, executive functions, memory, language, visuoconstructional skills, conceptual thinking, calculations, and orientation.

continues

Table 5–8. *continued*

Assessment	Age	Description	Skills Tested
Multiple Errands Test—Simplified Version and Hospital Version		Developed to assess the role of executive impairments in the context of everyday functioning.	Designed for people who performed within or above the normal range when tested using existing psychometric measures.
Prospective Memory Training Screening		Samples prospective memory involving responses to both time and event cues.	Attention and executive functions relevant to everyday memory demands.
Rey Auditory Verbal Learning Test	8–85+	Assesses word list learning.	Immediate recall, delayed recall, and recognition.
Rivermead Behavioural Memory Test	11–94	Identifies impairments of everyday memory functioning and monitors change following treatment for memory difficulties.	Memory for first and last names, remembering belongings, remembering appointments, picture recognition, face recognition, immediate and delayed recall (story, routes, messages), and orientation and date.
Rivermead Post Concussive Symptom Questionnaire		Measures the presence and severity of postconcussive symptoms.	Compares current symptoms with preinjury levels.
Speed and Capacity of Language Processing	16–65	A measure cognitive processing speed experienced by individuals with TBI.	Language processing.
Stroop Color and Word Test	5–90	A measure of selective attention and cognitive flexibility.	Cognitive flexibility, resistance to interference from outside stimuli, creativity, and psychopathology.
Test of Everyday Attention	18–80	Measures clinical and theoretical aspects of attention.	Selective attention, sustained attention, attentional switching, attentional switching, and divided attention.

Table 5–8. *continued*

Assessment	Age	Description	Skills Tested
Trail Making Test	15–89	Assesses cognitive impairment associated with TBI.	Assesses attention, speed, and mental flexibility, spatial organization, visual pursuits, recall, and recognition.
Wechsler Adult Intelligence Scale	16–89	Derived from the Digit Symbol Coding and Symbol Search subtests of the WAIS III.	Processing time, processing capacity.
Woodcock-Johnson-III	2–90	Assesses academic achievement in children and adults.	Short-term memory, long-term retrieval, processing speed, auditory processing, visual processing, comprehension-knowledge, fluid reasoning, visual/auditory learning, concept formation, and analysis-synthesis.

ADLs = activities of daily living; *IADLs* = instrumental ADLs.

Behavior Rating Inventory of Executive Function–Adult (BRIEF-A)

The BRIEF-A (Gioia, Isquith, Guy, & Kenworthy, 2000) is used to assess executive functioning in adults up to 90 years of age. Results are useful for evaluating and planning treatment strategies for a wide spectrum of developmental and acquired neurological conditions, including, attention deficit hyperactivity disorder, Tourette's disorder, TBI, and autism. It is suitable for individuals with diagnosed of developmental, systemic, neurological, or psychiatric disorders. The eight non-overlapping clinical scales form two broader indexes: Behavioral Regulation (three scales) and Metacognition (five scales). A Global Executive Composite score is also produced.

Behavioural Assessment of the Dysexecutive Syndrome (BADS)

The BADS (Wilson, Alderman, Burgess, Emslie, & Evans, 2003) specifically assesses the skills and demands involved in everyday life. It is sensitive to the capacities affected by frontal lobe damage, emphasizing those usually exercised in everyday situations, such as temporal judgment, thought flexibility, problem solving, strategy formation, and planning.

Brief Symptom Inventory (BSI-18)

The BSI-18 (Derogatis, 2001) is designed to provide a brief self-report measure of psychological distress and has three subscales (Depression, Anxiety, and Somatization), as well as a Global Severity Index. The self-report measure consists of 18 items rated on a 5-point scale and can be completed manually or by computerized administration. The BSI-18 provides a brief global assessment of common psychological issues in individuals with TBI and has sound psychometric characteristics. It can be used for initial assessment, as well as to monitor change in response to treatment.

California Verbal Learning Test (CVLT)

The CVLT (Delis, Kramer, Kaplan, & Ober, 2000) is similar to the RAVLT, and studies have shown high correlations of performances between the two tests for persons with TBI.

Comprehensive Assessment of Prospective Memory (CAPM)

The CAPM (Shum & Fleming, 2008) is a self-rating scale, designed to measure specific, everyday prospective memory lapses. The CAPM has three sections. Section A contains 39 items examining perceived frequency of failure. It contains two statistically derived components: basic activities of daily living and instrumental activities of daily living. Section B uses the same 39 items from Section A to assess concerns about failures. Section C contains 15 items focusing on reasons associated with successes/failures. The CAPM was originally developed for older people but has also been used with young people and people with TBI.

Craig Handicap and Assessment Reporting Technique (CHART-SF)

The CHART-SF (Whiteneck, Charlifue, Gerhart, Overholser, & Richardson, 1992; Whiteneck et al. 2011) is an easily administered tool developed as an objective measure of the degree to which impairments and disabilities impact participation. It consists of 19 items categorized into six subscales: Physical Independence, Cognitive Independence, Mobility, Occupation, Social Integration, and Economic Self Sufficiency. Each subscale has a maximum score of 100, corresponding to the level of performance typical for a person without a disability. Subscale scores can be added to obtain a total score (max = 600). It is best used with adults with moderate to severe disability and those who make a good recovery. It has demonstrated good reliability and validity in the TBI population.

Delis-Kaplan Executive Function System (D–KEFS™)

The D-KEFS (Delis, Kaplan, & Kramer, 2001) is a standardized set of tests to evaluate higher level cognitive functions in children and adults. It consists of nine stand-alone tests, comprehensively assessing the components of executive functions mediated primarily by the frontal lobe.

Doors and People

Doors and People (Nimmo-Smith, Emslie, & Baddeley, 2006) is a broad-based test of long-term explicit memory. It yields a single age-scaled overall score with separate measures available for visual and verbal memory, recall and recognition, and forgetting. It is designed for use both as a clinical tool and as a research instrument. The test has four subcomponents: visual recognition, visual recall, verbal recognition, and verbal recall. Factor analysis of an age-stratified sample of 238 normal subjects indicated a strong general memory factor, followed by a weaker visual/verbal factor. Studies indicate that the test is sensitive across a wide range of abilities, from elderly patients with Alzheimer's disease of low educational level to younger, graduate students.

Dysexecutive Questionnaire (DEX)

The DEX (Wilson, Alderman, Burgess, Emslie, & Evans, 1996) is a rating scale designed to sample everyday problems commonly associated with frontal system dysfunction. The DEX was used as a validation tool for BADS, although it is not a formal part of the BADS. The DEX can also be used as a measure of awareness, by calculating the discrepancy score between self and informant responses. The DEX comprises 20 items sampling four domains: emotional, motivational, behavioral, and cognitive.

Multiple Errands Test– Simplified Version (MET-SV) and Multiple Errands Test– Hospital Version (MET-HV)

The MET-SV (Shallice & Burgess, 1991) was developed to reflect how executive impairments are manifested in the context of everyday functioning. It was designed for people who performed

within or above the normal range when tested using existing psychometric measures. The procedures were administered and subjects tested in a public place. The Multiple Errands Test-Hospital Version (MET-HV: Knight, Alderman, & Burgess, 2002) is a shortened form of the MET-SV.

Prospective Memory Training Screening (PROMS)

The PROMS (Sohlberg & Mateer, 1989) samples prospective memory involving responses to both time and event cues. Prospective memory has been shown to relate to attention and to various other executive functions, especially relevant to everyday memory demands. A modification of this test was developed by Raskin and Buckheit (1998), includes a larger number of tasks, and provides a system for scoring different types of errors.

Repeatable Battery for the Assessment of Neuropsychological Status (RBANS)

The RBANS (Randolph, 1998) is a brief neurocognitive battery designed to detect and track declining neurocognitive deficits in dementia and other disorders. It is comprised of four alternate forms, that measure immediate and delayed memory, attention, language, and visuospatial skills.

Rey Auditory Verbal Learning Test (RAVLT)

A word list learning task that takes approximately 10 minutes to administer, the RAVLT (Strauss, Sherman, & Spreen, 2006) can be administered to individuals ranging in age between 7 and 85+ years. The RAVLT is one of the most extensively studied neuropsychological performance measures and consists of 15 unrelated words repeated five times with recall after each presentation. The test requires immediate recall and delayed recall and recognition. The instrument has extensive normative data and meta-norms and good psychometric properties and has been used in different languages, cultures, and ethnic groups.

Rivermead Behavioural Memory Test–Third Edition (RBMT-3)

The purpose of the RBMT and the RBMT-3 (Wilson, Cockburn, & Baddeley, 1985; Wilson et al., 2008) is to identify impairment of everyday memory functioning and to monitor change following treatment for memory difficulties. The test was initially standardized in the United Kingdom on a sample of brain-damaged patients and a sample of 118 healthy subjects aged 16 to 69 years with a mean IQ of 106. The RBMT has also been standardized with the elderly, aged 70 years and over, with healthy adolescents aged 11 to 14 years, and with children aged 5 to 10 years.

Rivermead Post Concussive Symptom Questionnaire (RPQ)

The RPQ (King, Crawford, Wenden, Moss, & Wade, 1995) is a 16-item self-report measure of the presence and severity of the 16 most commonly reported post concussive symptoms found in the literature. The scale compares current symp-

toms with pre-injury levels to account for potential symptom exacerbation due to TBI. The range of scores is 0 to 64, with values for each of the 16 items rated 0 (not experienced at all), 1 (no more of a problem than before the injury), 2 (mild problem), 3 (moderate problem), and 4 (severe problem). The total score is a summation of symptoms rated as >2, indicating postconcussion symptoms or an exacerbation of a symptom present pre-injury. It requires 5 to 10 minutes to complete. It is useful in assessing postconcussion symptoms in persons with mild to moderate TBI. The RPQ can be used for diagnostic and severity purposes, as well as to monitor change in response to treatment. The RPG is in public domain and is a widely used measure.

Speed and Capacity of Language Processing (SCOLP)

The SCOLP (Baddeley, Emslie, & Nimmo-Smith, 1992) is a measure of the slowing in cognitive processes often reported by individuals with TBI. It can be used to distinguish between individuals who have always been slow and individuals whose performance reflects impairment as a result of brain damage or some other stressor. It is sensitive to the effects of TBI, normal aging, Alzheimer's disease, schizophrenia, and to a wide range of drugs and stressors, including alcohol.

Stroop Color and Word Test

The Stroop test and the Western Stroop Color and Word Test (Golden, 1978; Golden & Freshwater, 2002) measures the Stroop effect, first described by Stroop in 1935, which shows how one area of the brain can dominate and inhibit other functional areas. The cognitive dimension measured is associated with cognitive flexibility, resistance to interference from outside stimuli, creativity, and psychopathology, all of which influence the individual's ability to cope with cognitive stress and to process complex input.

Test of Everyday Attention (TEA)

The TEA (Robertson, Ward, Ridgeway, & Nimmo-Smith, 1994) gives a broad-based measure of the most important clinical and theoretical aspects of attention. The TEA can be used analytically to identify different patterns of attentional breakdown. Originally standardized on 154 normal volunteers in Australia, ranging in age from 18 to 80, stratified into four age groups and two levels of educational attainment; in addition, 80 unilateral stroke patients were given TEA 2 months after a cardiovascular accident. The test has been validated successfully with closed head injury patients, stroke patients, and patients with Alzheimer's disease, including those of low educational level.

Trail Making Test (TMT)

The TMT (Reitan & Wolfson, 1985) is designed to evaluate attention, speed, and mental flexibility and is sensitive to cognitive impairment associated with TBI. It is a brief test with good reliability. Available in adult and child forms and demographically adjusted normative data are available for ages 20 to 85 years. Practice effects are found over short retest intervals but disappear after several administrations, and only modest change is seen among

healthy adults after longer intervals. Performance on TMT declines with aging.

Wechsler Adult Intelligence Scale Processing Speed Index (WAISPSI)

This index (Wechsler, 2008) is derived from the Digit Symbol Coding and Symbol Search subtests of the Wechsler Adult Intelligence Scale (WAIS III). This measure represents the amount of time it takes to process a set amount of information, or the amount of information that can be processed within a certain unit of time. As part of the WAIS, it has extensive normative data and excellent psychometric properties. It is clinically one of the most sensitive cognitive measures to neurologic conditions. It is culturally, racially, and ethnically sensitive.

Woodcock-Johnson-III (WJ-III)

The WJ-III (Woodcock, McGrew, & Mather, 2001) consists of 7 cognitive tests and 11 achievement tests that measure general intellectual ability and specific cognitive abilities; including short-term memory, long-term retrieval, processing speed, auditory processing, visual processing, comprehension-knowledge, and fluid reasoning. In addition, a few subtests evaluate performance in a controlled-learning context: visual/auditory learning, concept formation, and analysis-synthesis. Normative data are available for ages 2 through 90+ and have been used extensively in the educational model for evaluating students of all ages with learning disabilities, including those with acquired TBI. In a study of the relationship of the Automated Neuropsychological Assessment Metrics and the WJ-III, Jones, Loe,

Krach, Rager, and Jones (2008) demonstrated a strong relationship between these measures of cognitive function.

Table 5–9 gives the suggested assessments for cognitive functioning.

COGNITIVE-COMMUNICATION MEASURES

Cognitive-communication impairments are among the most common sequelae of TBI. Deficits in attention, orientation, memory, organization, reasoning, and problem solving can limit a patient's ability to integrate into society and return to pre-injury educational, social, and vocational activities. As part of the interdisciplinary rehabilitation team, speech-language pathologists assess and treat the cognitive-communication deficits of individuals with TBI. Following are brief descriptions of some of the tests that can be used with this population. Readers may also access survey results from speech-language pathologists on assessments provided by the Academy of Neurologic Communication Disorders and Sciences at http://www.ancds.org/pdf/CogComTable_SLP_survey_results.pdf

The American Speech-Language-Hearing Association Functional Assessment of Communication Skills (ASHA-FACS)

The ASHA-FACS (Frattali, Thompson, Holland, Wohl, & Ferketic, 1995) is a questionnaire that was designed to assess functional communication behaviors at the level of disability. It was standardized on a group of 54 individuals with cognitive-communication impairments from mild, moderate, and severe TBI. The overall score from the FACS is significantly correlated with other cognitive tests like the LOCF but contributes unique variance attributable to factors in daily living not captured by other standardized measures. The ASHA-FACS and other measurements of functional communication are described in Chapter 6.

Table 5–9. Suggested Tests of Cognitive-Communication Abilities

Assessment	Age	Description	Skills Tested
American Speech-Language-Hearing Association Functional Assessment of Communication Abilities for Adults (ASHA-FACS)	16–Adult	Assesses functional communication of adults with speech, language, and cognitive communication disorders resulting from left hemisphere stroke or TBI.	Social communication, communication of basic needs, reading, writing, number concepts, and daily planning.
Boston Naming Test-2 (BNT-2; Kaplan, Goodglass, & Weintraub, 2001)	Adult	60-item test of line drawings.	Assesses visual confrontational naming abilities.

Table 5–9. *continued*

Assessment	Age	Description	Skills Tested
Brief Test of Head Injury (BTHI; Helm-Estabrooks & Holz, 1991)	14–59+	Evaluates cognitive, linguistic and communication abilities in children, adolescents, and adults with severe head injury.	Orientation/attention, following commands, linguistic organization, reading comprehension, naming memory, and visual-spatial skills.
Burns Brief Inventory of Cognition and Language (Burns Inventory; Burns, 1997)	Adult	Neuropathological subtest.	See Table 4–3.
California Verbal Learning Test (CVLT-Second Edition, Adult Version; Delis, Kramer, Kaplan, & Ober, 2000)	16–89	Assesses word list learning. Similar to RAVLT.	Verbal memory: recall and recognition of word lists over immediate and delayed memory trials.
Cognitive-Linguistic Quick Test (CLQT; Helm-Estabrooks, 2001)	Adult	Screening assessment.	Evaluates cognition in 5 domains: attention, language, executive functions, and visuospatial skills.
The Discourse Comprehension Test (DCT; Brookshire & Nichols, 1993)	Adults	Assesses narrative comprehension.	Comprehension for explicit (stated or implied) and salient (main ideas and details) information.
Functional Assessment of Verbal Reasoning and Executive Strategies (FAVRES; MacDonald, 2005)	Adult	Simulates real-life situations.	Measures verbal reasoning, comprehension, discourse, and executive skills.

continues

Table 5–9. *continued*

Assessment	Age	Description	Skills Tested
Functional Linguistic Communication Inventory (FLCI; Bayles & Tomoeda, 1995)	Adult	Evaluates functional communication.	Greeting and naming, answering questions, writing, sign comprehension, object-to-picture matching, word reading and comprehension, following commands, pantomime, gesture, and conversation
LaTrobe Communication Questionnaire (LCQ; Douglas, O'Flaherty, & Snow, 2000; Douglas, Bracey & Snow, 2007)	13–64	Measures perceived cognitive-communication ability in adults after severe TBI.	Individual's self-perceptions and perceptions of others.
Measure of Cognitive Linguistic Abilities (MCLA; Ellmo, Graser, Krchnavek, Calabrese, & Hauck, 1995)	Adolescents & Adults	Provides a systematic evaluation of clients who have mild to moderate impairments caused by TBI. Identifies cognitive deficits that impact linguistic performance.	Measures linguistic abilities.
Pragmatics Rating Scale (PRS; MacLennan, Cornis-Pop, Picon-Nieto, & Sigford, 2002)	Adult	Pragmatic communication scale.	Measures nonverbal, verbal, and interactional aspects of communication.
Ross Information Processing Assessment-2 (RIPA-2; Ross-Swain, 1996)	15–90	Assesses cognitive-linguistic functioning in individuals with TBI.	Immediate memory, temporal orientation, spatial orientation, orientation to environment, recall of general information, problem solving and abstract reasoning, organization, auditory processing, and retention.
Scales of Cognitive Ability in Traumatic Brain Injury (SCATBI; Adamovich & Henderson, 1992)	Adolescents & adults	A comprehensive standardized test of cognitive abilities for use with head-injured patients.	Perception/discrimination, orientation, organization, recall, and reasoning.

Boston Naming Test–2 (BNT-2)

The BNT-2 (Kaplan, Goodglass, & Weintraub, 2001) consists of 60 black and white line drawings of objects, and it measures confrontation naming. This type of picture-naming vocabulary test is useful in the evaluation of adults with brain injury.

The Brief Test of Head Injury (BTHI)

The BTHI (Helm-Estabrooks & Holz, 1991) is designed for individuals ranging in age from 10 to 59 and older. The test probes cognitive, linguistic, and communicative abilities of patients with severe head trauma. It provides useful diagnostic information for immediate treatment and a baseline for charting recovery. Areas evaluated include Orientation and Attention, Following Commands, Linguistic Organization, Reading Comprehension, Naming, Memory, and Visual-Spatial Skills.

The Burns Brief Inventory of Communication and Cognition

The Burns (1997) Brief Inventory consists of three inventories: (a) Right Hemisphere, (b) Left Hemisphere, and (c) Complex Neuropathology. The third inventory is designed to assess the cognitive skills of individuals with neurological problems due to head injury. The standardization sample of the Burns Inventory comprised 333 individuals ranging in age from 18 to 80 years. English was the primary language spoken. Participants in the normative sample were diagnosed as having neurological damage due to head injury with an absence of dementia. All participants were from the Midwest and represented non-Hispanic whites ($n = 255$), African Americans ($n = 39$), and Hispanics ($n = 10$).

California Verbal Learning Test (CLVT-2, Adult Version)

The CLVT-2 (Delis, Kramer, Kaplan, & Ober, 2000) assesses verbal memory, retention and retrieval over immediate and delayed memory trials.

Cognitive-Linguistic Quick Test (CLQT)

The CLQT (Helm-Estabrooks, 2001) is a screening tool for use with individuals ages 18 to 89 and is designed to evaluate cognition in five domains: attention, memory, language, executive functions, and visuospatial skills. This CLQT version consists of two subtests: Symbol Cancellation and Clock Drawing. Symbol Cancellation is a nonlinguistic task that assesses visual attention, scanning, and visual discrimination. Clock Drawing is a commonly used screening tool for neurological dysfunction. The complete test battery provides a standardized scoring system for use in analysis of language, visuospatial planning skills, and conceptualization of time. The CLQT was normed on 171 nonclinical cases and 38 clinical cases, including TBI. It establishes criterion-referenced cutoff scores within each task and severity ratings based on the distribution of scores of the clinical and nonclinical subjects.

The Discourse Comprehension Test (DCT)

The DCT (Brookshire & Nicholas, 1993) is a test of narrative comprehension. Individuals listen or read narratives and answer yes/no questions that tap comprehension for explicit (stated or implied) and salient (main ideas and details) information.

The Functional Assessment of Verbal Reasoning and Executive Strategies (FAVRES)

The FAVRES (MacDonald, 2005) was developed to assess verbal reasoning, complex comprehension, discourse, and executive functioning with functional tasks that challenge even those with subtle cognitive-communication disorders. The test requires processing of "real life" amounts of verbal information, analysis of multiple facts and goals, integration of a variety of types of stimuli, and formulation of written and oral responses. Its strength is its ecological validity in that tasks simulate real-world communications and incorporate context using natural settings, roles, and conversation. It is standardized on healthy controls and individuals with brain injury, ages 18 to 79.

Functional Linguistic Communication Inventory (FLCI)

The FLCI (Bayles & Tomoeda, 1995) measures domains in functional and pragmatic skills. This instrument allows for developing therapy goals. Areas tested are greeting/naming, answering questions, writing, comprehension of signs/pictures, following commands, conversation, reminiscing, gesture/pantomime, and word reading/comprehension.

LaTrobe Communication Questionnaire (LCQ)

The LCQ (Douglas, O'Flaherty, & Snow 2000; Douglas, Bracey, & Snow, 2007) is a 30-item questionnaire that measures perceived cognitive-communication ability in adults after severe TBI. Information is collected from different sources, including the individual's self-perceptions and perceptions of others. Content and test-retest reliability and discriminant validity of the LCQ have been demonstrated with adults following TBI. The questionnaire has been shown to be sensitive to the effect of severity of injury.

Measure of Cognitive Linguistic Abilities (MCLA)

The MCLA (Ellmo, Graser, Krchnavek, Calabrese, & Hauck, 1995) is designed to provide a systematic evaluation of clients who have mild to moderate impairments caused by TBI. The MCLA has three major purposes: to assess linguistic abilities, to help identify cognitive deficits that have an impact on linguistic performance, and to recognize the important interrelationship between cognition and language. The test was standardized on 204 healthy, English-speaking adults ages 16 to 50 with no history of TBI or other neurologic disorder.

Pragmatics Rating Scale (PRS)

The PRS (MacLennan, Cornis-Pop, Picon-Nieto, & Sigford, 2002) is a pragmatic communication scale established and based on assessments of 144 subjects with TBI. The assessment is based on a rating scale of pragmatic behaviors developed for the Defense and Veterans Brain Injury Center. The scale measures nonverbal, verbal, and interactional aspects of communication, based on samples of conversation, narrative discourse, and procedural discourse.

Ross Information Processing Assessment-2 (RIPA-2)

The RIPA-2 (Ross-Swain, 1996) is one of the most commonly used tests for assessment of cognitive-linguistic functioning of individuals with TBI. It is standardized on a sample of 126 persons with TBI between 15 and 77 years of age from nine states, representative of TBI cases relative to gender, area of residency, geographic area, and ethnic background as described in TBI literature relative to demographic information. The RIPA-2 quantifies cognitive-linguistic deficits, determines severity levels for each skill area, and develops rehabilitation goals and objectives. Ten key areas basic to communicative and cognitive functioning are tested: Immediate Memory, Recent Memory, Temporal Orientation (Recent Memory), Temporal Orientation (Remote Memory), Spatial Orientation, Orientation to Environment, Recall of General Information, Problem Solving and Abstract Reasoning, Organization, and Auditory Processing and Retention.

Scales of Cognitive Ability for Traumatic Brain Injury (SCATBI)

The SCATBI (Adamovich & Henderson, 1992) provides a systematic method for assessing cognitive deficits associated with TBI. The normative sample included 244 patients with TBI from 26 sites in the United States and Canada. The sample primarily included patients who suffered closed head injuries.

LANGUAGE TESTS

Although many language deficits may resolve after TBI (Groher, 1977), others (LeBlanc, DeGuise, Feyz, & Lamou-reux, 2006) found that education and TBI severity as measured by GCS scores are predictive of language disorders in the acute care setting. Safaz, Yasar, Tok, and Yilmaz (2008) found that among 116 persons with TBI, 19% had aphasia, 30.2% had dysarthria, and 17.2% demonstrated dysphagia. Speech-language pathologists should, therefore, test for language competence during the recovery period and/or when the patient has: (1) a history of previous stroke, (2) complications from penetrating injuries in addition to blast or blunt force trauma, (3) a severe TBI, or (4) a history of repeated head injuries. A full description of the tests of aphasia may be found in Chapter 6.

GLOBAL MEASURES

Global measures provide additional information about the patient's perception of disability and how well the patient is coping with the physical and cognitive-communication changes since the TBI. Below are suggested global measures that are available.

Awareness Questionnaire (AQ)

Developed as a measure of impaired self-awareness after TBI, the AQ (Sherer, 2004) consists of three forms to be completed by the individual with TBI, a family member or significant other, and a clinician. Results of standardized tests provide valuable information critical for development of an effective treatment plan. Assessment is an ongoing component of the treatment process and helps determine specific areas to target with the goal of helping patients improve their cognitive and communication status to aid in reintegration into society and the workforce.

Community Integration Questionnaire (CIQ)

The CIQ (Dijkers, 2000) provides a measure of community integration after TBI that could be used in the TBI Model Systems program. Designed to be brief, it is administered in person or by telephone interview and is conducted with the person with TBI or with a proxy. The focus is on behaviors rather than feeling states, is without biases for age, gender, or socioeconomic status, is sensitive to a variety of living situations, and is value neutral. The CIQ consists of 15 items relevant to home integration, social integration, and productive activities. Subtotals are calculated for each of these domains as well as for community integration overall.

Mayo-Portland Adaptability Inventory, fourth edition (MPAI-4)

This 30-item inventory (Malec et al., 2003; Malec, 2004) is rated on a 5-point scale ranging from normal for age to severely restricted. Items selected represent key indicators in three interrelated subdomains represented by three subscales: Ability Index (physical and cognitive abilities), Adjustment Index (emotional and behavioral self-regulation, interpersonal activities), and Participation Index (community integration). An overall score and scores for each index may be obtained. Specified modifications to the rating scales allow the measure to be applied across the age span from children to adults.

Participation Assessment with Recombined Tools– Objective (PART-O)

This is a measure (Whiteneck et al., 2011) of community participation developed by the Traumatic Brain Injury Model Systems (TBIMS) that combines several primary measures found in the TBI literature (CIQ, original and revised; POPS; and CHART). The 24-item PART-O is an acceptable measure of objective participation for persons with moderate and severe TBI. It has been adopted as the measure of participation in the TBIMS.

Participation Objective/ Participation Subjective (POPS)

The POPS (Brown, 2006) consists of a list of 26 items designed to assess elements of participation (for example., going to the movies, housework, opportunities to meet new people). Two types of questions are presented: objective questions and subjective questions. The 26 items are sorted into five categories: Domestic Life, Major Life Activities, Transportation, Interpersonal Interactions and Relationships, and Community, Recreational, and Civic Life. The test was designed with the TBI population in mind but the items refer to normative activities.

Quality of Life After Brain Injury (QOLIBRI)

Developed as a disease-specific health-related quality of life tool, the QOLIBRI (Von Steinbuechel et al., 2010) is designed as a multidimensional instrument that contains 37 items on four satisfaction scales: cognition, self, daily life and autonomy, and relationships. Two additional scales assess emotions and physical problems. Responses on all scales yield a total score. There is an additional overall scale available with six items that can be used for screening purposes. Percent scores are available for the six subscales (with

100% indicating best quality of life) and one total score. Higher scores on all scales indicate higher health-related quality of life after TBI. The questionnaire is validated in German, Finnish, Italian, French, English, and Dutch and requires just 15 minutes to complete. Validation in eight additional countries is in progress. (Computer Adaptive Test [CAT] in preparation. http://www.qolibri-international.com)

Satisfaction With Life Scale (SWLS)

This assessment is a five-item self-reporting global measure of life satisfaction. The SWLS (Diener, Emmons, Larsen, & Griffin, 1985) has shown consistent differences between populations that would be expected to have different qualities of life (e.g., psychiatric patients, male prison inmates). The SWLS has been found to change in the expected directions in response to major life events and in patients receiving psychotherapy.

World Health Organization Quality of Life BRIEF Assessment (WHOQOL-BRIEF)

This assessment instrument (WHO, 1993; Murphy, Herrman, Hawthorne, Pinzone, & Evert, 2000) was developed as an international cross-culturally comparable quality of life assessment. It assesses individuals' perceptions in the context of their culture and value systems and their personal goals, standards, and concerns. The WHOQOL was developed in locations worldwide and has been widely field-tested. The WHOQOL-BREF instrument includes 26 items, which measure the broad domains of physical health, psychological health, social relation-

ships, and environment. This instrument is a shorter version of the original instrument, the Disability Rating Scale (DRS). A measure of general functioning over the course of recovery, the DRS assesses three areas of functioning, including level of arousal; cognitive ability to perform basic activities of daily living, including eating, grooming, and toileting; and level of functioning, including level of dependency and employability. It is applicable across a wide range of injury severity and recovery intervals. It may be useful in studies of moderate to severe TBI with serial measurement, particularly where initial measurement occurs in the acute post-injury interval.

COMPLICATIONS OF ASSESSMENT AND DIAGNOSIS

When speech-language pathologists provide assessments for returning military service personnel, concurrent physical, cognitive, and social-emotional symptoms of mTBI and PTSD indicate the need for a multidisciplinary/interdisciplinary approach in primary care. The assessment and treatment process at the VA is completed by an extensive and comprehensive polytrauma interdisciplinary team. Its purpose is to create an individualized, evidenced-based treatment program that will increase functionality and decrease disability related to mTBI (Schneider et al., 2009). Members of the polytrauma interdisciplinary team include professionals from the disciplines of speech-language pathology, physiatry (rehabilitation medicine), neurology, psychiatry, psychology, occupation and physical therapy, neuropsychology, audiology, optometry, orthodontics/prosthetics, social work case management, critical care nursing case management recreation therapy, drivers rehabilitation, and blind rehabilitation outpatient specialty.

Despite the ingenuity and effort of the team, Jones, Young, and Leppma (2010) indicate that there are three reasons that overlapping symptoms make assessment and diagnosis difficult:

1. The symptoms of mTBI and PTSD are subtle and not often recognized immediately, which leads to soldiers being overlooked in the military health care system.
2. Organic and psychological symptoms are difficult to differentially diagnose.
3. Service members may present with amnesia about the trauma and be unable to report a history of head injury during a case history.

Lawhorne and Philpott (2010) describe several barriers that may prevent service personnel from seeking care. Primarily, many of the OIF/OEF veterans are young adults and do not want a mental health stigma. They may want to continue serving in the military or continue on in their civilian lives without being labeled as having a disability. Also, persons who suffer depression may delay seeking care because of decreased motivation. In this case, medication or psychotherapy may be needed before other issues can be confronted. Depression should be managed to decrease risks for suicidal thoughts and drug and/or alcohol abuse. Finally, the symptoms may be dismissed because they are often too subtle to be recognized or may not present until weeks or months after injury.

There are also a number of external factors that complicate the assessment process and diagnosis outlined in the VA TBI Independent Study Course (U.S. Department of Veterans Affairs, 2010).

Assessment can be complicated by limited medical records. Delayed presentation for evaluation or treatment includes the risk of the veteran's not being able to remember details regarding the trauma. Unfortunately, there have been media reports about veterans who returned home and murdered their entire families. These persons are possibly those who were not identified as having TBI or PTSD and who, therefore, did not receive help. This is a particularly critical point because many armed services personnel have been exposed to daily polytrauma events in Iraq and Afghanistan, and many veterans have experienced multiple brain injuries. Finally, diagnosis of the presenting disorder may not take into consideration any preexisting physical or psychological problems that can complicate assessment and diagnosis.

Scarcity of interdisciplinary research data also complicates assessment (Capeheart & Bass, 2012). Research is extremely limited about this population, and the most current literature does not include sufficient empirical data. Most published reports are literature reviews and surveys. The largest studies have relied on medical records and self-report measures for both PTSD and TBI. Therefore, there is not enough known about blast brain trauma to rely on self-report instruments for diagnosis of either PTSD or TBI in combat veterans, and self-reporting measures may result in inappropriately high prevalence of PTSD (Capeheart & Bass).

The self-reported history of mTBI during deployment of military personnel, particularly when associated with altered mental status with LOC, lacks specificity in predicting post-deployment physical health problems (Hoge et al., 2008). For instance, Spencer, Drag, Walker, and Bieliauskas (2010) examined the association between self-reported cognitive functioning and performance of a sample of veterans by studying the relationship between formal neuropsychological assessments and self-reports. Self-reported ratings were significantly correlated to depression, anxiety, and PTSD in all domains. Conversely, the percentage of veterans who scored as impaired on the neuropsychological assessment ranged from 9% to 41%, although 88% to 94% of them reported impairments. On tests of attention, 91% performed within normal limits (WNL), while only 6% reported intact attention abilities. Only 9% reported normal memory abilities, and 67% performed WNL. Lastly, 73% performed WNL on tests of processing speed and organization, while only 8% reported intact functioning (Spencer et al., 2010). These results show severe discrepancies between the soldiers' self-reported cognitive skills and actual cognitive performance as determined by neuropsychological testing. It appears, therefore, that self-assessment of cognitive impairments may not be legitimate indicators of true cognitive functioning using objective measurement, Rather, data from objective measurements may be more closely associated with psychiatric symptoms. This finding was corroborated in the second part of the study, which confirmed an overestimation of a strong correlation between self-report and test performance.

Spencer and associates (2010) found that using a brief neuropsychological screening in addition to self-reporting can help to rule out cognitive dysfunction. Overall, this study indicates that the use of self-report alone should not be a preferred method of assessment. Clinicians should attempt to obtain a comprehensive picture of clients' abilities by including other methods of assessment along with self-reports, such as neuropsychological evaluations. Neuropsychological evaluations can assist with difficult diagnostic situations, including impaired attention in veterans with PTSD, suspected TBI, and a possible prior history of attention deficit hyperactivity disorder (Capeheart & Bass, 2012). Cognitive-linguistic assessments can assist with differential diagnosis in that the communicative symptoms seen in mTBI are not present in PTSD.

The Traumatic Brain Injury Screening Instrument (TBISI) was implemented in April 2007 to diagnose returning veterans with TBI. Test-retest reliability of the TBISI was studied by Van Dyke, Axlerod, and Schutte (2010) who found that none of the items on the TBISI had excellent reliability. and six had good/fair reliability. The questions related to symptoms included questions on the participant's history and current status. Study results also indicated that patient's statements regarding history may stay the same; however, responses for current symptoms can change between testing situations, which can lead to unreliable results. The veterans in the study were not identified as having any social-emotional disorders as a result of the TBISI. This may be due to the tendency of those with PTSD to block out traumatic events.

MANAGEMENT OF COGNITIVE-COMMUNICATION DISORDERS AFTER TBI

ASHA Position on Treatment Efficacy for Persons with TBI

ASHA's Treatment Efficacy Summary (American Speech-Language-Hearing Association, 2008) for cognitive-communication disorders secondary to traumatic brain injury indicates that persons with TBI benefit from therapeutic intervention from speech-language pathologists. Further, it is noted that intervention goals should follow the course of recovery for the patient in that:

> Early in recovery, intervention goals focus on providing sufficient environmental support and structure to facilitate reemergence of communication. Later in recovery, intervention goals focus on generalizing cognitive-communication skills across activities in various contexts. Ultimately, the goal of cognitive communication intervention is for the person to achieve the highest level of communicative participation in daily living.

Metacognitive and Direct Intervention

Polovoy (2011) reported that the Institute of Medicine, commissioned by the DOD, reviewed 90 articles on cognitive rehabilitation for persons with TBI and found modest collaboration that cognitive rehabilitation treatment was effective. Their findings included studies involving participants with mild, moderate, and severe TBI across acute, subacute, and chronic recovery phases. Treatment approaches were compensatory (internal or external), restorative, or a mixture.

The review of 90 studies that met these criteria found evidence of effectiveness in three narrowly defined categories:

- Immediate treatment benefit for language and social communication in patients with moderate to severe TBI in the chronic recovery phase (e.g.,

participants in small outpatient social skills groups showed immediate improvement in individualized targeted goal areas)
- Immediate treatment benefit for internal compensatory strategies for memory in moderate to severe TBI in the chronic recovery phase (e.g., scores improved on standard memory tests in which strategies such as mnemonics were likely used)
- Immediate treatment benefit for external compensatory strategies for memory in moderate to severe TBI in the chronic recovery phase (e.g., the use of diaries, notebooks, and other devices reduced the number of memory failures, with improved patient satisfaction)

These recommendations can serve as guidelines for selecting the most efficacious therapeutic strategies. Considerations for the individual needs of patients with TBI are important (Coehlo, DeRuyter, & Stein, 1996). What seems appropriate for mild or moderately impaired patients may not be as effective for severely impaired persons, as in the case of attention and memory training (Ryan & Ruff, 1988). Severely involved patients need more structure and reinforcement than mild to moderately impaired persons with TBI. Issues of self-realization are also critical. Patients need to be aware of their deficits in order to participate in decision making about goals for rehabilitation. Metacognitive strategy instruction means that additional emphasis will be given to instructing the patient to self-monitor or self-assess and to exert self-control in strategy decisions (Kennedy & Constantinidou, 2013; NINDS, 2005). In addition, patients can benefit from therapy long after the acute stage has passed.

To that end, several strategies have been proposed to manage cognitive communication disorders. One, developed by Ylvisaker and Szekeres (1986) and Hagen (1984), recommends managing cognitive disorders as a means to improve language abilities. Hagen (1984) proposed that the goal of treatment is to promote the conscious processing of language stimuli in an orderly, sequential manner through environmental manipulation and direct treatment. His postulates for treatment, upon which strategies for treatment are founded, are related to the cognitive levels of the patients. If there is no response, or only generalized or localized responses, the patient should be talked to in a calm and soothing manner. The clinician manages the environmental stimuli and determines which types of stimuli seem to encourage the patient to respond. At the next level of recovery, the patient may be confused and agitated. The clinician should then describe what is going on to the patient and modify the environment if the patient appears to become agitated.

When the patient progresses to responses that are nonagitated but confused and inappropriate or confused and appropriate, the tasks should be presented one at a time so that the patient has time to think about the task. Few words should be used at this stage. Instructions should incorporate gestures and demonstration. A routine should be established at this stage and followed closely. At the last stage, when patient responses have become automatic-appropriate and purposeful-appropriate, the goal is to assist the patient to conduct activities with minimal or no assistance.

Others (Adamovich, Henderson, & Auerbach, 1985; Butler-Hinz, Caplan, & Waters, 1990) recommend more direct intervention for disorders of language. See Table 5–10 for suggestions for direct intervention and recommended activities. Specific therapy for specific language deficits in aphasia are discussed more fully in Chapter 6. For persons with TBI, clinicians should pay particular attention to the following types of cognitive-communication disorders and target goals for therapy that are appropriate for the patient's level of severity.

Specific strategies in cognitive-communication intervention using errorless learning and spaced retrieval have been discussed extensively in Chapter 4.

Memory Disorders

Many persons recovering from TBI experience antero- or retrograde amnesia, particularly in the acute stage. There are those patients, however, whose memory problems persist after the acute stage. According to Kennedy (2006), these persons continue to be forgetful, are unable to remember the details from stories or conversation, have trouble remembering appointments the next day or tasks they need to plan for, may have difficulty remembering people's names, and may struggle to recall changes in procedures at work. These short-term memory problems are related to the injury and interfere with successful reintegration back to the community and work.

Being able to think about one's memory (metamemory) is critical to the improvement of memory problems. Kennedy (2006) suggests that several intervention

Table 5–10. Specific Language Areas for Direct Intervention and Suggested Activities

Language Area	Intervention Strategy
Syntactical comprehension	Activities for recognizing correct and incorrect syntax in phrases and sentences
Word-finding problems	Exercises for word retrieval and speed of retrieval
Discourse cohesion	Exercises in topic maintenance and topic shifting
Auditory comprehension	Activities in responding to direction of increasing length and complexity; recognizing environmental sounds.
Functional communication	Activities for daily living, such as banking and telephoning, ordering from menus, preparing grocery lists, functional readings, schedules, arranging for public transportation, bus and subway schedules, using maps, money management.
Orientation	Reality retraining in time, place, and person, community, country, family, hobbies, and leisure activities.
Pragmatics	Practice in conversation and listener demands, turn-taking, sharing the conversation burden.
Abstract language	Practice in recognizing and explaining meaning from proverbs, idioms, sarcasm, and humor.
Reading comprehension	Activities in word, phrase and sentence recognition; functional reading for consumer-related activities and communication.
Awareness of deficits	Activities in which patient predicts self-performance on activities based on feedback from the clinician; self-assessment activities and activities to interpret the intentions and feelings of others.

techniques are available that can facilitate accurate metamemory in survivors of TBI and thereby improve the likelihood that memory aids will be used. Her recommendations include:

- Individualizing educational information about the client's specific memory and cognitive disabilities.
- Involving the client in setting memory goals and in selecting memory aids.

- Creating opportunities for accurate self-monitoring.
- Integrating metacognitive strategies into training individuals to use memory aids. Make explicit the link between self-monitoring (e.g., predictions) and strategy decisions.
- Providing distributed practice at high levels of accuracy. Practice with strategy supports in a sequence of steps is critical

for individuals with memory impairment. Building in breaks in-between practice sessions (i.e., distributed practice) increases the likelihood that the person will use the memory strategy or recall the information.

Additionally, attention training using the Attention Process Training II program (APT II) developed by Sohlberg, Johnson, Paule, Raskin, and Mateer (2001) can be used to target improved concentration, followed by gradual transfer of improved skills to functional tasks, and generalization into different environments. Cognitive tasks are designed to be functional and relevant to the patient's daily life. These tasks ranged from reviewing standardized college entrance exams, such as the ACT and SAT tests, to researching local, state, or junior college academic requirements, to locating rehabilitation resources within the vicinity of their homes. As individual performance accuracy increases within structured tasks, therapy tasks can focus on transferring behaviors to less structured and more complex conditions, including introducing distracters (Schneider et al., 2009).

PTSD Treatment

The symptoms of PTSD will play a role in all areas of treatment for mTBI. This population struggles with the adjustment from military life to civilian life, and having injuries along with a stress disorder makes this adjustment even more difficult. Speech-language pathologists and other rehabilitation professionals should be mindful of certain behaviors and needs of a client with blast injury and PTSD. Over-

lapping symptoms can lead to confusion over what symptoms to treat and what intervention to utilize. The VA addresses PTSD first in an attempt to decrease emotional symptoms. If this approach is followed and re-experiencing subsides but increased arousal or depression persists, it is possible that the patient may have untreated TBI sequelae of a second psychiatric disorder (Capeheart & Bass, 2012).

Managing comorbid PTSD and TBI remains a challenge to VA clinicians in mental health, TBI/polytrauma, and primary care because no clear guidance exists on the simultaneous management of these two conditions (Capeheart & Bass, 2012). The VA/DOD Clinical Practice Guideline for Management of Post-traumatic Stress (U.S. Department of Veterans Affairs, 2009) outlines four general principles for outpatient care:

1. Treat PTSD with appropriate psychopharmacologic and psychotherapeutic modalities.
2. Identify and treat any comorbid neuropsychiatric conditions of substance use disorders.
3. Identify and treat any associated medical comorbidities.
4. Directly address cognitive sequelae.

PTSD and depression can be treated with psychiatric medications and psychotherapy (Schneider et al., 2009). The use of narcotics must be managed carefully because of the high risk for substance abuse, particularly for patients with chronic pain. If substance abuse should occur, this should be referred for immediate treatment to minimize the possible effects of anxiety, cognition disturbances, and sleep disorders. Programs such as Seeking Safety, a psychotherapeutic intervention for comorbid PTSD and substance use disorders, have been found to be effective in male and female veterans (Capeheart & Bass, 2012).

Harman and Kelly (2012), speech-language pathologists from the VA hospital, provide suggestions for effective treatment of service members with mTBI/PTSD. They emphasize that it is important to remember that in providing cognitive treatment of individuals who have mTBI/PTSD, the clinician must not move on to the next step until the patient is ready in order to decrease opportunities for anxiety, re-experiencing, and hyperarousal. Some activities, such as computer programs for attention, have distracters put in them. It is recommended that the clinician remain with the patient who is using a computer program with distracters in case the patient becomes anxious or frustrated. Seating positions should be carefully considered; many patients with PTSD will not sit with their back facing the door because they need to be able to watch their surroundings.

Good sleep hygiene should be encouraged for increased memory, attention, and overall performance. The speech-language pathologist should also encourage abstinence from caffeine or alcohol because these may increase anxiety and hypervigilance. Additionally, therapy sessions should be held in a quiet room and have structure. Sessions can be held individually or in groups depending on the needs of the client. Family and friends should be included in treatment as much as possible. Telehealth is also an option for treatment because the patient does not have to leave the familiar surroundings of home, which reduces anxiety and the risk of cancellations. It is also a convenient option for soldiers and veterans living in rural areas (Mashima, 2010).

Family and Community Reintegration

Wallace (2006) recommends that the speech-language pathologist's role is to facilitate restoration and wholeness for returning soldiers who have communication and swallowing impairments. Wallace advises that the intervention approach should focus on treating the symptoms of communication and swallowing disorders, because it is difficult to differentiate between TBI and PTSD. The combination of physical injury and psychological problems are of concern because many of the veterans are reentering civilian life and some are returning to duty. It is very important to monitor and provide strategies for readjustment to the workplace, family life, and/or school.

Returning to civilian life means reestablishing relationships with friends and family. The level of support from the family is important to the success of the client. Negative reactions from a spouse, family, or friends can significantly hinder and decrease functionality, whereas positive support can lead to an easier transition. Resources for caregivers and family members such as contacts for family/couples therapy should be provided because they too are experiencing readjustment. Spouses and family members need to have a safe forum in which they can express their feelings (Lawhorne & Philpott, 2010). Relationship counseling is beneficial for successful reintegration into the family structure. This support is also helpful for family members who must adjust to the service member's return and rehabilitation (Schneider et al., 2009).

To obtain additional perspectives of quality of life after brain injury, Degeneff and Lee (2010) interviewed siblings of individuals with brain injury to gain understanding on how siblings perceive the quality of life of their brothers and sisters who have sustained TBI. Overall the participants reported more negative responses than positive (Degeneff & Lee, 2010). Participants reported that family support and support from professionals increased the quality of life for their siblings. The second most mentioned aspect of quality of life was positive psychological adjustment, where siblings noted the ability and willingness of their injured siblings to accept the realities of their lives and the challenges they will face. Many discussed their sibling's recovery in terms of their level of independence post-injury (Degeneff & Lee, 2010). On the other hand, negative reports included role strain. This is related to high levels of frustration as well as a lack of awareness of how TBI has changed their sibling and how some had lost hope. A common theme was that the participants felt that unsatisfactory professional care may inhibit the quality of life of their injured siblings. A final concern was for the paucity of programs to assist in maintaining long-term recovery and community integration These results suggest that reports from family can enhance assessment by providing information that the patient may not be able to disclose (Degeneff & Lee, 2010).

Academic Re-entry

Because of the young ages of the returning soldiers, a number of them may enter college or pursue a trade or vocation. For this group, treatment should address note-taking skills, outlining, and reading strategies. They should focus on organizing notebooks and assignments and utilizing flashcards, as well as utilizing the varieties of computer programs and applications for phones and other technological devices designed to assist with daily tasks and assignments. The clinician should also make efforts to connect the patient with the special education liaison and teachers/professors on their campus to ensure that any necessary accommodations are met.

The option of returning to school and being successful can be a realistic goal for survivors of TBI with adequate support. Hux and colleagues (2010) were concerned with the learning strategies of student survivors of TBI between the ages of 20 and 28 years and explored the effects of their learning strategies and accommodations on social and academic aspects of their college experience. In-depth analysis of each student participant showed differences and similarities among them. The most common similarity was that each had formal accommodations provided by their institutions, although it was reported that a couple of them did not take full advantage of the accommodations. It is possible that, due to their cognitive difficulties, they would forget to bring the accommodation letters or felt that they could handle the class without the extra assistance. It was also found that much of their success in higher education was due to the support that they received at home and in school (Hux et al., 2010).

The survivors of severe TBI in this study are doing well in college even with their challenges. Each case was unique, and success depended on individual motivation. The information provided by Hux and associates (2010) is beneficial for speech-language pathologists who work with veterans who have mTBI and PTSD because success in college is possible with adequate support and strategies. The study includes a civilian population without PTSD who sustained injuries at young ages. Overall, study results provide a positive outlook for those who have sustained mTBI and would like to return to school.

Vocational Re-entry

For those who are resuming previous work assignments, adequate support is necessary to an individual with mTBI and PTSD to efficiently complete tasks, organize materials, and be punctual. Gilworth, Eyres, Carey, Bhakta, and Tennant (2008) conducted a survey of concussion/mTBI patients and reported that many respondents felt that their injuries were invisible, although persistent symptoms interfered with the ability to work effectively. Of concern was a perceived lack of guidance from the VA for returning to work. Respondents reported that they were in need of strategies and accommodations to successfully complete assigned tasks requested by their employer and to handle social interactions with coworkers.

The VA/DOD Clinical Practice Guideline for Management of Post-traumatic Stress (U.S. Department of Veterans Affairs, 2009) includes modifications for vocational reintegration. Gradual re-entry may be necessary, such as returning for 2 days a week and increasing as the comfort level and ability to complete multiple tasks increases. The length of the workday can also be modified to allow for readjustment. Additional time to complete tasks is another modification that assists with adjustment. Impaired attention and hypervigilance may indicate the need for a quiet work space or other environmental modifications. If the environment is too stressful or demanding, a job change may be necessary. For example, a factory job where there are a lot of loud noises is not advantageous to one who has sustained a blast injury and has a diagnosis of PTSD.

Using Augmentative and Alternative Communication with Persons Recovering From TBI

Persons with TBI can often regain much of the ability to communicate using augmentative and alternative communication (AAC) devices that are recommended by speech-language pathologists, regardless of age. Doyle and Fager (2011) report that there are three groups of patients with TBI who can benefit from AAC methods, techniques, and strategies. The three groups are: (1) emergent communicators, (2) transitional communicators, and (3) long-term augmentative communicators. These groups were developed from accepted TBI classification systems. In the Doyle and Fager model, each of the three groups has its own unique needs and abilities. The emergent group is unable to speak because of cognitive or medical status and in some cases, respiratory status. For this group, the suggested AAC methods are:

- A yes/no response system using whatever means the patient has to respond, for example, head nods, pointing to cards, hand or finger movements, eye blinks, eye movements
- Object choices (e.g., intervention tasks, clothing, and food items, if appropriate)
- Simple communication boards with two or three pictures (e.g., family members, activity choices, treatment task-specific boards)
- Single-message voice output devices to communicate yes/no or to request an item or activity within a structured context

Persons in the transitional stage have resumed using natural voice, but may have severe dysarthria and other limitations that make communication difficult. However, the patient desires a method of communication in order to participate in therapy and to make wants and needs known. For this patient, Doyle and Fager (2011) recommend the following AAC methods:

■ Writing or using an alphabet board to supplement speech. Writing is considered first because it is familiar and more automatic than pointing to letters. If writing is not an option because of motor impairment, then an alphabet board is considered. Most individuals will need cues to initiate use of these systems.

■ Low-tech alphabet or communication boards accessed by looking or gazing at messages with the eyes or using eye-safe laser pointers for those with severe motor impairment

■ Low-tech communication boards and books

■ Digitized, static-display speech generating devices (SGDs) for individuals with significant cognitive/language deficits and whose spelling has yet to reemerge to a functional level. These devices have a single display or overlay with messages prerecorded by the speech-language pathologist or caregiver.

■ Text-to-speech SGDs for individuals with functional spelling. Letters, words, or sentences are "spoken" as the individual types. Spelling and syntax errors may occur due to

impulsivity, perseveration, and poor self-monitoring.

■ Dynamic-display SGDs may be tried with individuals who have the attention, organization, and memory skills to navigate between displays or screens. One screen may have the alphabet for generating messages and another screen may contain preprogrammed words or phrases. The SLP may reduce the number of screens or simplify the navigation strategies to accommodate the individual's cognitive and language deficits.

The long-term augmentative communicator is the patient who is able to use natural speech and who may have cognitive and/or language impairments of long standing. The patient may have begun the re-entry into work and family and needs AAC to assist with the transition. For this patient, Doyle and Fager (2011) recommend the following:

■ Spelling-based text-to-speech SGD purchased through insurance that he or she is learning to use with new caregivers at home and with teachers at school. This is the preferred device because SGDs have built-in louder speakers for text-to-speech output.

■ Less costly options include communication software for commercially available devices, such as the iPad and iPod Touch by Apple®, or netbooks. This strategy is not as highly recommended as SGDs but appeal to some patients who are accustomed to using these devices.

Speech-language pathologists have a number of online resources that are useful for making technology-driven choices for patients with TBI. Doyle and Fager (2011) suggest the following AAC online resources: (1) AAC–RERC—Rehabilitation Engineering and Research Center on AAC; (2) Barkley AAC Center and the Munroe-Meyer Institute for Genetics and Rehabilitation at the University of Nebraska; and (3) International Society of Augmentative and Alternative Communication (ISAAC).

Currently, technology is playing a major role in the treatment of TBI. It is very common to see clinicians with laptops, tablets, and smartphones during treatment sessions. The use of everyday technology is beneficial, particularly with persons diagnosed with mTBI, for a number of reasons. Individuals with TBI typically appear to be functioning normally within society and want to continue to fit in with their peers. Because the phone and computer devices can be used, they do not have to stand out from everyone else at school or work or in other social settings.

Additionally, smaller devices are easier to carry than the traditional roller box with mountains of papers, activities, and workbooks. Applications or "apps" for assessment, treatment, and management have been developed to address most speech and communication impairments related to TBI. Apps can be downloaded directly onto the device, and some can be stored for access when changing devices. For example, athletes can be assessed right on the field for suspected concussion. These devices are cost-effective and within reach of persons regardless of socioeconomic status. Assistive technology, such as speech generating devices, has been costly even with the help of medical insurance and may be difficult to change when a patient ages or has a change of status. However, smartphones, tablets, and laptops can be purchased at most shopping centers with the opportunity to obtain insurance for theft, loss, damage, or upgrades.

There are some disadvantages to using these devices. There can be issues of ethics and privacy. Most apps can be downloaded by anyone, and concerns for professional ethics and competency may arise if assessment or treatment is being done by someone who is not a certified speech-language pathologist. Comfort with using devices may be complicated by vision or hearing disorders in an aging population. While some aging adults are accustomed to using digital technology, others may find the use of technology to be confusing or overwhelming.

Even the most advanced technology is not always dependable. The success of technology depends on the device, the quality of Internet service, and the applications being used. Programs can be discontinued or some upgrades can delete existing information if the clinician is tracking patient statistics using a device. If the Internet is necessary, slow connections can decrease valuable session time. Technology is constantly changing; therefore many of the apps and devices may not be available in the next few years. Follow-through of tasks can be difficult to track. Finally there can be an issue of cost. Although most devices are easily accessible and may not be as difficult to obtain as augmentative devices, purchasing devices and applications can become costly (Schwabacher, Lewis, Eshel, & Goudy, 2011).

There are, however, a number of excellent applications for use with patients with cognitive and communication disorders who are recovering from TBI

(Sutton, 2012). The reader is referred to an article by Sutton (2012) for suggestions.

Telehealth Rehabilitation

Telerehabilitation (telerehab) is the method of using technology to provide services at a distance. The modes and options for services range from traditional telephone consultations to satellite-based videoconferencing with live audio and video. Research has shown that videoconference-based rehab is a feasible, effective, and appropriate method for providing services to a broad range of clients. It has also been found to be effective for cognitive assessment of persons with brain injury (Schopp, Johnstone, & Merveille, 2001).

Telehealth or telepractice has been a mode of service delivery within the field of speech-language pathology for a little more than 30 years, beginning with the use of telephones to provide services (Georgeadis, Brennan, Barker, & Baron, 2004). More recently, as technology has advanced, telepractice is now utilized with computers, laptops, tablets, and even cell phones through virtual videoconferencing. This type of service is especially beneficial for individuals who are in remote or rural locations. It is now suggested that this mode is sufficient for those who are extremely busy and have difficulty maintaining a schedule for therapy. ASHA's (2010) position statement on telehealth states:

> The use of telepractice does not remove any existing responsibilities in delivering services, including adherence to the Code of Ethics, Scope of Practice, state and federal laws (e.g., licensure, HIPAA, etc.), and ASHA policy documents on professional practices. Therefore, the quality of ser-

vices delivered via telepractice must be consistent with the quality of services delivered face-to-face.

To date, there is limited published empirical research on telehealth for cognitive-linguistic assessment and treatment of TBI in speech-language pathology. Research in this area is needed to settle the ethical debates of validity and reliability. Most literature on telerehabilitation has included small samples and typically focuses on technical feasibility. Some researchers have found no differences between face-to-face service and telerehabilitation (Mashima, Birkmire-Peters, Syms, Holtel, & Burgess, 2003) and have found that current standardized assessments are valid and reliable when administered remotely (Waite, Theodoros, Russell, & Cahill, 2010). The limitation is that these studies have been in the areas of audiology and child language.

Georgeadis and colleagues (2004) administered a story-retelling task to three groups: TBI, left-hemisphere cerebrovascular accidents, and right-hemisphere cerebrovascular accident, in both face-to-face (FF) and telerehabilitation (T) settings to determine whether performance was affected by either setting. Across all participants the T settings were slightly better than the FF settings; however, there were no significant differences between performances across settings. In terms of groups, the TBI group performed more poorly in the T setting. Decreased attention is a common symptom of TBI and very likely played a role in the group's performance. Some participants in the groups reported that it was "difficult to pay attention in the T setting." The participants in the study showed a strong preference for the FF setting for the feedback; although they also responded "yes" when asked if they would use videoconferencing in the future (Georgeadis et al., 2004). It appeared that the TBI participants were accepting of telerehab; however, there were challenges with maintaining attention. Future use of videoconferencing with the TBI population will have to make considerations for attentional impairments.

The Defense and Veterans Brain Injury Center Tele-TBI Clinic and Remote Assessment Center provides screening, assessment, and consultation to remote military medical centers and troop-intensive sites. Video teleconferencing is also used for professional education, including monthly multidisciplinary grand rounds and remote speech-language pathology services from Brooke Army Medical Center. The U.S. Veterans Administration and the Department of Defense are also collaborating with civilian and academic organizations to develop technologies to improve care. There is presently an ongoing grant to develop reading comprehension strategies that will be utilized with active duty service members and veterans with mTBI who plan to reenter the workforce, school, or other programs (Mashima, 2010).

The goals of telemedicine and innovative technologies are to:

- connect patients remotely with providers and specialist,
- identify concussion and mTBI using electronic cognitive assessment systems,
- provide real-time video visits with family members,
- share information that enables clinical teams to collaborate on TBI care,
- manage medication, and
- provide interactive video programs and Web-based

courses to train medics, physician assistants, nurses, and other providers in civilian and military settings. (Doarn, 2009)

Innovative Approaches to Managing Patients with Special Needs

The Sport as a Laboratory Assessment Model (SLAM) is used with athletes to collect brief baselines of cognition and compare with data with repeat concussions. The model suggests that there is a quick recovery curve in healthy, young, motivated athletes when they are allowed to rest and other complicating psychosocial or medical factors are not present. SLAM is currently incorporated in high schools, universities, and professional sports teams with the intention of protecting players from returning to play before they are completely ready. The program has also been adopted by the military to assist with determining when a service member is able to return to duty.

The VA has developed polytrauma centers to better serve returning OIF/OEF veterans. *Polytrauma* is a term that has been popularized in Military Treatment Facilities and VA Medical Centers. Currently, there are five Polytrauma Rehabilitation Centers, four Polytrauma Transitional Rehabilitation Programs, 23 Polytrauma Network Sites, and 87 Polytrauma Support Clinic Teams.

Polytrauma System of Care

Polytrauma Rehabilitation Centers provide acute, comprehensive, inpatient rehabilitation. They maintain a full team of professionals and consultants from other specialties related to polytrauma and provide information to other facilities in the system of care.

Polytrauma Transitional Rehabilitation Programs offer structured residential programs in a therapeutic, real-world setting with a focus on progressive return to independent living. Individual and group-based treatment is provided with focus on physical and emotional health and wellness, cognitive therapy, successful community reintegration, return to work, and return to school.

Polytrauma Network Sites provide continued medical care and rehabilitation for veterans and service members transitioning closer to home following discharge from a Polytrauma Rehabilitation Center. This type of care is an entry point for rehabilitation services for those who have sustained mild to moderate TBI or polytraumatic injury.

Polytrauma Support Clinic Teams provide continued, specialized outpatient care. An advantage of these teams is that they may offer continued medical and rehabilitation care and support closer to the patient's home community. This management approach can also be an entry point for outpatient rehabilitation services for those who have sustained mild to moderate TBI or polytraumatic injury.

The VA has developed a five-part approach to treating the cognitive and social symptoms of mTBI to assist service members and veterans in everyday life situations (Schwabacher et al., 2011). The treatment includes developing compensatory strategies, the use of technology, projects, applied learning, and group therapy. Metacognitive Strategy Instruction consists of teaching individuals to regulate their own behavior by breaking complex tasks into steps while thinking strategically and is a practice standard for

young to middle-aged adults with TBIs who have difficulty with problem solving, organization, and planning (Kennedy et al., 2008)

Technology in treatment includes aids for reading, writing, listening, and cognition. Reading aids include Screen Readers (listening while reading), E-reader devices (Kindle, Nook), and audio books. Writing aids assist with spelling and grammar and error detection/correction. Voice recorders and personal FM listening systems aid in listening. For example, the Live Scribe pen is helpful for students who take class notes because it can record lectures as notes are written and has memory capability to play back portions of the lectures when the pen is placed on the written note. The cognitive aids used include smart phones/personal digital assistants that often are preinstalled with calendars, maps/navigation, contacts with pictures, notes, alarms/reminders. If not preinstalled, there are applications that can be downloaded, such as voice recorders and apps for personal/daily management of functional tasks (e.g., appointments, notetaking, finances). Cognitive brain games are also beneficial for individuals with mTBI (Schwabacher et al., 2011).

Computer-based programs and websites can also be used that function similarly to Google Calendar, Google Voice, Google Health, IGoogle, Outlook calendars, and OneNote. Computer projects are advantageous for treatment because they increase skills for organization, attention, and task completion, which are all necessary for tasks/assignments in school, work, and in the military. The VA enforces applied learning by taking the skills learned in the previous treatments and applying them to tasks such as scavenger hunts and evacuation routes (Schwabacher et al., 2011).

The final part is group therapy, which helps the patient with social skills. In the military, particularly, the completion of tasks/jobs depends on how well one works with others. Group therapy includes training for executive function, memory, attention, communication, and social pragmatics. Functional activities such as cooperative gaming (e.g., Pandemic) and mock missions (e.g., Geocaching) engage all areas of cognition and communication (Schwabacher et al., 2011). Cooperative games such as Pandemic allow two to five people to work as a team. Each player has a different role with a special ability to help the player find cures for four diseases that are spreading around the world. The advantages of this activity are that it is cooperative, strategic, tactical, flexible, dynamic, and instructional and has multiple steps. Geocaching is a type of scavenger hunt or "hide and seek" that utilizes a Global Positioning System (GPS). A geocache can be placed anywhere in the world, and the geocacher must locate the geocache using GPS technology and share the geocache's existence and location online (Schwabacher et al., 2011).

Group Therapy

Group-based interventions seem to address different needs and may be more appropriate at varying stages in treatment than individual therapies. There are several group therapy strategies that offer remediation for cognitive-communication disorders. Groups can be task oriented, that is, the group works together to solve a group problem or provide a service, as for example, groups that focus on memory, orientation, vocational training, or independent living. Groups can also be thematic, for example, sharing stories, gardening, or travel, to name a few. Importantly, group therapy offers opportunities for increased socialization and role-playing situations for practicing pragmatic, social, behavioral management, cognitive, and communication skills.

Perna, Bubier, Oken, Snyder, and Rouselle (2004) identified eight reasons for establishing group therapy for adults with TBI:

1. Groups provide opportunities for participants to work on social skills and elicit behaviors that are often not readily apparent in individual sessions. These encounters can give the clinician additional insight into areas that should be treated.

2. Groups allow participants to engage in safe interpersonal exchanges and obtain social support from their peers.

3. Groups are a cost-effective format in which to treat cognitive disorders such as those that affect attention, memory, and problem solving.

4. Feedback from peers may be more palatable than that from a therapist and may function to heighten self-awareness of deficits in patients.

5. Groups enable patients to model participants and facilitators and see exemplars of desirable social behavior.

6. Groups can serve to increase member self-esteem and decrease feelings of isolation as group participants identify with others with similar concerns. Skills learned in individual sessions can be carried over in groups.

7. Groups can more likely simulate real-world situations, giving participants more opportunities to practice and encouraging overlearning with multiple partners.

8. Groups also provide opportunities for socialization and bonding, helping participants to develop friendships and communication partners.

Family Education

TBI is a catastrophic event for which most families are ill-prepared. Families will want to know the possible outcomes for their patient's cognitive and communication problems. Speech-language pathologists should provide realistic information about the patient's progress, the effect of TBI on cognitive and language skills, and the methodologies for treatment of these disorders.

The suddenness of head injury, unlike the gradual onset of dementia or stroke, which is somewhat predictable from an older adult's health history, has a deleterious effect on family relations and equilibrium. Martin (1990) described four stages in family adaptation to the head-injured person. The most common initial stage is shock and its emotions of numbness and disorientation. As these reactions subside, denial or disbelief follows. When the family realizes the magnitude of the injury and the process of recovery, profound sorrow may follow and may last for weeks or months. There may be expressions of anger at the injustice of the injury, particularly if the injury has occurred from a criminal assault. Finally, as the family begins to reach some form of acceptance, the last stage of adaptation is reached.

As clinicians develop strategies for family education, these stages are important to recognize and include in an ongoing program of family information, involvement, and support. Information on the impact of head injury, on the patient's ability to maintain family relations and responsibilities, cognitive and language deficits, stages of language recovery, and behavioral changes that typically accompany head injury, is vitally important to share with the family. A realistic prognosis should be shared with the family also, which takes into consideration the patient's age, health, head injury complications, motivation, and residual capacities.

Chapter 4 provides guidelines for questions to ask in order to develop an appropriate program of family education. Clinicians should be prepared to advise families about alternative solutions in case there are concerns that the customary treatment options are ineffective, too costly, or both (Walker, Kreutzer, & Witol, 1996). For example, computer software that the patient can use at home, AAC devices that help to make communication at home more manageable, or telerehab services may be viable alternatives for patients that are unable to get to outpatient treatment regularly.

As repeated head injuries are a major concern for persons with head injuries, clinicians can advise families on measures to take to ensure home safety. Persons who sustain TBIs as a result of falls do somewhat poorer compared with those injured due to a transportation accident (Rosenthal et al., 1996).

A home safety checklist may be used to modify the environment for patients both in the institutional and in the home setting. Low-cost adjustments in the home, for example, can decrease the possibility of falls from environmental hazards. Honaker, Criter, and Patterson (2013) recommend that clinicians recommend that patients should shoes with nonskid soles. Other suggestions for home modifications are to keep the home be well-lit, use night lights around the house, place nonslip mats in the bathtub or shower, repair loose flooring and carpets, arrange commonly used items within easy reach, remove obstacles from the floor, and install glow switches in room entrances.

Additional programming may be needed for successful community re-entry. Persons with poor or no work history have continuing problems with community integration. One source of difficulty is that the individual will be unable to apply skills to a practical situation for carry-over, like the work environment. Another is that a return to living situations in which there is no income is demoralizing and counterproductive to the therapy process. Patients should be referred to vocational rehabilitation counselors and social workers, who can assist in finding employment that is suitable to the level of functioning.

The Brain Injury Association of America offers the following suggestions to provide for families as they begin to cope with the changes they see in their loved ones:

1. Learn about your family member's deficits by close involvement in the rehabilitation process. Have a clear understanding about ways your family member's deficits will affect his abilities and ask about compensatory strategies you can implement in your home to lessen the impact of these deficits. Start planning for homecoming as far in advance of discharge as possible.

2. Plan the room arrangement so the individual can function as independently as possible. This may mean that drawers are thoughtfully arranged with stickers on the outside to describe the contents; a divided tray, properly labeled to hold wallet, watch, coins, glasses, and so forth placed on the nightstand to ensure that personal items are not misplaced; and a notebook or cue cards are available with steps for completing tasks as simple as showering or other personal care routines.

3. Establish a schedule that includes as much activity as the individual can tolerate without becoming overly fatigued. This may mean an outpatient therapy schedule, a day activity program in the community, or even a volunteer "job." Everyone needs a reason to get up in the morning and something satisfying to look forward to. Many families complain that the individual never wants to do anything. However, the problem may be an inability to initiate and plan, so the family should help with planning activities. Deciding on the plan is the first step, but reminders, written and verbal, keep the plan in motion. Equally important is the follow-up, which may require cueing to help the person "remember" the event. Don't make the mistake of asking, "What did you do last night?" Instead ask, "Did you enjoy the concert last night? Tell me about it." By cueing, you are helping the person retrieve the information from long-term storage and integrate it into the conversation.

4. If social problems such as drugs/alcohol were a problem before the injury, they are likely to be a problem afterward. As long as the family member is dependent on the family, then the family is in the best position to prevent this from happening. A hard-line approach now may make life easier later. It is important to be aware that use of medication, such as anti-seizure medication, can be a dangerous combination with the use of other nonprescription substances.

5. External cueing is very helpful. If the individual is constantly faced with situations in which he has no recall and those around him constantly remind him of his lack of memory, it may eventually cause an erosion of self-esteem. Family members should create some strategies for compensating for this problem by developing lists, Post-it notes, or cue cards or any other strategies that help the person feel more independent and less likely to make mistakes and be nagged or scolded.

6. Structure, structure, structure and consistency! The importance of a structured environment cannot be overemphasized. There's nothing more frustrating and frightening than being an adult and not knowing what you're supposed to be doing. Structuring helps offset some problems by giving the individual a consistent and dependable way of life.

7. Always check with the person's physician when behavioral changes occur. Seizures can develop after brain injury and it is not uncommon that they occur some months or years after the injury. They are frequently called "silent seizures" because they do not involve convulsions; however, they often create changes in behavior. Symptoms include random and restless pacing, staring into space, complaints of foul odors or taste changes, and/or hallucinations. These symptoms can indicate seizure activity and warrant testing to determine if there is abnormal electrical activity in the brain, which is commonly controlled with the use of anti-seizure medications.

The Brain Injury Association of America can be accessed at http://www.biausa .org/brain-injury-family-caregivers.htm and is invaluable for families seeking answers about resources, treatment, living with brain injury, and caregiver stress. Support groups, a source of information and encouragement to patients and their families, can be identified through state offices of the Brain Injury Association of America. Additional resources include:

Brain Trauma Foundation
523 E. 72nd St.
New York, NY 10021
Phone: 212-772-0608
Fax: 212-772-0357
http://www.braintrauma.org/

National Institute on Disability and Rehabilitation Research
400 Maryland Ave., S.W.
Washington, DC 20202-7100
Phone: 202-245–7640
TTY: 202-245–7316
http://www.ed.gov/about/ offices/list/osers/nidrr/index .html?src=mr/

Summary

Many valid and reliable standardized assessments are available to assist speech-language pathologists in determining residual skills in mental status, cognition, communication, functional independence, life satisfaction, and self-perception for persons with TBI. Clinicians are encouraged to select the most appropriate tests and to supplement them with their own observations of the patient in the daily living setting and with other informal assessments to get the best picture of the patient's motivation and residual skills.

Therapeutic intervention should be both therapist directed and client centered. Clinicians can select from metacognitive and metamemory strategies, from direct intervention for cognitive communication problems, and from a variety of low- and high-tech devices that assist the patient at various levels to communicate.

Persons who sustained TBI from sports injuries and those who sustained TBI from missile blast injuries have a number of resources available to provide specialized intervention. New research on sports injuries hold promise in the prevention and early identification of these injuries in athletes who play football, box, or play soccer. Returning military personnel have highly individualized programs that provide treatment for both PTSD and cognitive-communication disorders associated with TBI.

Technological advances are also available for patients with TBI who live in remote regions or who are unable to commute to therapy because of limited access to transportation. Telehealth and telerehab are two ways by which therapists can reach those who cannot meet with them in face-to-face sessions. Evidence indicates that telehealth and telerehab are as effective as face-to-face clinical encounters and can be considered as a viable alternative for patients.

Group-based rehabilitation is effective in providing carryover from individual sessions. In addition, group therapy is a cost-effective approach to treatment and one that provides group members with opportunities to practice their skills in real-world situations with multiple partners. This type of therapy for persons with TBI has the advantage of providing opportunities for socialization and the development and maintenance of friendships and communication partners (Shorland & Douglas, 2010).

Family education and counseling are critical to successful rehabilitation. TBI is a catastrophic event that upsets family relations. Family members are often at a loss and will go through four stages of grieving until successful adaptation occurs. Clinicians are asked to be mindful of this process and provide support and realistic information to families. Suggestions from the Brain Injury Association of America will be helpful to assist families to cope with the changes brought about by TBI, including the need to structure the patient's home environment, the importance of cueing to assist with memory retrieval, the importance of alerting the patient's physician when behavioral changes occur, and the importance of being involved in the rehabilitation process. Support groups are invaluable for families to come together around the challenges of TBI. Information about support groups can be accessed through state offices of the Brain Injury Association of America.

STUDY QUESTIONS

1. What is the difference between a closed head injury and an open or penetrating head injury?

2. In a closed head injury, what is diffuse axonal injury?

3. What neuropathological factors occur during a closed head injury?

4. How does alcohol use worsen a TBI?

5. What is the most prevalent cause of head injury in older adults? Why?

6. Why are older adults susceptible to pedestrian accidents and TBI?

7. What is PTSD?

8. What is a missile blast injury?

9. What is a skull fracture? What are the types of skull fractures?

10. What are the stages of recovery from TBI?

11. What is amnesia? What are the types of amnesia seen after TBI?

12. Why are older drivers at risk for vehicular accidents?

13. What are low-tech AAC devices? For whom are they most appropriate?

14. What are speech generating devices (SGDs)? For whom are they most appropriate?

15. What are some commonly used devices that can be used to assist persons with TBI to navigate and to communicate?

16. What long-term effects does repeated head injuries have on cognition?

17. What are the reasons that re-entry into school or work can be difficult for persons with TBI?

18. What advances in neuroimaging are used to diagnose TBI?

19. Why is the prevalence of assaults different in urban versus rural areas?

20. Why is length of coma significant for predicting outcome after TBI? and what is TADD and how does it relate to coma?

21. In what ways can the computer be useful to persons with TBI and their families? What other high-tech devices can be used?

22. What tests are most appropriate to use at bedside to evaluate cognitive communication disorders?

23. What assessments identify discourse and pragmatic problems after TBI?

24. What assessments measure executive function in a person with TBI?

25. What is meant by the term *metacognitive*?

26. Why is self-assessment important for persons with TBI in therapy?

27. In what ways is group therapy helpful to persons with TBI?

28. What professionals can assist with determining appropriate employment for a person with TBI?

29. What are some of the direct intervention strategies for cognitive and communication disorders?

30. What are the four stages that families go through as they learn to cope with the effects of TBI?

REFERENCES

Adamovich, B. B., & Henderson, J. (1992). *Scales of cognitive ability for traumatic brain injury*. Austin, TX: Pro-Ed.

Adamovich, B. B., Henderson, J. A., & Auerbach, S. (1985). *Cognitive rehabilitation of closed head injured patients: A dynamic approach*. Austin, TX: Pro-Ed.

American Speech-Language-Hearing Association. (2004). *Preferred practice patterns for the profession of speech-language pathology* [Preferred practice patterns]. Retrieved from http://www.asha.org/policy

American Speech-Language-Hearing Association (2008). *Treatment efficacy summary. Cognitive-communication disorders resulting from traumatic brain injury*. Retrieved from http://www.asha.org/uploadedFiles/public/TESCognitiveCommunicationDisordersFromTBI.pdf

American Speech-Language-Hearing Association. (2010). *Professional issues in telepractice for speech-language pathologists* [Professional issues statement]. Retrieved from http://www.asha.org/ policy

Aoki, Y., Inokuchi, R., Gunshin, M., Yahagi, N., & Suwa, H. (2012). Diffusion tensor imaging studies of mild traumatic brain injury: A meta-analysis. *Neuropsychiatry, 83*, 870–876. doi:10.1136/jnnp-2012-302742

Arciniegas, D. B., Held, K., & Wagner, P. (2002). Cognitive impairment following traumatic brain injury. *Current Treatment Options in Neurology, 4*, 43–57.

Armed Forces Health Surveillance Center. (2012a). *Department of Defense numbers for traumatic brain injury: Worldwide—totals 2000–2012Q3.* Retrieved from http://www.dvbic.org/dod-worldwide-numbers-tbi

Armed Forces Health Surveillance Center. (2012b) *Incidence by branch.* Retrieved from http://www.dvbic.org/dod-worldwide-numbers-tbi

Armed Forces Health Surveillance Center. (2012c) *Incidence by severity.* Retrieved from http://www.dvbic.org/dod-worldwide-numbers-tbi.

Aschkenasy, M. T., & Rothenhaus, T. C. (2006). Trauma and falls in the elderly. *Emergency Medical Clinics in North America, 24*, 413–432.

Atkinson, R. M., Tolson, R. L., & Turner, J. A. (1990). Late versus early onset problem drinking in older men. *Alcoholism: Clinical Experimental Research, 14*, 574–579.

Auerbach, S. H. (1986). Neuroanatomical correlates of attention and memory disorders in traumatic brain injury: An application of behavioral subtypes. *Journal of Head Trauma Rehabilitation, 1*, 1–12.

Baddeley, A., Emslie, H., & Nimmo-Smith, I. (1992). *Speed and capacity of language processing.* San Antonio, TX: Pearson Assessment.

Balestreri, M., Czosnya, M., & Hutchinson, P. (2006). Impact of intracranial pressure and cerebral perfusion pressure on severe disability and mortality after head injury. *Neurocritical Care, 4*, 8–13.

Barber, J. B., & Webster, J. C. (1974). Head injuries: Review of 150 cases. *Journal of the National Medical Association, 66*, 201–204.

Bayles, K. A., & Tomoeda, C. (1995). *Functional linguistic communication inventory.* Austin, TX: Pro-Ed.

Bazarian, J. J., Pope, C., McClung, J., Cheng, Y. T., & Flesher, W. (2003). Ethnic and racial disparities in emergency department care for mild traumatic brain injury. *Academic Emergency Medicine, 10*, 1209–1217.

Beukelman, D. R., & Yorkston, K. M. (1991). *Communication disorders following traumatic brain injury: Management of cognitive, language and motor impairments.* Austin TX: Pro-Ed.

Biros, M. H., & Heegaard, W. G. (2009). Head injury. In J. A. Marx (Ed.), *Rosen's emergency medicine: Concepts and clinical practice* (7th ed.). Philadelphia, PA: Mosby.

Bittner, R. M., & Crowe, S. F. (2005). The relationship between naming difficulty and FAS performance following traumatic brain injury. *Brain Injury, 20*, 971–980.

Blachstein, H., Vakil, E., & Hoofien, D. (1993). Impaired learning in patients with closed-head injuries: An analysis of components of the acquisition process. *Neuropsychology, 7*, 530–535.

Bowman, S. M., Martin, D. P., Sharar, S. R., & Zimmerman, F. J. (2007). Racial disparities in outcomes of persons with moderate to severe traumatic brain injury. *Medical Care, 45*, 686–690.

Brain Injury Association of America. (2013). *Traumatic brain injury.* Washington, DC: Author.

Brooks, D. N. (1983). Disorders of memory. In M. Rosenthal, E. R. Griffith, M. Bond, & J. D. Miller (Eds.), *Rehabilitation of the head injured adult* (pp. 185–197). Philadelphia, PA: F. A. Davis.

Brooks, J., Fos, L. A., Greve, K. W., & Hammond, J. S. (1999). Assessment of executive function in patients with mild traumatic brain injury. *Journal of Trauma, 46*, 159–163.

Brookshire, R. H., & Nicholas, L. E. (1993). *Discourse comprehension test.* Tucson, AZ: Communication Skill Builders.

Brown, M. (2006). Introduction to the participation objective, participation subjective. *Center for Outcome Measurement in Brain Injury.* Retrieved from http://www.tbims.org/combi/pops

Burns, M. S. (1997). *Burns brief inventory of communication and cognition.* San Antonio, TX: Pearson Education.

Butler-Hinz, S., Caplan, D., & Waters, G. (1990). Characteristics of syntactic comprehension deficits following closed head injury versus left cerebrovascular accident. *Journal of Speech and Hearing Research, 33*, 269–280.

Canteen, K. (2011). Traumatic brain injury and blast injuries: From assessment and treatment to community re-integration. *District of Columbia Speech and Hearing Association Discussion,*Washington, DC.

Capeheart, B., & Bass, D. (2012). Review: Managing posttraumatic stress disorder in combat veterans with comorbid traumatic brain injury. *Journal of Rehabilitation Research Development, 49*, 789. doi:10.1682/JRRD.2011.10.0185

Cavanna, A. E. (2010). The neural correlates of impaired consciousness in coma and unresponsive states. *Discovery Medicine*. Retrieved from http://www.discovery medicine.com/Andrea-Eugenio

Centers for Disease Control and Prevention. (2003). *Mass causalities*. Retrieved from http://www.bt.cdc.gov/masscasualties/pdf/glasgow-coma-scale.pdf

Centers for Disease Control and Prevention. (2010a). *Concussion: What are the signs and symptoms of concussion?* Retrieved from http://www.cdc.gov/concussion/signs_symptoms.html

Centers for Disease Control and Prevention. (2010b, March). *Traumatic brain injury in the United States. Emergency department visits, hospitalizations and deaths, 2002–2006.* Retrieved from http://www.cdc.gov/traumaticbraininjury/factsheets_reports.html

Cernak, I. (2007). Blast injuries: Importance, basic mechanisms and consequences. *Johns Hopkins University Applied Physics Laboratory Biomedicine*, pp. 1–11.

Cernak, I., Wang, Z., Jiang, J., Bian, X., & Savic, J. (2001). Ultrastructural and functional characteristics of blast injury–induced neurotrauma. *Journal of Trauma, 50*, 695–706.

Channon S., & Watts, M. (2003). Pragmatic language interpretation after closed head injury: Relationship to executive functioning. *Cognitive Neuropsychiatry, 8*(4), 243–260.

Chapel, B. (2013). U.S. military's suicide rate surpassed combat death in 2012. *The two-way: NPR.* Retrieved from https://www.npr.org/blogs/the two-way/2013/01/14/16936733/u-s-militarys-suicide-rate-surpassed-combat-deaths-in-2012

Clark, M. E., Scholten, J. D., Walker, R. L., & Gironda, R. J. (2009). Assessment and treatment of pain associated with combat-related polytrauma. *Pain Medication, 10*, 456–469. doi:10.1111 /j.1526-4637.2009.00590.x

Coelho, C. A., DeRuyter, F., & Stein, M. (1996). Treatment efficacy: Cognitive-communication disorders resulting from traumatic brain injury in adults. *Journal of Speech and Hearing Research, 39*, S5–S17.

Collins, M. W., Grindel, S. H., Lovell, M. R., Dede, D. E., Moser, D. J., Phalin, B. R., . . . McKeag, D. B. (1999). Relationship between concussion and neuropsychological performance in college football players. *Journal of the American Medical Association, 282*, 964–970.

Constantinidou, F., & Kennedy, M. (2012). Traumatic brain injury in adults. In I Papathanasiou, P. Coppens, & C. Potagas (Eds.), *Aphasia and related neurogenic communication disorders* (pp. 365-392). Burlington, MA: Jones & Bartlett Learning.

Council on Scientific Affairs. (1996). American Medical Association. Alcoholism in the elderly. *Journal of the American Medical Association, 275*, 797–801.

Crosson, B., Novak, A. T., Trenerry, M. R., & Craig, P. L. (1988). California verbal learning test (CLVT) performance in severely head-injured and neurologically normal adult males. *Journal of Clinical and Experimental Neuropsychology, 10*, 754–768.

Cullum, C. M., & Bigler, E. D. (1986). Ventricle size, cortical atrophy and relationship with neuropsychological status in closed head injury: A quantitative analysis. *Journal of Clinical and Experimental Neuropsychology, 8*, 437–452.

Czosnyka, M., Balestreri, M., Steiner, L., Smielewski, P., Hutchinson, P. J., Matta, B., & Pickard, J. D. (2005). Age, intracranial pressure, autoregulation, and outcome after brain trauma. *Journal of Neurosurgery, 102*, 450–454.

Czosnyka, M., Smielewski, P., Timofeev, I., Lavinio, A., Guazzo, E., Hutchinson, P., & Pickard, J. D. (2007). Intracranial pressure: More than a number. *Neurosurgery Focus, 22*, E10.

Dawodu, S. T., & Campagnolo, D. I. (2013). *Traumatic brain injury (TBI): Definition, epidemiology, pathophysiology.* MedScape reference retrieved from http://emedicine.medscape.com/article/326510-overview#showal.l

Degeneff, C. E., & Lee, G. K. (2010). Quality of life after traumatic brain injury: perspectives of adult siblings. *Journal of Rehabilitation, 76*(4), 27–36. doi:10.1002/j.15566678.2010. tb00036.x

Delis, D. C., Kaplan, E., & Kramer, J. H. (2001). *Delis–Kaplan Executive Function System*™ (D–KEFS™). San Antonio, TX: Pearson Assessments.

Delis, D. C., Kramer, J. H., Kaplan, E., & Ober, B. A. (2000). *California Verbal Learning Test, second edition.* San Antonio, TX: Pearson Education.

Demetriades, D., Murray, J. A., Martin, M., Velmahos, G., Salim, A., Alo, K., & Rhee, P. (2004). Pedestrians injured by automobiles: Relationship of age to injury type and severity. *Journal of the American College of Surgeons, 119,* 324.

Dennis, K. (2009). Current perspectives on traumatic brain injury. Vol. 8, No. 4. *ASHA Access Audiology.*

Derogatis, L. R. (2001). *Brief symptom inventory 18: Administration, scoring and procedures manual,* Minneapolis, MN: NCS Pearson.

Diener, E., Emmons, R., Larsen, J., & Griffin, S. (1985). The Satisfaction with Life Scale. *Journal of Personality Assessment, 49,* 71–75.

Dijkers, M. (2000). *The community integration questionnaire.* Center for Outcome Measurement in Brain Injury. Retrieved from http://www .tbims.org/combi/ciq

DiRusso, S. M., DiRusso, S. M., Risucci, D., Nealon, P., Cuff, S., Haider, A., & Benzil, D. (2002). Traumatic brain injury in the elderly: increased mortality and worse functional outcome at discharge despite lower injury severity. *Journal of Trauma, 53,* 19–23.

Disabled World News. (2011). *Concussion—Signs, symptoms and treatment.* Retrieved from http:// www.disabled-world.com/health/neurol ogy/tbi/signs-of-concussion.php

Doarn, C. R. (2009, September). *Symposium report of innovative new technologies to identify and treat traumatic brain injuries: Crossover technologies and approaches between military and civilian application.* Symposium sponsored by U.S. Army Medical Research & Material Command and Telemedicine and Advanced Technology Research Center, hosted by the American Telemedicine Association, Indian Wells, CA.

Douglas, J., Bracey, C., & Snow, P. (2007). Measuring perception of communicative ability: Reliability and validity of the La Trobe communication questionnaire. *Journal of Head Trauma Rehabilitation. 22,* 31–38.

Douglas, J., O'Flaherty, C., & Snow, P. (2000). Measuring perception of communicative ability: The development and evaluation of the La Trobe communication questionnaire. *Aphasiology, 14,* 251–268.

Douglas, J. M. (2010). Relation of executive functioning to pragmatic outcome following severe traumatic brain injury. *Journal of Speech, Language and Hearing Research, 53,* 365–382. doi:10.1044/1092-4388(2009/08-0205)

Doyle , M., & Fager, S. (2011, February 15). Traumatic brain injury and AAC: Supporting communication through recovery. *ASHA Leader.* Retrieved from http://www.asha.org/Publi cations/leader/Traumatic-Brain-Injury-and-AAC-Supporting-Communication-Through-Recovery.htm

Elder, G. A., & Cristian, A. (2009). Blast-related mild traumatic brain injury: Mechanisms of injury and impact on clinical care. *Mount Sinai Journal of Medicine, 76,* 111–118. doi:10.1002/ msj.20098

Ellmo, W. J., Graser, J. M., Krchnavek, E. A., Calabrese, D. B., & Hauck, K. (1995). *Measure of cognitive linguistic abilities.* Norcross, GA: The Speech Bin.

Farrer, T. J., & Hedges, D. W. (2011). Prevalence of traumatic brain injury in incarcerated groups compared to the general population: a meta-analysis. *Progress in Neuropsychopharmacol Biological Psychiatry, 35*(2), 390–3944. Advance online publication. doi:10.1016/j .pnpbp.2011.01.007

Faul, M., Xu, L., Wald, M. M., & Coronado, V. G. (2010). *Traumatic brain injury in the United States: Emergency department visits, hospitalizations, and deaths.* Atlanta, GA: Centers for Disease Control and Prevention, National Center for Injury Prevention and Control.

Finkelstein, E., Corso, P., & Miller, T. (2006). *The incidence and economic burden of injuries in the United States.* New York, NY: Oxford University Press.

Folstein, M., Folstein, S. E., & McHugh, P. R. (1975). Mini-mental state: A practical method for grading the cognitive state of patients for the clinician. *Journal of Psychiatric Research, 12*(3), 189–198.

Frattali, C., Thompson, C., Holland, A., Wohl, C., & Ferketic, M., (1995). *Functional Assessment of Communication Skills for Adults (ASHA-FACS).* Rockville, MD: American Speech Language Hearing Association.

Frost, R. B., Farrer, T. J., Primosch, M., & Hedges, D.W. (2012). Prevalence of traumatic brain injury in the general adult population: A meta-analysis. *Neuroepidemiology, 40,* 154–159.

Georgeadis, A. C., Brennan, D. M., Barker, L. M., & Baron, C. R. (2004). Telerehabilitation and its effect on story retelling by adults with neurogenic communication disorders. *Aphasiology, 18*(5/6/7), 639–652. doi:10.1080/ 02687030444000075

Giacino, J. T. Kalmar, K., & Whyte, J. (2000). The JFK Coma Recovery Scale-Revised: Measurement characteristic and diagnostic utility. *Archives of Physical Medicine and Rehabilitation, 85*(12), 2020–2029.

Gibson, C. (2012). Review of posttraumatic stress disorder and chronic pain: The path to integrated care. *Journal of Rehabilitation Research Development, 49*(5), 753–776. doi:10.1682/JRRD.2011.09.0158

Gilworth, G., Eyres, S., Carey, A., Bhakta, B. B., & Tennant, A. (2008). Working with a brain injury: Personal experiences of returning to work following a mild or moderate brain injury. *Journal of Rehabilitative Medicine, 40*(5), 334–339.

Gioia, G., Isquith, P. K., Guy, S. C., & Kenworthy, L. (2000). Test review: Behavior rating inventory of executive function. *Child Neuropsychology, 6*, 235–238.

Godunsky, J. S., & Reiter, M. P. (2005). Protecting military convoys in Iraq: An examination of battle during Operation Iraqi Freedom II. *Military Medicine, 170*, 546–549. Retrieved from http://www.ncbi.nlm.nih.gov/pubmed/16001610

Golden, C. (1978). *The Stroop Color and Word Test*. Lutz, FL: Psychological Assessment Resources.

Golden, C. J., & Freshwater, S. M. (2002). *Western Stroop Color and Word Test*. Torrence, CA: Western Psychological Services.

Goozée, J. V., Murdoch, B. E., Theodoros, D. G., & Stokes, P. D. (2000). Kinematic analysis of tongue movements in dysarthria following traumatic brain injury using electromagnetic articulography. *Brain Injury, 14*, 153–174.

Graham, D. P., & Cardon, A. L. (2008). An update on substance use and treatment following traumatic brain injury. *Annals of the New York Academy of Sciences, 1141*, 148–162. doi:10.1196/annals.1441.029

Grieve, M. W., & Zink, B. J. (2009). Pathophysiology of traumatic brain injury. *Mount Sinai Journal of Medicine, 76*, 97–104. doi:10.1002/msj.20104

Groher, M. (1977). Language and memory disorders following closed head trauma. *Journal of Speech and Hearing Disorders, 20*, 212–223.

Groot, Y., Wilson, B. A., Evans, E., & Watson, P. (2002). Prospective memory functioning in people with and without brain injury. *Journal of International Neuropsychological Society, 8*, 645–654.

Guskiewicz, K. M., Marshall, S.W., Bailes, J., McCrea, M., Cantu, R. C., Randolph, C., & Jordan, B. D. (2005). Association between recurrent concussion and late-life cognitive impairment in retired professional football players. *Neurosurgery, 57*, 719–726.

Gutierrez, E., Huang, Y., Haglid, K., Bao, F., Hansson, H. A., Hamberger, A., & Viano, D. (2001). A new model for diffuse brain injury by rotational acceleration: I model, gross appearance, and astrocytosis. *Journal of Neurotrauma, 18*, 247–257.

Haacke, E. M. (2013, January). The future present: A new way to look at traumatic brain injury. *The ASHA Leader*.

Hagelson, S. R. (2010). Identifying brain injury in state juvenile justice, corrections and homeless populations: Challenges and promising practices. *Brain Injury Professional, 7*, 18–21.

Hagen, C. (1984). Language disorders in head trauma. In A. L. Holland (Ed.), *Language disorders in adults: Recent advances* (pp. 245–282). San Diego, CA: College-Hill Press.

Hagen, C. (1998). *The Rancho levels of cognitive functioning–Revised* (3rd ed). Downey, CA: Ranchos Los Amigos Medical Center.

Hagen, C., Malkmus, D., & Durham, P. (1972). *Levels of cognitive functioning*. Downey, CA: Rancho Los Amigos Hospital.

Hagen, C., Malkmus, D., & Durham, P. (1979). Levels of cognitive functioning. In *Rehabilitation of the head injured adult: Comprehensive physical management*. Downey, CA: Professional Staff Association of Rancho Los Amigos Hospital.

Haijar, E. R., Cafiero, A. C., & Hanlon, J. T. (2007). Polypharmacy in elderly patients. *American Journal of Geriatric Pharmacotherapy, 5*, 345–351.

Hammeke, T. A., & Gennarelli, T. A. (2003). Traumatic brain injury. In R. B. Schiffer, S. M. Rao, & B. S. Fogel (Eds.), *Neuropsychiatry* (p. 1150). Hagerstown, MD: Lippincott Williams & Wilkins.

Harman, P., & Kelly, M. (2012). *Traumatic brain injury in veteran populations: From assessment to community re-integration*. Rockville, MD: District of Columbia Speech and Hearing Conference.

Haut, M. W., & Shutty, M. S. (1992). Patterns of verbal learning after closed head injury. *Neuropsychology, 6*, 51–58.

Hegde, M. N. (2008). *Hegde's Pocket Guide to Assessment in Speech-Language Pathology* (3rd ed.). Independence, KY: Cengage Learning.

Helfer, M. T., Jordan, N. N., Lee, R. B., Pietrusiak, P., Cave, K., & Schairer, K. (2011). Noise- induced hearing injury and comorbidities among post-deployment U.S. Army soldiers: April 2003–June 2009. *American Journal of Audiology, 20*, 33–41. doi:10.1044/1059-0889(2011/1000033)

Helm-Estabrooks, N. (2001). *Cognitive Linguistic Quick Test*. San Antonio, TX: Psychological Corporation.

Helm-Estabrooks, N., & Holz, G. (1991). *Brief test of head injury*. Austin, TX: Pro-Ed.

Hoge, C. W., McGurk, D., Thomas, J. L., Cox, A. L., Engel, C. C., & Castro, C. A. (2008). Mild traumatic brain injury in US soldiers returning from Iraq. *New England Journal of Medicine, 358*, 453–463. doi:10.1056/NEJMoa072972

Honaker, J. A., Criter, R. E., & Patter, J. N. (2013). *Life in balance*. Retrieved from http://www.asha.org/Publications/leader/2013/131201/Life-in-Balance.htm

Honsinger, M. J., & Yorkston, K. M. (1991). Compensation for memory and related disorders following traumatic brain injury. In D. R. Beukelman & K. M. Yorkston (Eds.), *Communication disorders following traumatic brain injury: Management of cognitive, language and motor impairments* (pp. 103–121). Austin, TX: Pro-Ed.

Hoofien, D., Gilboa, A., Vakil, E., & Donovick, P. J. (2001). Traumatic brain injury (TBI) 10-20 years later: A comprehensive outcome study of psychiatric symptomatology, cognitive abilities and psychosocial functioning. *Brain Injury, 15*, 189–209.

Huang, A. R., Mallet, L., Rochefort, C. M., Eguale, T., Buckeridge, D. L., & Tamblyn, R. (2012). Medication-related falls in the elderly: Causative factors and preventive strategies. *Drugs & Aging, 29*, 359–376.

Huckens, M., Pavawalla, S., Demadura, T., Kolessar, M., Seelye, A., Roost, N., & Storzbach, D. (2010). A pilot study examining effects of group-based cognitive strategy training treatment on self-reported cognitive problems, psychiatric symptoms, functioning, and compensatory strategy use in OIF/OEF combat veterans with persistent mild cognitive disorder and history of traumatic brain injury. *Journal of Rehabilitation Research & Development, 47*, 43–60. doi:10.1682/JRRD.2009.02.0019

Human Service Transportation Delivery (HSTD). (2010). Retrieved from http://www.ncsl.org/document/transportation/ky-HSTCpublic.pdf

Hux, K., Bush, E., Zichefosse, S., Holmberg, M., Henderson, A., & Simanek, G. (2010). Exploring the study skills and accommodations used by college student survivors of traumatic brain injury. *Brain Injury, 24*(1), 13–26. doi:10.3109/02699050903446823

Ivancevic V. G. (2009). New mechanics of traumatic brain injury. *Journal of Cognitive Neurodynamics, 3*, 281–293.

Jaeger, M., Hertrich, I., Stattrop, U., Schönle, P. W., & Ackermann, H. (2000). Speech disorders following severe traumatic brain injury: Kinematic analysis of syllable repetitions using electromagnetic articulography. *Folia Phoniatric Logopedics, 52*, 187–196.

Jennett, B., & Bond, M. (1975). Glasgow outcome scale: Assessment of outcome after severe brain injury: A practical scale. *Lancet, 1*, 480–484.

Jett, S. (October-December, 2010). Combat-related blast-induced neurotrauma: A public health problem. *Nursing Forum, 45*, 237–245. doi:10.1111/j.1744-6198.2010.00195.x

Jones, W. P., Loe, S. A., Krach, S. K., Rager, R. Y., & Jones, H. M. (2008). Automated neuropsychological assessment metrics (ANAM) and Woodcock-Johnson III tests of cognitive ability: A concurrent validity study. *The Clinical Neuropsychologist, 22*, 305–320.

Jones, K. D., Young, T., & Leppma, M. (2010). Mild traumatic brain injury and posttraumatic stress disorder in returning Iraq and Afghanistan war veterans: Implications for assessment and diagnosis. *Journal of Counseling & Development, 88*, 372–376. Retrieved from http://search.proquest.com.ezproxy.lib.uh.edu/docview/518721310?accountid=7107

Jordan, B. D., Relkin, N. R., Ravdin, L. D., Jacobs, A. R., Bennett, A., & Gandy, S. (1997). Apolipoprotein E ε4 associated with chronic traumatic brain injury in boxing. *Journal of the American Medical Association, 278*, 136–140.

Joynt, R. J. (1975). Human memory. In D. B. Tower (Ed.), *The nervous system* (pp. 441–448). New York, NY: Raven Press.

Kaplan, E., Goodglass, H., & Weintraub, S. (2001). *Boston Naming Test* (2nd ed.). Austin, TX: Pro-Ed.

Keith, R. A., Granger, C. V., Hamilton, B. B., & Sherwin, F. S. (1987). The functional independence measure: A new tool for rehabilitation. In M. G. Eisenberg & R. G. Grzesiak (Eds.), *Advances in clinical rehabilitation* (pp. 6–18). New York, NY: Springer-Verlag.

Kennedy, M. (2006, October 17). Managing memory and metamemory impairments in individuals with traumatic brain injury. *The ASHA Leader.*

Kennedy, M. R., Coelho, C., Turkstra, L., Ylvisaker, M., Moore Sohlberg, M. M., Yorkston, . . . Kan, P. F. (2008). Intervention for executive functions after traumatic brain injury: A systematic review, meta-analysis and clinical recommendations. *Neuropsychological Rehabilitation, 18,* 257–299. doi:10.1080/09602010701748644

Kennedy, M. R. T., & DeRuyter, F. (1991). Cognitive and language bases for communication disorders. In D. R. Beukelman & K. M. Yorkston (Eds.), *Communication disorders following traumatic brain injury: Management of cognitive, language, and motor impairments* (pp. 123–190). Austin, TX: Pro-Ed.

Kennedy, M. R .T., & Nawrocki, M. D. (2003). Delayed predictive accuracy of narrative recall after traumatic brain injury: Salience and explicitness. *Journal of Speech, Language and Hearing Research, 46,* 98–112.

Kennedy, M. R. T., & Yorkston, K. M. (2000). Accuracy of metamemory after traumatic brain injury: Predictions during verbal learning. *Journal of Speech, Language, and Hearing Research, 43,* 1072–1086.

Kerr, C. (1995). Dysnomia following traumatic brain injury: An information-processing approach to assessment. *Brain Injury, 9,* 777–796.

Kessler, R. C., Sonnega, A., Bromet, E., Hughes, M., & Nelson, C. B. (1995) Posttraumatic stress disorder in the national comorbidity survey. *Archives of General Psychiatry, 52,* 1048–1060. doi:10.1001/archpsyc.1995.03950240066012

King, N. S., Crawford S., Wenden, F. J., Moss, N. E., & Wade, D. T. (1995). The Rivermead post concussion symptoms questionnaire: A measure of symptoms commonly experienced after head injury and its reliability. *Journal of Neurology, 242,* 587–592.

Klatzo, I. (1979). Brain edema. In G. L. Odom (Ed.), *Central nervous system trauma research status report* (pp. 110–113). Rockville, MD: National Institutes of Health.

Knight, C., Alderman, N., & Burgess, P. W. (2002). Development of a simplified version of the multiple errands test for use in hospital settings. Development of a simplified version of the multiple errands test for use in hospital settings. *Neuropsychological Rehabilitation, 12,* 231–255. doi:10.1080/09602010244000039

Langlois, J. S., Rutland-Brown, W., & Wald, M. M. (2006). The epidemiology and impact of traumatic brain injury: A brief overview. *Journal of Head Trauma Rehabilitation, 21,* 375–378.

LaPointe, L. L., Murdoch, B. E., & Stierwalt, J. A. G. (2010). *Brain-based communication disorders* (pp. 106–110). San Diego, CA: Plural.

Lawhorne, C., & Philpott, D. (2010). *Combat-related traumatic brain injury and PTSD: A resource & recovery guide.* Lanham, MD: Government Institutes.

LeBlanc, J., DeGuise, E., Feyz, M., & Lamoureux, J. (2006). Early prediction of language impairment following traumatic brain injury. *Brain Injury, 20,* 1391–1401.

Levin, H. S. (1985). Outcome after head injury. Part II: Neurobehavioral recovery. In D. P. Becker & J. T. Povlishock (Eds.), *Central nervous system trauma. Status report, 1985.* Washington, DC: National Institutes of Health.

Levin, H. S., Benton, A. L., & Grossman, R. G. (Eds.). (1982). *Neurobehavioral consequences of closed head injury.* New York, NY: Oxford University Press.

Levin, H. S., Grossman, R. G., & Kelly, P. J. (1976). Aphasic disorders in patients with closed head injury. *Journal of Neurology, Neurosurgery, and Psychiatry, 39,* 1062–1070.

Levin, H. S., O'Donnell, V. M., & Grossman, R. G. (1979). The Galveston Orientation and Amnesia Test. A practical scale to assess cognition after head injury. *Journal of Nervous and Mental Diseases, 167,* 675–684.

Lezak, M. D. (1995). *Neuropsychological assessment* (3rd ed.). New York, NY: Oxford University Press.

Li, J., Brown, J., & Levine, M. (2001). Mild head injury, anticoagulants, and risk of intracranial injury. *Lancet, 357,* 771–772.

Lishman, W. A. (1978). *Organic psychiatry.* Oxford, UK: Blackwell Scientific.

MacDonald, S. (2005). *Functional assessment of verbal reasoning and executive strategies.* Guelph, Ontario: CCD Publishing.

MacGregor, A. J., Dougherty, A. L., Morrison, R. H., Quinn, K. H., & Galarneau, M. R. (2011). Repeated concussion among U.S. military personnel during Operation Iraqi Freedom. *Journal of Rehabilitation Research and Development, 48*(10), 1269–1278. doi:10.1682/JRRD.201.01.0013.

MacLennan, D. L., Cornis-Pop, M., Picon-Nieto, M., & Sigford, B. (2002). The prevalence of pragmatic communication impairments in traumatic brain injury. *Premier Outlook, 3,* 38–45. Retrieved from http://www.premier outlook.com/winter_2002/prevelance_prag matic_communication.html

Malec, J. F. (2004). The Mayo-Portland participation index: A brief and psychometrically sound measure of brain injury outcome. *Archives of Physical Medicine Rehabilitation, 85,* 1989–1996. Retrieved from http://www .tbims.org/combi/mpai

Malec, J. F., Moessner, A. M., Kragness, M., & Lezak, M. D. (2003). Refining a measure of brain injury sequelae to predict post-acute rehabilitation outcome: Rating scale analysis of the Mayo-Portland Adaptability Inventory. *Journal of Head Trauma Rehabilitation, 15,* 670–682.

Malik, A. M., Dal, N. A., & Talpur, K. A. H. (2012). Road traffic injuries and their outcome in the elderly patients (60 years and above). Does age make a difference? *Journal of Trauma and Treatment, 1,* 129–133. doi:10 .4172/2167-1222.1000129.

Malkamus, D., &. Stenderup, K. (1974). *Rancho Los Amigos Cognitive Scale–Revised.* Downey, CA: Rancho Los Amigos Hospital.

Martin, D. A. (1990). Family issues in traumatic brain injury. In E. D. Bigler (Ed.), *Traumatic brain injury* (pp. 381–394). Austin, TX: Pro-Ed.

Mashima, P. A. (2010, November). Using telehealth to treat combat-related traumatic brain injury. *The ASHA Leader.*

Mashima, P. A., Birkmire-Peters, D. P., Syms, M. J., Holtel, M. R., & Burgess, L. P. A. (2003). Voice therapy using telecommunications technology. *American Journal of Speech, Language, Pathology, 12,* 432–439. doi:1058-0360/ 03/1204-0432

Matser, E. J. T., Kessels, A. G., Lezak, M. D., Jordan, B. D., & Troost, J. (1999). Neuropsychological impairment in amateur soccer players. *Journal of the American Medical Association, 282,* 971–979.

McCoy, G. F., Johnstone, B. A., & Duthie, R. B. (1989). Injury to the elderly in road traffic accidents. *Journal of Trauma, 29,* 494–497.

McCrary, M. B. (1992, April). Urban multicultural trauma patients. *ASHA, 34,* 37–40.

McDonald, S. (1993). Pragmatic language skills after closed injury: Ability to meet the informational needs of the listeners. *Brain and Language, 44,* 28–46.

McDonald, S. (1998) Communication and language disturbances following traumatic brain injury. In B. Stemmer & H. A. Whitaker (Eds,). *Handbook of Neurolinguistics* (pp. 487–495). San Diego, CA: Academic Press.

McDonald, S. (2007). The social and neuropsychological underpinnings of communication disorders after traumatic brain injury. In M. J. Ball & J. Damico (Eds.), *Clinical aphasiology—future directions* (pp. 42–71). Sussex, UK: Psychology Press.

McKee, A. C., Cantu, R. C., & Nowinski, C. J. (2009). Chronic traumatic encephalopathy in athletes: Progressive tauopathy after repetitive head injury. *Journal of Neuropathology and Experimental Neurology, 68,* 709–735. doi:10.1097/NEN.0b013e3181a9d503

Menon, D. K., Schwab, K., Wright, D. W., & Maas, A. I. (2010). Position statement: Definition of traumatic brain injury. *Archives of Physical Medicine and Rehabilitation, 91,* 1637–1640.

Miller, J. D. (1983). Early evaluation and management. In M. Rosenthal, E. R. Griffith, M R. Bond, & J. D. Miller (Eds.), *Rehabilitation of the head injured adult* (pp. 37–58). Philadelphia, PA: F. A. Davis Company.

Millis, S. R., & Ricker, J. H. (1994). Verbal learning patterns in moderate and severe traumatic brain injury. *Journal of Clinical and Experimental Neuropsychology, 16,* 498–507.

Milton, S., Prutting, C., & Binder, G. (1984). Appraisal of communication competence in head injured adults. In R. H. Brookshire (Ed.), *Clinical aphasiology conference proceedings* (pp. 114–123). Minneapolis, MN: BRK.

Moore, D. F., & Jaffe, M. S. (2010). Military traumatic brain injury and blast. *NeuroRehabilitation, 26,* 179–181. doi:10.3233/NRE-2010-0553

Morris, G. F., & Marshall, S. B. (2000). Head injury. In C. Goldman, *Textbook of Medicine,* (21st ed.). Philadelphia, PA: W.B. Saunders Company, 2000. Retrieved from Harvard Medical School Head Injury in the Elderly http://symptom-checker.about.com/od/Diagnoses/head-injury-in-adults.htm on January 12, 2013

Mungas, D., Marshall, S. C., Weldon, M., Haan, M, & Reed, B. R. (1996). Age and education correction of Mini-Mental State Examination for English and Spanish-speaking elderly. *Neurology, 46,* 700–706.

Murphy, B., Herrman, H., Hawthorne, G., Pinzone, T., & Evert, H. (2000). *Australian WHOQoL instruments: User's manual and interpretation guide.* Melbourne, Australia: Australian WHO-QoL Field Study Centre.

Nasreddine, Z. S., Phillips, N. A., Bedirian, V., Charbonneau, S., Whitehead, V., Collin, I., . . . Chertkow, H. (2005). The Montreal cognitive assessment, MoCA: A brief screening tool for mild cognitive impairment. *Journal of the American Geriatric Society, 53,* 695–699.

National Center on Elder Abuse. (1998). *National elder abuse incidence study: Final report.* Washington, DC: American Public Human Services Association in collaboration with Westat.

National Center for Health Statistics. (2012). *Vital statistics mortality data, multiple cause of death detail* (machine-readable public-use data file). Hyattsville, MD: U.S. Department of Health and Human Services, Public Health Service (annual).

National Healthcare Quality and Disparities Reports. (2010). Rockville, MD: Agency for Healthcare Research and Quality. http://www.ahrq.gov/research/findings/nhqrdr/nhqrdr10/qrdr10.html

National Highway Traffic Safety Administration (2012). *2012 Motor vehicle crashes.* Retrieved from http://www.nrd.nhtsa.dot.gov/Pubs/811856.pdf

National Institute on Alcohol Abuse and Alcoholism. (1988). *Alcohol alert.* Retrieved from http://www.pubs.Niaaa.nih.gov/publications/aa02.htm

National Institute on Alcohol Abuse and Alcoholism. (2011). *Alcohol and aging.* Alcohol Alert, No. 40. Updated October 2000, Retrieved from http://pubs.niaaa.nih.gov/publications/aa40.htm.

National Institute of Neurological Disorders and Stroke (NINDS). (2005). *Cognitive rehabilitation interventions: Moving from bench to bedside.* NINDS Workshop and Conference Proceedings. Retrieved from http://www.ninds.nih.gov/news_and_events/proceedings/execsumm07_19_05.htm

National Institute of Neurological Disorders and Stroke (NINDS). (2012). *Traumatic brain injury: Hope through research.* Retrieved from http://www.ninds.nih.gov/disorders/tbi/detail_tbi.htm

National Institute of Neurological Disorders and Stroke (NINDS). (2013). *Coma information.* Retrieved from http://www.ninds.nih.gov/disorders/coma/coma.htm#

Nayback, A. M. (2008). Health disparities in military veterans with PTSD: Influential sociocultural factors. *Journal of Psychosocial Nursing, 46*(6), 43–51. doi:10.3928/02793695-20080601-08

Neselius, S., Brisby, H., Theodorsson, A., Blennow, K., Zetterberg, H., & Marcusson, J. (2012). CSF-Biomarkers in Olympic boxing: Diagnosis and effects of repetitive head trauma. *PLoS ONE, 7*(4), 1–8. doi:10.1371/journal.pone.0033606

NIH Senior Health. (2011, January). *Falls and older adults: Causes and risk factors.* Retrieved from http://nihseniorhealth.gov/falls/causesandriskfactors/01.html

Nimmo-Smith, I., Emslie, H., & Baddeley, A. (2006). *Doors and people.* San Antonio, TX: Pearson Assessment.

Niogi, S. N., Mukherjee, P., Ghajar, J., Johnson, C. E., Kolster, R., Lee, H., & McCandliss, B. D. (2008). Structural dissociation of attentional control and memory in adults with and without mild traumatic brain injury, *Brain, 131,* 3209–3221. doi:10.1093/brain/awn247

Nordell, E., Jarnlo, G. B., Jetsen, C., Nordstrom, L., & Thorngren, K.G. (2000). Accidental falls and related fractures in 65–74 year olds: A retrospective study of 332 patients. *Acta Orthopaedica Scandinavica, 71,* 175–179.

O'Halloran, R. T., Worrall, L. E., Toffolo, D., Code, C., & Hickson, L. M. H. (2004). *IFCI: Inpatient Functional Communication Interview.* Oxon, UK: Speechmark.

Okie, S. (2005). Traumatic brain injury in the war zone. *New England Journal of Medicine, 352,* 2043–2047. doi:10.1056/NEJMp058102

Olson, D., & Henig, E. (1983). *A manual of behavioral management strategies for traumatically brain-injured adults.* Chicago, IL: Rehabilitation Institute of Chicago.

Olver, J. H., Ponsford, J. L., & Curran, C. A. (1996). Outcome following traumatic brain injury: A comparison between 2 and 5 years after injury. *Brain Injury 10,* 841–848.

Omalu, B., Bailes, J., Hamilton, R. L., Kamboh, M. I., Hammers, J. L., Case, M., & Fitzsimmons, R. (2011a). Emerging histomorphologic phenotypes of chronic traumatic encephalopathy in American athletes. *Neurosurgery, 69,* 173–183. doi:10.1227/NEU.0b013e318212bc7b

Omalu, B. I., Hamilton, R. L., Kamboh, M. I., DeKosky, S. T., & Bailes, J. (2010). Chronic traumatic encephalopathy (CTE) in a National Football League player: Case report and emerging medicolegal practice questions. *Journal of Forensic Nursing, 6,* 40–46.

Omalu, B., Hammers, J. L., Bailes, J., Hamilton, R. L., Kamboh, M. I. Webster, G., & Fitzsimmons, R. P. (2011b). Chronic traumatic encephalopathy in an Iraqi war veteran with posttraumatic stress disorder who committed suicide. *Neurosurgical Focus, 31*(5), E3. doi:10.3171/2011.9.FOCUS11178

Ommaya, A. K. (1979). Reintegrative action of the nervous after trauma. In A. J. Popp (Ed.), *Neural trauma* (pp. 371–378). New York, NY: Raven Press.

Ommaya, A. K. (1995). Head injury mechanisms and the concept of preventive management: A review and critical synthesis. *Journal of Neurotrauma, 12,* 527–546.

Ommaya, A. K. (1997). Why neurobehavioral sequelae do not correlate with head injury severity: A biomechanical explanation for the traumatic disturbances of consciousness. *Seminars in Clinical Neuropsychiatry, 2,* 163–178.

Ommaya, A. K., & Gennarelli, T. (1974). Cerebral concussion and traumatic unconsciousness, *Brain, 97,* 833–654.

Ommaya, A. K., Goldsmith, W., & Thibault, L. (2002). Biomechanical neuropathology of adult and paediatric head injury. *British Journal of Neurosurgery, 16,* 220–242.

Ommaya, A. K., Salazar, A. M., Dannenberg, A. L., Chervinsky, A B., Stewart, W., & Drachman, D. (1996). *Behavioral sequelae of traumatic brain injury: A longitudinal study in the U. S. Army.* Unpublished manuscript.

Parrish, C., Roth, C., Roberts, B., & Davie, G. (2009). Assessment of cognitive-communicative disorders of mild traumatic brain injury in combat. *Perspectives on Neurophysiology and Neurogenic Speech & Language Disorders, 19,* 47–57.

Payne, J. C., & Ommaya, A. K. (1997). Traumatic brain injury in the older adult. In J. C. Payne (Ed.), *Adult neurogenic language disorders: Assessment and treatment. A comprehensive ethnobiological approach.* San Diego, CA: Singular.

Peach, R. K. (2013). The cognitive basis for sentence planning difficulties in discourse after traumatic brain injury. *American Journal of Speech-Language Pathology, 22,* S285–S297. doi: 10.1044/1058-0360(2013/12-0081)

Perna, R. B., Bubier, J., Oken, M., Snyder, R., & Rouselle, A. (2004). *Brain injury rehabilitation: Activity based and thematic group treatment.* Retrieved from http://www.neuropsychonline.com/loni/jcrarchives/vol22/V22I3Perna.pdf

Polovoy, C. (2011, December). National report points to CRT effectiveness for TBI. *The ASHA Leader.*

Porth, C. (2007). *Essentials of pathophysiology: Concepts of altered health states.* Hagerstown, MD: Lippincott Williams & Wilkins.

"Practice parameter: The management of concussion in sports summary." (1997, March). *Neurology, 48*(3), 581–585. doi:10.1212/WNL.48.3.581

Randolph, C. (1998). *Repeatable Battery for the Assessment of Neuropsychological Status.* San Antonio, TX: Pearson Assessment.

Rappaport, M., Hall, K. M., Hopkins, K., Belleza, T., & Cope, D. N. (1982). Disability rating scale for severe head trauma patients: Coma to community. *Archives of Physical Medicine and Rehabilitation, 63,* 118–123.

Raskin, S., & Buckheit, C. (1998). *Prospective memory in traumatic brain injury.* San Francisco, CA.: Cognitive Neuroscience Society.

Reitan, R., & Wolfson, D. (1985). *The Halstead-Reitan Neuropsychological Test Battery.* Tucson, AZ: Neuropsychology Press.

Ribbers, G. M. (2013). Brain injury: Long term outcome after traumatic brain injury. In J. H. Stone & M. Blouin (Eds.), *International encyclopedia of rehabilitation.* Retrieved from http://cirrie.buffalo.edu/encyclopedia/en/article/338/

Robertson, I. H., Ward, T., Ridgeway, V., & Nimmo-Smith, I. (1994). *Test of Everyday Attention.* Bury St. Edmonds, UK: Thames Valley Test Company.

Roseberry-McKibben, C., & Hegde, M. N. (2006). *An advanced review of speech-language pathology* (2nd ed.). Austin, TX: Pro-Ed.

Rosenthal, M., Dijkers, M., Harrison-Felix, C., Nabors, J., Witol, A. D., Young, M. E., & Englander, J. S. (1996). Impact of minority status on functional outcome and community integration following traumatic brain injury. *Journal of Head Trauma Rehabilitation, 11,* 40–45.

Ross-Swain, D. (1996). *Ross Information Processing Assessment* (2nd ed.). Austin TX: Pro-Ed.

Roth, C. R. (2007). Mechanisms and sequelae of blast injuries. *Perspectives on Neurophysiology and Neurogenic Speech & Language Disorders, 3,* 20–24.

Rutland-Brown, W., Langlois, J. A., & Thomas, K. E. (2006). Incidence of traumatic brain injury in the United States, 2003. *Journal of Head Trauma Rehabilitation, 21,* 544–548.

Ryan, T. V., & Ruff, R. M. (1988). The efficacy of structured memory retraining in a group comparison of head trauma patients. *Archives of Clinical Neuropsychology, 3,* 165–179.

Safaz, I., Yasar, A. R., Tok, F., & Yilmaz, B. (2008). Medical complications, physical function and communication skills in patients with traumatic brain injury: A single centre 5-year experience. *Brain Injury, 22,* 733–739.

Santora, T. A., Schinco, K. A., & Trooskin, S. Z. (1994). Management of trauma in the elderly patient. *Surgical Clinics of North America, 74,* 164–186.

Schneider, S. L., Haack, L., Owens, J., Herrington, D. P., & Zelek, A. (2009). An interdisciplinary treatment approach for soldiers with TBI/PTSD: Issues and outcomes. *Perspectives on Neurophysiology and Neurogenic Speech & Language Disorders, 19,* 36–46.

Schopp, L. H., Johnstone, B. R., & Merveille, O. C. (2001) Multidimensional telecare strategies for rural residents with brain injury. *Journal of Telemedicine and Telecare, 6*(Suppl. 1), S146–S149. Retrieved from http://www.ncbi.nlm.nih.gov/pubmed/10794002

Schwabacher, S., Lewis, B., Eshel, I., & Goudy, L. (2011). *Metacognition and executive functioning in mTBI: Apps to cognitive gaming.* Paper presented at the 2011 American Speech and Hearing Association convention in San Diego, CA.

Scott, S. G., Belanger, H. G., Vanderploeg, R. D., Massengale, J., & Scholten, J. (2006). Mechanism-of-injury approach to evaluating patients with blast-related polytrauma. *Journal of the American Osteopathic Association, 106,* 265–270. Retrieved from http://www.jaoa.org/content/vol106/issue5/

Shafi, S., de la Plata, C. M., Diaz-Arrastia, R. B. A., Frankel, H., Elliott, A. C., Parks, J., & Gentilello, L. M. (2007). Ethnic disparities exist in trauma care. *Journal of Trauma-Injury Infection & Critical Care, 63,* 1138–1142.

Shallice,T., & Burgess, P. W. (1991). Multiple errands test: Deficits in strategy application following frontal lobe damage in man. *Brain, 114,* 727–741.

Sherer, M. (2004). The awareness questionnaire. *Center for Outcome Measurement in Brain Injury.* Retrieved from http://www.tbims.org/combi/aq

Sherer, M., Nick, T. G., Sander, A. M., Hart, T., Hanks, R., Rosenthal, M., . . . Yablon, S. A. (2003). Race and productivity outcome after traumatic brain injury: Influence of confounding factors. *Journal of Head Trauma Rehabilitation, 18,* 408–424.

Shively, S. B., & Perl, D. P. (2012). Traumatic brain injury, shell shock, and posttraumatic stress disorder in the military—past, present, and future. *Journal of Head Trauma Rehabilitation, 27,* 234–239. doi:10.1097/HTR.0b013e318250e9dd

Shorland, J., & Douglas, J. M. (2010). Understanding the role of communication in maintaining and forming friendships following traumatic brain injury. *Brain Injury, 24,* 569–580.

Shum, D. H., & Fleming, J. M. (2008). *Comprehensive assessment of prospective memory: Manual.* Brisbane, Australia: Applied Cognitive Neuroscience Research Center.

Shum, D., Valentine, M., & Cutmore, T. (1999). Performance of individuals with severe long-term traumatic brain injury on time- event- and activity-based prospective memory tasks. *Journal of Clinical and Experimental Neuropsychology, 21,* 49–58.

Sjogren, H., & Bjornstig, U. (1991). Injuries to the elderly in the traffic environment. *Accident Analysis and Prevention, 23,* 77–86.

Sklar, D. P., Demarest, G. B., & McFeeley, P. (1989). Increased pedestrian mortality among the elderly. *American Journal of Emergency Medicine, 7,* 87–90.

Slone, L. B., & Friedman, M. J. (2008). *After the war zone: A practical guide for returning troops and their families.* Philadelphia, PA: Da Capo Press Life Long.

Snow, P., Douglas, J., & Ponsford, J. (1997). Conversational assessment following traumatic brain injury: A comparison across two control groups. *Brain Injury, 11,* 409–429.

Snow, P., Douglas, J., & Ponsford, J. (1998). Conversational discourse abilities following severe traumatic brain injury: A follow-up study. *Brain Injury, 12,* 911–935.

Sohlberg, M., Johnson, L., Paule, L., Raskin, S., & Mateer, C. (2001). *Attention process training II.* Wake Forest, NC: Lash & Associates.

Sohlberg, M., & Mateer, C. (1989). *Prospective memory training screening. Introduction to cognitive* rehabilitation: Theory and practice. New York, NY: Guilford Press.

Sohlberg, M. M., & Mateer, C. A. (2001). Cognitive rehabilitation: An integrative neuropsychological approach. New York, NY: Guilford Press.

Spelman, J. F., Hunt, S. C., Seal, K. H., & Burgo-Black, L. (2012). Post deployment care for returning combat veterans. Journal of General Internal Medicine, 27, 1200–1209. doi:10.1007/s11606-012-2061-1

Spencer, R. J., Drag, L. L., Walker, S. J., & Bieliauskas, L. A. (2010). Self-reported cognitive symptoms following mild traumatic brain injury are poorly associated with neuropsychological performance in OIF/OEF veterans. Journal of Rehabilitation Research and Development, 47, 521–530. doi:10.1682/JRRD.2009.11.0181

Spoont, M. R., Hodges, J., Murdoch, M., & Nugent, S. (2009). Race and ethnicity as factors in mental health service use among veterans with PTSD. Journal of Traumatic Stress, 22, 6, 648–653. doi:10.1002/jts.20470

Squire, L. R. (2004). Memory systems of the brain: A brief history and current perspective. Neurobiology of Learning and Memory, 82, 171–177.

Squire, L. R., Stark, C. E. L., & Clark, R. E. (2004). The medial temporal lobe. Annual Review of Neuroscience, 27, 279–306.

Stanczak, D. E., White, J. G., Gouview, W. D., Moehle, K. A., Daniel, M., Novack, T., & Long, C. J. (1984). Assessment of level of consciousness following severe neurological insult. A comparison of the psychometric qualities of the Glasgow Coma Scale and the Comprehensive Level of Consciousness Scale. Journal of Neurosurgery, 60, 955–960.

Stevens J. A. (2006). Fatalities and injuries from falls among older adults—United States, 1993–2003 and 2001–2005. MMWR, 2006a, 55(45) cited in CDC (2012), Falls among the elderly: an overview. Retrieved from http://www.cdc.gov/homeandrecreationalsafety/falls/adultfalls.html

Stierwalt, J. A., & Murray, L. L. (2002). Attention impairment following traumatic brain injury. Seminars in Speech and Language, 23, 129–138.

Strauss, E., Sherman, E., & Spreen, O. (2006). Rey auditory verbal learning test. A compendium of neuropsychological tests: Administration, norm, and commentary (3rd ed., pp. 776–807). New York, NY: Oxford University Press.

Subramanian, R. (2012). Motor vehicle traffic crashes as a leading cause of death in the United States, 2008 and 2009. U.S. Department of Transportation. National Highway Traffic Safety Administration. Retrieved from http://www-nrd.nhtsa.dot.gov/Pubs/811620.pdf

Susman, M., DiRusso, S. M., Sullivan, T., Risucci, D., Nealon, P., Cuff, S., . . . Benzil, D. (2002). Traumatic brain injury in the elderly: Increased mortality and worse functional outcome at discharge despite lower injury severity. Journal of Trauma, 53, 219–224.

Sutton, M. (2012, July). APP-titude: Apps for brain injury rehab. Retrieved from http://www.asha.org/Publications/leader/2012/120703/APP-titude-for-Brain-Iijury-Rehab.htm

Teasdale, G., & Jennett, B. (1974). Assessment of coma and impaired consciousness. Lancet, 2, 81–84.

Teasdale, G. M., Pettigrew, L. E., Wilson, J. T., Murray, G., & Jennett, B. (1998). Analyzing outcome of treatment of severe head injury. A review and update on advancing the use of the Glasgow Outcome Scale. Journal of Neurotrauma, 15, 587–597.

Thompson, H. J., McCormick, W. C., & Kagan, S. H. (2006). Traumatic brain injury in older adults: Epidemiology, outcomes, and future implications. Journal of the American Geriatrics Society, 54, 1590–1595.

Thompson, H. J., Weir, S., Rivara, F. P., Wang, J., Sullivan, S. D., Salkever, D., & Mackenzie, E. J., (2012). Utilization and costs of health care after geriatric traumatic brain injury. Journal of Neurotrauma, 29, 1864–1871. doi:10.1089/neu.2011.2284

Timmons, T., & Menaker, J. (2010).Traumatic brain injury in the elderly. Clinical Geriatrics, 18, 20–24.

Turkstra, L., McDonald, S., & Kaufmann, P. (1995). Assessment of pragmatic communication skills in adolescents after traumatic brain injury. Brain Injury, 10, 329–345.

Turkstra, L., Ylvisaker, M., Coehlo, C., Kennedy, M., Sohlberg, M. M., & Avery, J. (2005). Practice guidelines for standardized assessment for persons with traumatic brain injury. Journal of Medical Speech-Language Pathology, 13, ix–xxviii.

U.S. Department of Transportation. (2010). Highway statistics, 2008. Washington, DC: Federal Highway Administration. Retrieved from

http://www.fhwa.dot.gov/policyinforma
tion/statistics/2008/dl20.cfm

U.S. Department of Veterans Affairs. (2009). *VA/
DOD clinical practice guideline: Management of
post-traumatic stress.* Retrieved from http://
www.healthquality.va.gov/PostTraumatic
Stress_Disorder_PTSD.asp

U.S. Department of Veterans Affairs. (2010). *Traumatic brain injury: Independent study course.*
Washington, DC: Author. Retrieved from
http://www.publichealth.va.gov/doc/vhi/
traumatic-brain-injury-vhi.pdf

U.S. Department of Veterans Affairs/Department
of Defense (VA/DOD). (2009). *Clinical practice
guidelines for management of concussion/mild TBI
(mTBI).* Retrieved from http://www.healthqual-
ity.va.gov/mtbi/concussion_mtbi_full_1_0.pdf

Uzzel, B. P., Obrest, W. D., Dolinkas, C. A., &
Langfitt, T. W. (1986). Relationship of acute
CBF and ICP findings in neuropsychological
outcome in severe head injury. *Journal of Neurosurgery, 65*, 630–635.

Van Dyke, S. A., Axelrod, B. N., & Schutte, C.
(2010). Test-retest reliability of the Traumatic
Brain Injury Screening Instrument. *Military
Medicine, 175*, 947–949. Retrieved from http://
www.ncbi.nlm.nih.gov/pubmed/21265299

Vogel, F. S. (1979). Pathology of trauma of the
nervous system. In G. L. Odom (Ed.), *Central
nervous system trauma research status report,
1979* (pp. 114–123). Rockville, MD: National
Institutes of Health.

Von Steinbuechel, N., Wilson, L., Gibbons, H.,
Hawthorne, G., Hofer, S., Schmidt, S., . . .
Truelle, J. L. (2010). Quality of life after brain
injury–Scale validity and correlates of quality
of life. *Journal of Neurotrauma, 27*, 1167–1185.
doi:10.1089/neu.2009.1076

Waite, M. C., Theodoros, D. G., Russell, T. G., &
Cahill, L. M. (2010). Internet-based telehealth
assessment of language using the CELF-4.
*Language, Speech, and Hearing Services in
Schools, 41*, 445–458. doi:10.1044/0161-1461
(2009/08-1031).

Walker, W. C., Kruetzer, J. S., & Witol, A. D. (1996).
Level of care options for the low-functioning
brain injury survivor. *Brain Injury, 10*, 65–75.

Wallace, G. (2006, June). Blast injury basics:
A primer for the medical speech-language
pathologist. *The ASHA Leader.*

Waller, P. F. (1996). Accidents: Traffic. In J. E.
Birren (Ed.), *Encyclopedia of gerontology: Age,*
aging, and the aged (pp. 19–25). San Diego, CA:
Academic Press.

Waller, P. F. (1998). Alcohol, aging, and driving.
In E. S. L. Gomberg, A. M. Hegedus, & R.
A. Zucker (Eds.), *Alcohol problems and aging.*
NIAAA Research Monograph No. 33. NIH
Pub. No. 98-4163. Bethesda, MD: NIAAA.

Wechsler, D. (2008). *Processing speed index,
Wechsler Adult Intelligence Scale IV.* San Antonio, TX: Pearson Education.

Werner, C., & Engelhard, K. (2007). Pathophysiology of traumatic brain injury. *British Journal of
Anaesthesia, 99*, 4–9.

Whiteneck, G., Charlifue, S., Gerhart, K., Overholser, J., & Richardson, G. (1992). Quantify-
ing handicap: A new measure of long-term
rehabilitation outcomes. *Archives of Physical
Medicine and Rehabilitation, 73*, 519–526.

Whiteneck, G. G., Djikers, M. P., Heinemann,
A.W., Bogner, J. A., Bushnik, T., Cicerone,
K. D., . . . Millis, S. R. (2011). Development
of the participation assessment with recom-
bined tools-objective for use after traumatic
brain injury. *Archives of Physical Medicine
and Rehabilitation, 92*, 542–551. doi:10.1016/j.
apmr.2010.08.002

Wilson, B. A., Alderman, N., Burgess, P., Emslie,
H., & Evans, J. (1996). *Behavioural Assess-
ment of the Dysexecutive System including the
DEX questionnaire.* San Antonio, TX: Pearson
Assessment.

Wilson, B. A., Alderman, N., Burgess, P. W., Emslie,
H., & Evans, J. (2003). Behavioural Assessment
of the Dysexecutive Syndrome (BADS). San
Antonio, TX: Pearson Assessment.

Wilson, B. A., Cockburn, J., & Baddeley, A. (1985).
Rivermead behavioural memory test. London,
UK: Pearson Assessment.

Wilson, B. A., Greenfield, E., Clare, L., Bad-
deley, A., Cockburn, A., Watson, P., Tate, R.,
. . . Crawford, J. (2008). *Rivermead Behavioural
Memory Test-Third edition (RBMT-3).* Oxford,
UK: Pearson Assessment:

Wilson, J. T. L., Pettigrew, L. E. L., & Teasdale,
G. M. (1998). Structured interviews for the
Glasgow outcome scale and the extended
Glasgow outcome scale: Guidelines for their
use. *Journal of Neurotrauma, 15*, 573–585.

Wilson, J. T., Slieken, F. J., Legrand, V., Murray, G.,
Slocchetti, N., & Maas, A. I. (2007). Observer
variability in the assessment of outcome in
traumatic brain injury: Experience from a

multicenter, international randomized clinical trial. *Neurosurgery, 61*, 123–128; 128–129.

Woodcock, R. W., McGrew, K. S., & Mather, N. (2001). *Woodcock-Johnson-III.* Itasca, IL: Riverside.

World Health Organization. (1993). Study protocol for the World Health Organization project to develop a quality of life assessment instrument (WHOQOL). *Quality of Life Research, 2,* 153–159.

World Health Organization (2011). *Elder maltreatment.* Retrieved from http://www.who.int/mediacentre/factsheets/fs357/en/index.htm

Wright, J. (2000). *The Disability Rating Scale.* The Center for Outcome Measurement in Brain Injury. Retrieved from http://www.tbims.org/combi/drs

Yee, W. Y., Cameron, P. A., & Bailey, M. J. (2006). Road traffic injuries in the elderly. *Emergency Medicine Journal, 232,* 42–46.

Yeh, P., Oakes, T. R., & Riedy, G. (2012). Diffusion tensor imaging and its application to traumatic brain injury: Basic principles and recent advances. *Open Journal of Medical Imaging, 2,* 137–161. doi:10.4236/ojmi.2012.24025

Ylvisaker, M., & Szekeres, S. (1986). Management of the patient with closed head injury. In R. Chapey (Ed.), *Language intervention strategies in adult aphasia* (pp. 474–491). Baltimore, MD: Williams & Wilkins.

Youse, K. M., Le, K. N., Cannizzaro, M. S., & Coelho, C. A. (2002, June 25). *Traumatic brain injury: A primer for professionals.* Retrieved from http://www.asha.org/Publications/leader/2002/02065/02065a.htm

CHAPTER 6

Aphasia and Right-Hemisphere Disorders

I. APHASIA

Aphasia is an acquired language impairment in all four modalities, spoken language, auditory comprehension, reading, and writing, which is caused by neurological damage. Aphasia may co-occur with other disorders, such as apraxia, speech disorders such as dysarthria, impaired swallowing, difficulty recalling words, and cognitive deficits. Approximately 1 million people, or 1 in 250 in the United States today, suffer from aphasia, and it is estimated that approximately 80,000 individuals acquire aphasia each year (National Stroke Association, 2008). Fifteen percent of individuals under the age of 65 experience aphasia from first-time strokes; this percentage increases to 43% for individuals 85 years of age and older (Engelter et al., 2006). Based on population growth estimates (Lingraphica, n.d.), the incidence of aphasia in the United States is expected to rise to 180,000 cases per year by 2020, with the prevalence then being 2 million persons living with aphasia.

The majority of persons with aphasia (80%) are diagnosed with cerebrovascular accidents, or strokes. Approximately 15% of persons with aphasia have diagnoses of other disorders: traumatic brain injury (TBI), brain tumors, degenerative and chronic diseases, and medical procedures.

Cerebrovascular Accidents

Stroke-induced aphasia is associated with twice the mortality from stroke compared with nonaphasic stroke (36% vs. 16%). This likely reflects underlying cardiovascular pathology, rather than an effect of aphasia itself (Laska, Hellblom, Murray, Kahan, & Von Arbin, 2001). According to the World Health Organization (n.d.), a cerebrovascular accident (CVA), or stroke, is caused by the interruption of the blood supply to the brain, usually because a blood vessel bursts or is blocked by a clot. This cuts off the supply of oxygen and nutrients, causing damage to the brain tissue. The most common symptom of a stroke is sudden weakness or numbness of the face, arm, or leg, most often on one side of the body. Other symptoms include: confusion, difficulty speaking or understanding speech, difficulty seeing with one or both eyes, difficulty walking, dizziness, loss of balance or coordination, severe headache with no known cause, fainting, and unconsciousness.

Types of Stroke

The National Stroke Association (2012) identifies the two major types of strokes as ischemic and hemorrhagic:

Ischemic Stroke. Ischemia occurs when blood clots block arteries and cut off blood flow to the brain. About 85% of all strokes are ischemic (CDC, 2012). Figure 6–1

shows a CT scan of an infarct caused by blockage to the middle cerebral artery.

Thrombotic Stroke. In the second type of blood-clot stroke, a clot, called an embolus, blocks blood flow to one or more of the arteries supplying blood to the brain. The process leading to this blockage is a thrombosis. Blood-clot strokes can also happen as the result of unhealthy blood vessels clogged with a buildup of fatty deposits and cholesterol. Figure 6–2 shows an MRI of a venous thrombosis. Two types of thrombosis can cause stroke: large vessel thrombosis and small vessel disease (or lacunar infarction).

Large Vessel Thrombosis. Thrombotic stroke occurs most often in the large arteries. Large vessel thrombosis is the

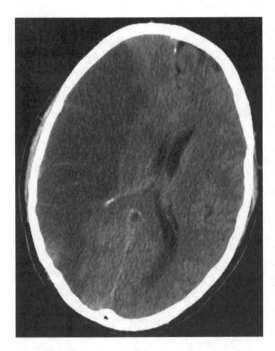

Figure 6–1. CT scan of middle cerebral artery infarct. (Lucien Monfils/Wikimedia Commons/GFDL 1.2; CC-A-SA-3.0 Unported, 2.5 Generic, 2.0 Generic, 1.0 Generic)

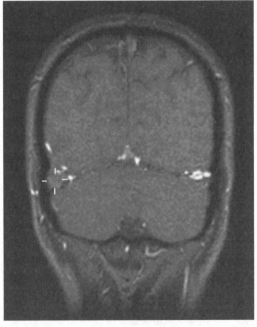

Figure 6–2. MRI of sinus vein thrombosis. (User: Mbq/Wikimedia Commons/Public Domain)

most common and best understood type of thrombotic stroke. Most large vessel thrombosis is caused by a combination of long-term atherosclerosis followed by rapid blood clot formation. Thrombotic stroke patients are also likely to have coronary artery disease, and heart attack is a frequent cause of death in patients who have suffered this type of brain attack.

Small Vessel Disease/Lacunar Infarction. Small vessel disease, or lacunar infarction, occurs when blood flow is blocked to a very small arterial vessel. The word *lacunar* comes from the Latin word *lacuna*, which means hole, and describes the small cavity remaining after the products of deep infarct have been removed by other cells in the body. Little is known about the causes of small vessel disease, but it is closely linked to hypertension.

Watershed Strokes. A watershed stroke is an ischemia, or blood flow blockage, that is localized to the border zones between the territories of two major arteries in the brain (internal carotid and vertebral/basilar). Insufficient blood flow to the brain may cause these strokes, which are usually the result of poor blood flow to the brain from occlusion of the arteries in the neck from atherosclerosis or from periods of poor cardiac function, such as during a heart attack. Watershed locations are those border-zone regions in the brain supplied by the major cerebral arteries where blood supply is decreased. Watershed strokes are a concern because they comprise approximately 10% of all ischemic stroke cases (Torvik, 1984).

Hemorrhagic Stroke. Strokes caused by the breakage or bursting of a blood vessel in the brain are called hemorrhagic strokes. Hemorrhages can be caused by a number of disorders that affect the blood vessels, including long-standing high blood pressure and cerebral aneurysms. An aneurysm is a weak or thin spot on a blood vessel wall. These weak spots are usually present at birth. Aneurysms develop over a number of years and may not cause detectable problems until they break. Figure 6–3 shows a lateral view of the cerebrum with aneurysms.

There are two types of hemorrhagic stroke: subarachnoid and intracerebral.

Subarchanoid Hemorrhage. In a subarachnoid hemorrhage, an aneurysm bursts in a large artery on or near the meninges. Blood spills into the area around the brain, which is filled with cerebral spinal fluid (CSF), causing the brain to be surrounded by blood-contaminated fluid.

Intracerebral Hemorrhage. In an intracerebral hemorrhage, bleeding occurs from vessels within the brain itself. Hypertension is the primary cause of this type of hemorrhage. Figure 6–4 shows an intracerebral hemorrhage.

Traumatic Brain Injury

Penetrating head injuries may result in focal damage and aphasia. Aphasia associated with blunt force head injuries can develop hours or even weeks after the initial precipitating event of right blunt orbitofrontal trauma with a contrecoup left temporoparietal injury. This type of impact imparts a shearing force to the head, which causes motion of the cerebral hemispheres within the closed cranium. In blunt force trauma, peripheral areas are more susceptible to direct impact with the cranium (Groher, 1977). Language disturbances associated with

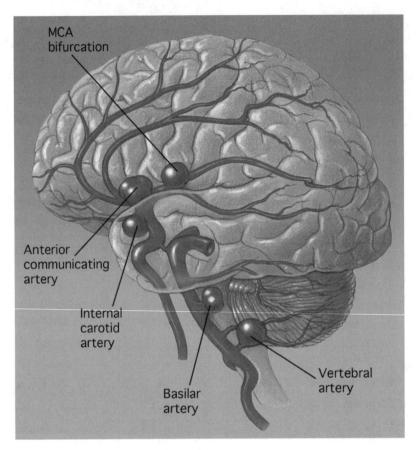

Figure 6–3. Lateral view of cerebrum showing aneurysms. © 2013 Medical Art Studio. Reprinted with permission.

TBI are termed the language of confusion because of the diffuse effect of blunt force TBI on pragmatics and higher cognitive and executive functions. Research, however, has shown that cognitive rehabilitation frequently results in improvement of language (Kavanagh, Lynam, Düerk, Casey, & Eustace, 2010; Nishio, Takemura Ikai, & Baba, 2004; Vukovic, Vuksanovic, & Vukovic, 2008).

Brain Tumors

Brain tumors may cause a wide range of neurological dysfunctions, including apha-sia (Shafi & Carroza, 2012). This largely depends on the where the tumor is developing. The specific area(s) of the brain that are affected by the tumor will determine the nature of any language disorders. The U.S. prevalence rate of primary brain tumors is 130.8 per 100,000 individuals, which translates to 359,000 people affected, based on current population estimates. It is additionally estimated that 100,000 cancer patients per year will be diagnosed with metastatic brain tumors (i.e., tumor cells from other body systems that spread to the brain) (Mayer, 2008).

A brain tumor is a mass of abnormal cells that can be benign (noncancer-

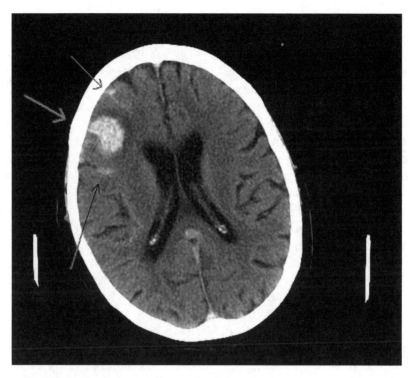

Figure 6–4. CT scan of intracerebral hemorrhage. (Lucien Monfils/Wikimedia Commons/GFDL 1.2; CC-A-SA-3.0 Unported, 2.5 Generic, 2.0 Generic, 1.0 Generic)

ous) or malignant (cancerous). A primary brain tumor emerges in the brain; a metastic tumor begins in another part of the body before spreading to the brain. Primary brain tumors are typically gliomas and are derived from glial cells, the non-neuronal, supportive tissue in the central nervous system. The majority of primary brain tumors are fast-growing and rapidly spreading high-grade gliomas. About 30% to 50% of patients with primary brain tumors experience aphasia (Davie, Hutcheson, Barringer, Weinberg, & Lewin, 2009).

Aphasia secondary to cancer is referred to as neoplastic aphasia (Paratz, 2011). The most common subtype of language disorder in cancer-related aphasia is anomic aphasia (Davie et al., 2009).

Brain tumor–related aphasia is generally transient, but if the tumor is inoperable or recurrent, symptoms may continue to develop and worsen over time.

Degenerative and Chronic Diseases

Primary progressive aphasia (PPA) is associated with frontotemporal dementia (Pick's disease), which has been discussed extensively in Chapter Four. Kirshner, Tanridag, Thurman, and Whetsell (1987) describe two cases of progressive aphasia without dementia resulting from focal spongiform degeneration. Both patients showed a focal spongiform change involving primarily layer 2 of the left inferior frontal gyrus (and temporal cortex in Patient 1) and a mild astrocytosis in layer 2 and deeper cortical layers.

Spongiform degeneration is characterized by vacuolation (small cavities) in nervous tissue accompanied by neuronal death and gliosis (Henics & Wheatley, 1999). Spongiform degeneration is a hallmark of prion diseases. Prion diseases are transmissible spongiform encephalopathies and are from a family of rare progressive neurodegenerative disorders that affect both humans and animals, as for example, in Creuzfeldt–Jakob disease (Belay & Schoenberger, 2005; Tzeng et al., 1997; Whatley, Li, & Chin, 2008). This pathology is also present in the brains of patients suffering from Alzheimer's disease, diffuse Lewy body disease, and human immunodeficiency virus (HIV) infection. These diseases present with disturbances in language such as loss of semantic content, word finding difficulties, and cognitive disturbances.

HIV infection can result in stroke via several mechanisms, including opportunistic infection, vasculopathy, cardioembolism, and coagulopathy. However, the occurrence of stroke and HIV infection might often be coincidental. HIV-associated vasculopathy describes various cerebrovascular changes, including stenosis and aneurysm formation, vasculitis, and accelerated atherosclerosis, and might be caused directly or indirectly by HIV infection (Benjamin et al., 2012). Ortiz, Koch, Romano, Forteza, and Rabinstein (2007) found that among 82 persons diagnosed with HIV and acute stroke, the mechanism of ischemic stroke was large artery atherosclerosis in 12%, cardiac embolism in 18%, small vessel occlusion in 18%, other determined etiology in 23%, and undetermined in 29% (including 19% with incomplete evaluation). Vasculitis was deemed responsible for stroke in 10 patients (13%) and hypercoagulability in 7 (9%). There was no difference in stroke rate for those on combination antiretroviral treatment (CART) and those not on the treatment.

Sickle cell disease (SCD), a blood disorder in which blood platelets become deformed into sickle shapes that injure vital organs, is a major cause of strokes among African Americans. Of the many severe consequences of SCD, acute stroke and chronic cerebral ischemia are among the most disabling. Hematologically normal African Americans have twice the stroke risk of non-Hispanic whites. This suggests that there is a subset of African Americans who may have particularly vulnerable cerebral blood vessels. The risk is enormous in SCD. Approximately 11% of SCD patients have clinically apparent strokes before the age of 20. That risk increases to 24% by the age of 45 (Verduzco & Nelson, 2009). Persons with SCD are living longer into adulthood and may have a history of repeated strokes and stroke sequelae that began in childhood. Several types of intracranial hemorrhage have been observed but usually in older children and adults. Cerebrovascular diseases restricted to small vessels may go unrecognized but are associated with cognitive and learning problems (Gebreyohanns & Adams, 2004).

Medical Procedures

Medical procedures to evacuate brain tumors or hematomas may cause a disruption in language functioning in the dominant left cerebral hemisphere or right hemisphere, may cause anoxia, or may cause an ischemia or watershed stroke within the major arteries that supply the brain.

APHASIA CLASSIFICATIONS

Aphasia is classified into fluent and non-fluent aphasias according to their neuroanatomical substrates. Lesions of the left hemisphere often result in specific language deficits across the modalities of speaking, listening, reading, and writing, which are collectively termed *aphasia*.

Left-Hemisphere Nonfluent Aphasias

Broca's Aphasia

If damage occurs in the left posterior portion of the third frontal convolution (F3) in area 44 (Brodmann classification), the result is nonfluent Broca's aphasia. See also Chapter 2 for other areas around Broca's area 44 that may be implicated in Broca's aphasia.

Broca's aphasia is characterized by effortful, poorly articulated speech, telegraphic speech, impaired repetition and naming, relatively intact reading comprehension, inability to read aloud, difficulty comprehending written materials, abnormal writing, and relatively intact auditory comprehension. The clinical picture may vary from a complete loss of speech to a mild deficit characterized simply by word-finding difficulties. In the case of telegraphic speech, all small, function words, for example, prepositions, are absent, and the patient uses primarily nouns and verbs (Potagas, Kasselimis, & Evdokimidis, 2013). The patient may omit small words such as "is," "and," and "the." For example, a person with Broca's aphasia may say, "Walk dog," meaning, "I will take the dog for a walk," or "book book two table," for "There are two books on the table" (National Institute

of Deafness and Other Communication Disorders, n.d.). A marked deficiency or absence of syntactical, structural words, or functors, make the output strikingly abnormal (Benson, 1979).

Broca's aphasia is an agrammatic aphasia because patients exhibit deficits in using and understanding syntactic structures. Persons with Broca's aphasia suffer from a pathological limitation in their ability to recognize correct grammatical structures. This limitation results in a quick decay of their ability to process syntactic information. Haartman and Kolk (1994) found that patients with Broca's aphasia were able to respond correctly only on tasks of subject-verb agreement violations when the sentences were simple rather than complex. Druks and Marshall (1995) also found that patients with Broca's aphasia experience agrammatic comprehension and described two clinical cases of patients who demonstrated better comprehension of passive rather than active cases of verbs.

Chronic, agrammatic aphasia is produced by lesions extending from Broca's area to the anterior insula and neighboring anterior temporal and inferior parietal areas. Damage in deeper structures also seems necessary to produce this aphasia, including the posterior internal capsule of tracts between the thalamus and basal ganglia (Davis, 2000). Lesions restricted to area 44 can cause an acute Broca's aphasia that may resolve quickly into something else, although patients with left basal ganglia lesions may suffer from both fluent and nonfluent aphasia (Robin & Schienberg, 1990).

Global Aphasia

Global aphasia, also a nonfluent aphasia, is the result of large lesions to anterior and posterior language areas and subcortical structures, including both Broca's and Wernicke's areas. The lesions extend in depth to the insula and lenticular nucleus, and even to the internal capsule (Vignolo, 1988). Global aphasia is characterized by a severe depression of all language modalities. Speech is typically nonfluent and comprehension is severely impaired (Mateer, 1989). Some patients speak noncommunicatively with verbal stereotypes. Patients can, however, be alert and aware of their surroundings and may be able to express their feelings and thoughts through facial and manual gestures (Davis, 2000).

Left-Hemisphere Fluent Aphasias

Wernicke's Aphasia

Wernicke's aphasia is caused by a lesion to the posterior portion of the first temporal gyrus (TI). Wernicke's area is area 22 (Brodmann classification). The supramarginal and lower temporal gyri may be included as part of Wernicke's area (Goodglass & Kaplan 1983). Superior temporal and middle temporal gyri are less involved in patients with good language recovery. Structures posterior or adjacent to Wernicke's area are important for compensation in Wernicke's aphasia and in the accompanying comprehension deficit. Persistent Wernicke's aphasia usually involves the supramarginal and angular gyri in addition to the superior temporal lobe area (Kertesz, Lau, & Polk, 1993). See Chapter 3 for the discussion on the possible involvement of the parietal lobe in Wernicke's aphasia.

Wernicke's aphasia is the most severe form of fluent aphasia and is also termed *sensory aphasia, receptive aphasia,* and *jargon aphasia.* The patient with Wernicke's aphasia has poor language comprehension, produces jargon, and often lacks awareness of semantic or neologistic paraphasias. A patient with Wernicke's aphasia may say something like, "You know that smoodle pinkered and that I want to get him round and take care of him like you want before" (National Institute of Deafness and Other Communication Disorders, n.d.). Lesions causing neologistic jargon extend more posteriorly than lesions producing semantic jargon (Kertesz, 1982).

The written output is different from the agraphia (writing deficit) in Broca's aphasia. The patient with Wernicke's aphasia can use the dominant hand for writing, and the output consists of well-formed, legible letters combined in the appearance of words. The letters are often combined in a meaningless manner (Benson, 1979).

Conduction Aphasia

Conduction aphasia is caused by lesions in the supramarginal gyrus and the arcuate fasciculus, a band of cortical fibers connecting anterior and posterior speech areas that separate Broca's area from Wernicke's area. The arcuate fasciculus is an association tract beneath the left parietotemporal juncture and carries impulses from Wernicke's area for listening to Broca's area for speaking (Davis, 2000).

Comprehension is good and spontaneous speech is fluent but may contain phonemic paraphasias (sound substitutions), and repetition is severely impaired. The repetition disorder is the result of damage to the posterior superior temporal cortex along with infarction of deep white matter below (Damasio & Damasio, 1980). Seddoh and his colleagues (1996) studied speech timing deficits in conduction aphasia and found that the underlying factors in these deficits were at the phonological level. Relatively preserved comprehension distinguished the patient with conduction aphasia from the patient with Wernicke's aphasia.

Most patients with conduction aphasia have difficulty with confrontational naming because of the inability to find a word. Reading aloud is abnormal and the patient experiences a rapid breakdown into severely paraphasic output. Reading comprehension is usually good to normal. Writing is disturbed to some degree. The patient may be able to write some words and produce well-formed letters, but spelling is poor and words in sentences are frequently interchanged, misplaced, or omitted (Benson, 1979).

The Transcortical Aphasias

The relatively rare transcortical aphasias are distinctive in that repetition is much better than would be expected from comprehension and spontaneous speech (Davis, 2000). These aphasia classifications result from an isolation of the speech areas from the rest of the cortex caused by multiple infarcts or diffuse lesions (Potagas, Kasselimis, & Evdokimidis, 2013).

Transcortical Motor Aphasia

Transcortical motor aphasia (TMA) is associated with frontal lobe lesions either in front of Broca's area or above Broca's area on the lateral surface at the supplementary area or at the cingulate gyrus (Cummings & Mega, 2003). Lichthelm was the first to recognize this symptom complex and described a patient with gross impairment of spontaneous speech and writing, but with preservation of spoken and written material. Lichthelm's patient had good comprehension to repeat words and sentences that could be uttered spon-

taneously (Rubens, 1979). The characteristics of TMA are strongly similar to Broca's aphasia. Patients have difficulty reading aloud, and writing is almost always defective (Benson, 1979). The basal ganglia are the involved subcortical structures, or there may be other lesions in the white matter beneath the frontal lobe (Damasio & Geschwind, 1984).

Transcortical Sensory Aphasia

In transcortical sensory aphasia (TSA), speech is fluent but in many cases meaningless or unintelligible, with many neologisms and paraphasias. The site of lesion is the border zone region of the parietotemporal junction. TSA symptoms bear a striking similarity to Wernicke's aphasia. Reading and writing are defective. Repetition of utterances ranges from good to excellent.

In TSA, the thalamus may be the subcortical structure involved. The basal ganglia and the thalamus are known to be directly connected to Broca's area and Wernicke's area, respectively (Mateer, 1989). Between 1979 and 1990, Servan, Verstichel, Catala, Yakovleff, and Rancurel (1995) studied 75 patients who suffered from an occipitotemporal infarction located in the superficial territory of the posterior cerebral artery. Aphasia was prominent in 18 cases and three patients showed features of TSA. Although computed tomography localization showed internal lobe and thalamic involvement of the dominant hemisphere, the dominant internal temporal lobe was always implicated.

Mixed Transcortical Aphasia

Mixed transcortical aphasia (MTA) is a rare disorder that combines symptoms and signs of motor and sensory transcortical aphasias. Speech is nonfluent, and comprehension, naming, writing, and reading are severely impaired. Repetition, however, is spared for words and sentences, often in the form of echolalia. MTA is, therefore, a global aphasia with the ability to repeat. Diffuse or multifocal pathologies in the frontal and parietal lobes can produce MTA while sparing the language area (Davis, 2000).

Pulvermüller and Schonle (1993) described a case of a patient with MTA stemming from destruction of the perisylvanian language area and adjacent structures. Hypothetically, neuronal changes in the damaged areas and associative cortex strengthen synaptic connections with other centers. In the patient studied, however, all language modalities were affected except for repetition. Comprehension

and expressive language improved after 5 years of intensive therapy because the patient was able to develop appropriate communication strategies.

A summary of the major characteristics of the aphasias described may be found in Table 6–1.

Other Aphasia Types

Pure Aphasias

Vignolo (1988) described two forms of pure aphasia, which he defined as a defect that is virtually confined to only one aspect of language. The two forms are alexia without agraphia and agraphia without alexia.

Table 6–1. Clinical Features of the Aphasia Syndromes

Syndrome	Spontaneous Speech	Auditory Comprehension	Repetition	Naming
Global	Nonfluent	Impaired	Impaired	Severely impaired
Broca's	Nonfluent	Spared	Impaired	Occasionally impaired
Wernicke's	Nonfluent	Mixed	Spared	Impaired
Conduction	Fluent	Spared	Impaired	Occasionally impaired
Transcortical Aphasias				
Transcortical motor	Nonfluent	Spared	Spared	Impaired
Transcortical sensory	Fluent	Impaired	Spared	Impaired
Mixed transcortical	Nonfluent	Severely impaired	Spared	Severely impaired

Source: Adapted from Mateer, C. A. (1989). Neural correlates of language function. In D. P. Kuehn, M. L. Lemme, & J. M. Baumgartner (Eds.), *Neural bases of speech, hearing, and language* (pp. 259–291). Boston, MA: College-Hill. Reprinted with permission.

Alexia without agraphia is associated with destruction of a large portion of the occipital lobe, specifically in the territory of the left posterior cerebral artery. This deficit is also called occipital alexia, pure alexia, pure word blindness, agnosic alexia, and optic aphasia (Benson, 1979). The definitive findings are a severe inability to read contrasted with a preservation of writing abilities. The patient is unable to read what has just been written. Most patients eventually regain the ability to read many or all of the individual letters and can read them aloud.

Agraphia is the loss of the inability to produce written language. Usually writing disturbances mirror the complexities of the language loss. However, isolated agraphia with alexia is a disturbance involving two small lesions. One lesion is in the upper half of the central region; the other is in the upper part of the posterior parietal (Vignolo, 1988).

Crossed Aphasia

Crossed aphasia is an aphasia that occurs when a right-handed person has lesions in the right hemisphere. Abnormal dominance for at least some language functions in the right hemisphere underlies the syndrome of crossed aphasia (Walker-Batson, Wendt, Devous, Barton, & Frederick, 1988). Three patients studied for crossed aphasia showed diaschisis, or a functional depression of the anatomically normal left hemisphere during the acute phase. One patient, however, did not evidence crossed aphasia once recovery began (Bakar, Kirshner, & Wertz, 1996).

There is some involvement of the left hemisphere in crossed aphasia. Cappa and colleagues (1993) examined two cases of right-handed persons with aphasia after right hemispheric strokes. The first patient had a severe MTA, apraxia, and neglect because of a lesion involving the right lenticular nucleus and periventricular white matter. Aphasia was still present after 3 months. The second patient had a mild, transient fluent aphasia after a small right hemispheric periventricular lesion. Neuroimaging studies showed functional depression extending to the structurally unaffected left hemisphere in both patients in the acute stage. After 3 months, in the patient with persistent aphasia, metabolism was still reduced in the right hemisphere, with some recovery of hypometabolism on the left; however, metabolic values eventually returned to normal with full language recovery. The researchers concluded that there may be a close parallel between glucose metabolism and the clinical course in crossed aphasia. Study results also indicated that the left hemisphere is functionally involved in the acute stage.

Anomic Aphasia

Anomic aphasia, often the mildest form of aphasia, frequently appears with Broca's aphasia. This aphasia is characterized by the inability to find names of people or objects. Patients with anomic aphasia are usually aware of the nature of the object but cannot name it upon request. Patients with anomic aphasia have slightly impaired comprehension and fluent, syntactically coherent utterances that are weakened by the disturbance in word retrieval (Davis, 2000).

Although identifying a specific site for naming storage has been elusive, anomic aphasia may be associated with lesions in the posterior language areas, particularly the angular gyrus in the left parietal lobe near the superior edge of the temporal lobe or the middle temporal gyrus.

Word-finding difficulties, or anomia, may coexist with aphasia or may exist independently from aphasia. Anomia is a selective impairment of lexical repertoire, primarily nouns and verbs, but adjectives and adverbs can be affected as well (Goodglass & Geschwind, 1976). Although naming sites are thought to be located in the immediate perisylvanian cortex, naming errors have been demonstrated with stimulation of a broad area of the lateral dominant cortex (Ojemann, 1979).

Geschwind (1967) distinguished aphasic anomia from word-finding problems in that in aphasic anomia, a patient with an aphasic language disorder has a demonstrable disturbance in confrontation naming. Contrastively, word-finding problems occur when a patient can perceive auditory or visual stimuli but cannot send this information to the language area of the dominant hemisphere to produce the name.

Benson (1979) identified nine varieties of word-finding disturbances, five of which can be associated with aphasia. *Word production anomia* is characterized by the patient's inability to produce the name of an object presented. With cueing, a patient may be able to use the cue and produce the appropriate name. This type of anomia is seen in nonfluent aphasia. *Word selection anomia* is the inability to name an object, although the patient can demonstrate or explain its use. In *semantic anomia*, the patient is unable to retrieve the appropriate word from the lexicon and may also have difficulty understanding his or her own name when spoken or written. *Category-specific anomia* is characterized by the patient's inability to name items in some categories while being able to name items in other categories. *Modality specific anomia* is the inability of the

patient to name objects presented to one sensory modality (vision, for example) but not others.

Subcortical Aphasias

Basal Ganglia Lesion Effects on Language

Both the basal ganglia and the thalamus have significant roles in language (Robin & Shienberg, 1990). A relationship between basal ganglia connections to the cortex has been largely observed in patients who present with nonfluent aphasias. Several clinical findings emerge from stereotactic surgery for the relief of Parkinsonian symptoms, CT scans, cerebral blood flow studies, MRI, and single-photon emission computed tomography imaging (Cappa et al., 1993; Cappa et al., 1997; Damasio, Damasio, Rizzo, Varney, & Gersh, 1982; D'Esposito & Alexander, 1995; Mega & Alexander, 1994; Okuda, Tanaka, Tachibana, Kawabata, & Sugita, 1994). These findings suggest:

◆ Anterior choroidal infarction of the globus pallidus results in a nonfluent aphasia.
◆ Left putamental hemorrhage results in nonfluent aphasia, impaired comprehension, and perhaps impaired repetition.
◆ Large lesions to the capsulostriatal region are associated with impaired executive and generative language functions.
◆ Hemorrhages in the head of the left caudate nucleus may result in nonfluent aphasia.
◆ Transcortical motor aphasia occurring with lentiform nucleus

lesions more closely resembles the speech disturbances seen after lesions of the supplementary motor area with relative sparing of repetition.

◆ Global aphasia has been observed in patients with subcortical lesions in the basal ganglia, posterior internal capsule, temporal isthmus, and pariventricular white matter in the left hemisphere.

Robinson and Schienberg (1990) found that their patients with left basal ganglia lesions suffered from both fluent and nonfluent aphasia. Disconnection of the basal ganglia from cortical language zones may have contributed to the observed aphasia. There was variability of aphasic symptoms across the patients in their study, which was likely caused by different patterns of disconnection, which disrupted the flow of information from the cortical centers. This and other clinical findings cited earlier strongly suggest that the basal ganglia may play a direct role in language.

Thalamic Lesions and Effects on Language

Subcortical lesions in the thalamus cause abnormal processing of language or indirectly influence language processing through mediating other systems such as attention and arousal. Language deficits result from left paramedian lesions and from left tuberothalamic lesions to the thalamus that include the ventrolateral nucleus (Schmahmann, 2003). A thalamic aphasia syndrome was described by Ozeren, Sarica, and Efe (1994) in which fluent aphasia, paraphasia, and reduced

comprehension are present while repetition and naming are well preserved. This type of aphasia has a rapid recovery and differs considerably from the classical aphasias. Hebb and Ojemann (2012) found that three distinct language effects of thalamic stimulation were established: anomia from posterior ventrolateral (VL) and pulvinar regions; perseveration from mid-VL regions; and a memory and acceleratory effect from anterior VL, described as a "specific alerting response." In general, thalamic lesions are found to produce the following language errors with relative preservation of repetition. The aphasias may or may not be persistent (Ojemann, 1979; Kennedy & Murdoch, 1993) and may be seen as:

◆ Word finding difficulty
◆ Reduced verbal output
◆ Disturbances in rhythm and modulation of speech
◆ Short-term memory disturbances
◆ Naming errors
◆ Neologisms

Cerebellar Lesions and Effects on Language

In addition to coordinating and smoothing fine motor movements, the cerebellum may play a role in language through its intricate circuitry to and from the neocortex (Baillieux et al., 2010; Baillieux, De Smet, Lasage, Paquier, & Mariën, 2008; Highnam & Bleile, 2011; Stoodley & Schmahmann, 2009). The language impairment secondary to cerebellar lesions is more subtle than a frank aphasia, however, and there is evidence that the cerebellum actively participates in language recovery after a CVA. Connor and her colleagues (2006) found that among controls and persons with mild aphasia, their functional MRI results indicated that the right posterolateral cerebellum participates with the left frontal lobe in the selection and production of words. Among their subjects with mild aphasia, the right frontal cortex and left cerebellar circuits participated in learning-related effects, which indicated transfer of function during recovery. Their findings supported the hypothesis that the right frontal cortex and the left cerebellar circuits participate in recovery of residual verbal functions.

Fiez, Petersen, Cheney, and Raichle (1992) have argued that the right posterolateral cerebellum is also involved in error detection in word generation tasks. Their primary evidence comes from a detailed analysis of performance of an individual with a right posterolateral cerebellar stroke and subtle language disturbance. Despite nearly normal performance in several cognitively demanding tasks, their patient showed an unusual degree of difficulty in learning repeated items on several different word generation tasks and failed to spontaneously correct his errors.

Evidence of verbal fluency deficits among patients with cerebellar lesions comes from several single-case reports (e.g., Baillieux, De Smet, Lesage, Paquier, & Marien, 2006; Paulus et al., 2004; Silveri, Leggio, & Molinari, 1994). Other research on cerebellum lesions and language disturbances suggest that aphasia symptoms may include mild anomia (Schmahmann & Sherman, 1998; Schmahmann, Weilburg, & Sherman 2007); agrammatism variously displayed as reduced sentence length, simplification of syntactic structures, and substitution/omission of grammatical morphemes (Gasparini et al., 1999; Marien et al., 1996; Silveri et al., 1994); mutism (Wells, Walsh, Khademian, Keat-

ing, & Packer, 2008) and problems with auditory verbal comprehension (Fabbro, Moretti, & Bava, 2000; Marien et al., 2009).

Associated Disorders

Coma

Altered consciousness is a strong predictor of adverse outcomes after stroke and is more likely when brain damage is extensive. Indications of severe brain damage are brainstem involvement, evidence of cerebral edema, or increased intracranial pressure. For additional information on levels of consciousness, see Chapter 4 on TBI. A prolonged deep coma after a stroke is rare and is more likely to complicate intracranial hemorrhage than infarction (Gresham et al., 1995).

Disorders of Vision

Strokes can cause visual field deficits, most commonly homonymous hemisanopsia. Homonymous hemisanopsia is a visual field defect involving either the two right or the two left halves of the visual field of both eyes caused from damage to the visual pathway where the optic nerve crosses at the optic chiasma (Oczna, 2012). Stroke can also lead to complex visual field defects. A visual field defect in the nondominant field needs to be differentiated from visual neglect, as the latter often improves spontaneously, whereas visual field defects usually do not. Stroke can also lead to complex visual deficits or disturbances in color vision. Paralysis of conjugate gaze is an unfavorable prognostic signal for survival but usually improves spontaneously in survivors (Gresham et al., 1995). Severe visual disturbances increase the complexity for rehabilitation, particularly as assessment instruments for aphasia and treatment formats often include the presentation of visual stimuli.

Disturbances of Verbal Memory

Severity of verbal memory impairment is independent of the language impairment and related to the site of lesion (Beeson, Bayles, Rubens, & Kaszniak, 1993). Greater impairment of long-term memory is associated with left-hemisphere anterior lesions, whereas greater impairment of short-term memory is observed with more posterior lesions.

Cognitive and Affective Disorders

Depression, seizure disorders, and cognitive impairment commonly occur in some adults after brain damage (Butzkueven et al., 2001; El, Annegers, Hauser, O'Brien, & Whisnant, 1996; Horner, Ni, Buft, & Lechner, 1995; National Stroke Association, 2012). For some persons, seizure disorders and depression can result in cognitive impairment. The effect of poststroke seizures on cognition was studied by De Reuck, De Clerck, and Van Maele (2006), who investigated 125 patients with late-onset seizures following an ischemic stroke. Patients who had a history of repeated seizures performed more poorly on a test for cognitive status than those who had no history of seizures or who had one seizure episode. This finding led the investigators to conclude that repeated seizures following an ischemic stroke may decrease cognitive function.

A decline in cognitive functioning related to brain damage frequently coexists with aphasia. Serrano, Domingo, Rodriguez-Garcia, Castro, and del Ser (2007) found that their patients evidenced cognitive impairment without dementia (CIND) before and after stroke and that the percentage of CIND in the subject population increased up to the 24 months of the study. Delayed dementia was higher for those persons with a diagnosis of CIND. Cognitive impairment was highly prevalent up to 3 years after a first-time stroke (Patel, Coshall, Rudd, & Wolfe, 2003). From a sample of 580 community-dwelling older persons, Aggrawal and colleagues (2012) found that the number and location of cerebral infarcts were predictable for the presence of dementia. Cortical and multiple infarcts in multiple regions increased the likelihood of dementia and lower cognitive performance, particularly in the area of processing speed.

Verbal memory is considered to be among the cognitive functions necessary for language competence. Beeson and associates (1993) found that severity of verbal memory impairment is independent of the language impairment and related to the site of lesion. Greater impairment of long-term memory is associated with left-hemisphere anterior lesions, while greater impairment of short-term memory is observed with more posterior lesions.

Depression in persons after stroke is also related to the type of lesions sustained (Kauhanen et al., 2002). Patients with chronic aphasia may exhibit major depressive disorders associated with subcortical lesions. Hermann, Bartels, and Wallesch (1993) identified three stages of poststroke depression that occur during the course of rehabilitation: primary depression resulting from structural neural change, secondary depression from neuropsychological sequelae of stroke, and tertiary depression arising from maladaptive coping strategies for long-term social change. Poststroke depression has also been linked to cognitive impairment.

Narushima, Chan, Kosler, and Robinson (2003) studied treatment effects on poststroke depression for 17 patients with cognitive impairment. They concluded that cognitive function, once improved after remission of poststroke depression, may remain stable over 2 years provided there is no further injury to the central nervous system. In their view, cognitive decline due to poststroke depression is remediable, unlike cognitive impairment associated with ischemic brain damage.

In a study of 106 adults with a diagnosis of first-time ischemic infarcts, Kauhanen and associates (2000) found that 34% of their patients had a diagnosis of aphasia in the acute stage and that over 60% of these persons were symptomatic for aphasia 12 months later. Seventy percent of patients with aphasia had a diagnosis of depression 3 and 12 months after their strokes. Those patients with aphasia were most likely to have depression and nonverbal cognitive deficits. Although the prevalence of depression in patients with aphasia decreased in the long term, the proportion of patients suffering from major depression tended to increase.

Poststroke depression can compromise language intervention. Speech-language pathologists can help to define the disorder and promote psychological well-being. Deficiencies in norepinephrine and cortisol or abnormal activities of the contralateral hemisphere, usually the right hemisphere, can cause depression. According to Swindell and Hammons (1991):

> Lesion locus and time poststroke appear to be two critical variables that influence the prevalence of poststroke depression. Patients at the greatest risk for becoming depressed are those who are within 2 years post onset of a stroke in the anterior portion of the left hemisphere. Moreover, if the lesion is close to the frontal pole, the depression is likely to be of greater severity. Several other factors that influence the development and severity of depression include premorbid social adjustment and social support, functional physical impairment, cognitive impairment and the patient's age. Without treatment, the depression typically lasts 7 to 8 months. The disorder may also resurface in patients who are more than 10 years post onset. (pp. 329–330)

Other emotional or behavioral disturbances, such as catastrophic reaction, anxiety, mania, outbursts of uncontrolled behavior, emotionless affect, and hostility, can occur in patients after stroke but are much less common than depression (Gresham et al.,1995). Emotional liability, also called pseudobulbar affect, consists of emotional outbursts (crying, laughing) due to brain damage that is uncontrolled and inappropriate to the person's mood or situation. Emotional liability is common after stroke and treatable. Morris, Robinson, and Raphael (1993) surveyed 66 patients 2 months poststroke for the presence of emotional liability. Demographic, clinical, psychiatric, and stroke lesion characteristics were also assessed. Emotional liability was present in 12% of the 66 patients, or 18. Single lesions located in anterior regions of the cerebral hemispheres were four times more likely to cause emotional liability than lesions located anywhere else.

APHASIA SEVERITY

No significant differences have been found in the incidence of aphasia in men and women. However, some data suggest differences may exist by type and severity of aphasia. For example, Wernicke's and global aphasia occur more commonly in women, and Broca's aphasia occurs more commonly in men (Hier, Yoon, Mohr, Price & Wolf, 1994; National Aphasia Association, 2011). Of the aphasias, global aphasia is the most severely affected type (Kang et al., 2010).

Stroke severity and subsequent aphasia are determined in part by the metabolic activity in the injured and collateral areas and the size and site(s) of lesions. Metabolic rate and size and site of lesions have a mitigating and negative influence on language. Cortical lesions are more likely to affect language function than subcortical lesions, although severity of aphasia is associated with both cortical and subcortical lesions.

Linebaugh (1984), Horner (1984), and Helm-Estabrooks (1984) described the clinical profiles of mild, moderate, and severe aphasia. In mild aphasia, patients tend to resemble normal speakers, except that they tend to place more of the communication burden on their conversational partners. Persons with mild aphasia also tend to use more compensation strategies than normal speakers and more nonlinguistic aids, such as head movements, to compensate for reduced lexicon and word-finding problems. Persons with moderate aphasia are fundamentally different from normal speakers, which is perhaps most obvious from their relative inability to recognize errors and correct them. Moderately involved speakers exhibit phonemic errors, reduced lexicon, impaired vigilance, and paucity of speech acts.

Persons with severe aphasia are markedly deficient in their access to the modalities of language and may demonstrate severe impairments in all modalities. Nicholas and Brookshire (1993) inves-

tigated the evolution of severe aphasia in the first 2 years post-onset. Severe and global aphasics were tested at 6-month intervals with the *Boston Assessment of Severe Aphasia*. Significant improvements were observed for up to 18 months post-onset. The greatest improvement occurred in the first 6 months poststroke. However, most subjects did not change aphasia classification during the 2-year period. The investigators concluded that the scores obtained at 6 months poststroke may be a reliable predictor for scores after 2 years.

FACTORS IN LANGUAGE RECOVERY

According to Thompson (2000), recovery is a complex process that is dependent on neurophysiological processes, environmental factors, and other variables. Reorganization processes begin soon after damage to the neural networks that subserve language, The greatest improvement in communication function generally occurs in the first 6 months post-onset (Nicholas & Brookshire, 1993). During this period, aphasia frequency decreases by half, from 24% within 7 days poststroke to 12% 6 months later.

Recovery of language function in the subacute stage following brain damage is aided by a neurophysiological process associated with spontaneous recovery. Left-hemisphere brain regions involved in language function rendered temporarily dysfunctional by brain damage (most commonly, stroke) contribute to early recovery (Cappa et al., 1997). This physiological restitution may be complemented by reorganization of brain function, the more likely mechanism of change, particularly at later stages of aphasia recovery.

Neuroimaging studies have provided evidence for two mechanisms of functional reorganization of language in aphasia: (1) recruitment of residual left-hemisphere structures that may have been premorbidly involved in language function and (2) recruitment of right-hemisphere regions, typically homologous to left-hemisphere language areas (Thompson et al., 2004). Recruitment of residual perilesional left-hemisphere regions for recovery has been documented in functional imaging studies in patients with aphasia and other neurogenic communication disorders (Pataraia et al., 2005; Price & Crinion, 2005; Rosen et al., 2000; Weiller et al., 1995).

Studies using newer technologies, such as structural MRI, have provided evidence of aphasia recovery. Fridriksson, Baker, and Richardson (2010) observed that most neuroimaging research on aphasia recovery can be divided into two categories: studies of early, spontaneous recovery, including the acute and/or subacute phases of stroke, and studies of treated recovery, usually occurring in the chronic phase of stroke. Most studies targeting the early phases of spontaneous recovery have used structural- and perfusion-weighted MRI to examine how structural damage or compromised cerebral perfusion influences early aphasia progression. In the case of treated recovery from chronic aphasia, the bulk of research has used functional MRI to identify functional brain changes

In addition to involvement of spared regions within the left-hemisphere language network, a shift of language function to right-hemisphere regions has also been documented in individuals with aphasia with corroboration that there is increased participation of the nondominant right hemisphere during language

recovery (Weiller et al., 1995). Right-hemisphere contributions to aphasia recovery may reflect recruitment of attention, memory, or executive functions to support language recovery rather than restoration of language functions (Crosson et al., 2009).Whether patients develop intrahemispheric left-hemisphere reorganization or atypical right-hemisphere dominance may be influenced by factors such as the age of lesion onset and etiology of the lesion (Pataraia et al., 2005).

Other brain regions may contribute to language recovery. Lesions in the deep subcortical white matter areas may be predictive for recovery of meaningful speech for as long as 10 years following stroke onset (Naesar & Palumbo, 1994). Patients with lesions to left temporobasal regions show less improvement during the first year poststroke and less total spontaneous recovery compared with patients without such lesions. It has been suggested that temporobasal lesions cause a disconnection between the hippocampal formation and perisylvanian language areas, which hinders linguistic knowledge and compensatory strategies (Goldenberg & Spatt, 1994).

Other factors in recovery include premorbid structural variations in the cerebrum. Increasing left occipital width asymmetry is associated with faster rate of language recovery and higher final language scores during the first year poststroke. There is also a tendency for increasing left occipital width asymmetry to be associated with less initial impairment (Burke, Yeo, Delaney, & Conner 1993). Those aspects of neural organization that enhanced premorbid language skills may be the same factors that confer greater recovery of language skills.

Prognostic variables to be considered in recovery of language are dependent, also, on a number of factors, such as the age of the patient at stroke onset, history of previous stroke, history of earlier treatment, the patient's premorbid health status, education, handedness, post-onset time, stimulability, and the patient's support networks. These factors may contribute to the patient's neurologic resiliency and motivation to recover. However, the initial severity of the aphasia is one of the most clinically relevant predictors of aphasia outcome (Pedersen, Jorgen, Nakayama, Raaschou, & Olsen, 1994).

Recovery may be associated with treatment effects. Research in neuroplasticity associated with aphasia has primarily focused on natural recovery processes but less commonly on the effects of behavioral treatment. Several case studies have examined changes associated with behavioral treatment. These studies provide promising evidence that functional brain reorganization underlies language improvement associated with specific treatments (Adair et al., 2000; Cornelissen et al., 2003; Legar et al., 2002; Pulvermüller, Hauk, Zohsel, Neininger, & Mohr, 2005; Vindiola & Rapp, 2005; Weirenga et al., 2006).

Summary

Aphasia is a language impairment in all modalities of language. Several disorders can cause aphasia: CVA, TBI, brain tumors, degenerative diseases, and medical procedures.

CVAs are either ischemic, where there has been an interruption in blood flow to the brain, or hemorrhagic, where blood flow has leaked from a ruptured blood vessel or from blood vessels into the brain. The majority of CVAs are from ischemia. TBIs can disrupt language either from closed or penetrating head injuries.

In closed head injuries (CHI), diffuse, bilateral damage can impair cognitive processes, like memory, that interfere with semantic recall. Disorders of pragmatics and discourse cohesion are also characteristic of language impairment in CHI. In many cases of CHI, aphasia symptoms will subside, but cognitive impairments tend to persist. Aphasia is more apparent in penetrating head injuries and CHI where there has been associated damage to the skull (resulting in penetrating bone fragments or shrapnel into the brain) or development of hematomas. Cancerous tumors can also produce aphasia depending on whether the tumors occur as primary or secondary cancers. Degenerative diseases, for example PPA and spongiform encephalopathies as seen in Cruetzfeldt–Jakob disease, can impair language as well. Finally, medical procedures that evacuate masses in the brain or that may result in anoxia (oxygen deprivation to the brain) may be implicated in aphasia.

Aphasia classifications include the nonfluent (anterior) and fluent aphasias (posterior). The transcortical aphasias are rare but do occur and include transcortical motor and transcortical and mixed transcortical aphasias. All three transcortical aphasias involve a disconnection of the speech areas. Crossover aphasia occurs when right-handed persons suffer a right-hemisphere stroke.

Severity of aphasia may be predicated on a number of factors. Related disorders in vision, length, and duration of coma, depression, and other affective disorders, impairment of verbal memory, and cognitive decline are prognostic indicators for severity. The type of aphasia, extent of lesion damage, and treatment effects are other important indicators for severity of aphasia. Global aphasia is considered to be the most severe category of aphasia because all four modalities are impaired from wide-spread anterior and posterior damage.

Aphasia recovery is a complex process that depends on the revitalization of injured neurons in the left hemisphere and activation of right-hemisphere areas to take over lost functions. Prognostic indicators for rehabilitation include age at stroke onset, premorbid health status, education, handedness, post-onset time, stimulability, and the patient's support networks.

APHASIA ASSESSMENT

The Case History

The case history format has been discussed previously in Chapters 4 and 5. For the person with aphasia, several areas should be covered to develop a comprehensive case history:

1. General health status and prescription medicines
2. History of previous strokes, head injuries, brain tumors, dementia, seizures, or degenerative diseases
3. History of depression or other affective disorders
4. History of previous speech-language therapy
5. History of disorientation
6. Type and location of brain damage
7. Hearing or visual impairment
8. Results of neuroimaging reports
9. Demographic variables: age, gender, native language, education, national origin, and occupation
10. HIV status and antiviral drug regimen, if applicable
11. Support network: friends, family, paid caregivers

Evidence-Based Assessment Recommendations

Assessment is critical to the development of an appropriate plan for rehabilitation of persons diagnosed with aphasia. The National Center for Evidence-Based Practice in Communication Disorders (asha.org) makes the following recommendations to guide clinicians in conducting evidence-based evaluations:

◆ Individuals identified with aphasia through screening should receive a formal assessment of language and communication by a speech-language pathologist. The nature of the impairment should be explained to the patient, family, and treatment team.
◆ Reassessment should be completed at appropriate intervals to determine the ongoing nature and severity of aphasia.
◆ Alternate means of communication such as gestures, drawing, writing, and use of communication aids should be evaluated in individuals who exhibit aphasia persisting for more than 2 weeks.

A comprehensive assessment should be completed to determine the communication strengths and weaknesses of the individual with aphasia. Assessment should identify the nature and extent of the communication disorder, level of preserved abilities, functional and pragmatic aspects of communication abilities, psychosocial well-being, and perception of communication impairment from the individual with aphasia and family; identify treatment goals based on the specific needs of the individual; and establish a baseline to measure improvement.

Recommended Assessments

There are a wide variety of assessment instruments that can be used to measure overall recovery and functioning after stroke, cognition, and auditory comprehension and expressive language abilities. Some of the language assessments can be given at bedside to patients in the acute

care facility. Table 6–2 provides information on these bedside assessments that can be used to measure neurologic status, disabilities, and independence.

Measures of Neurologic Status, Disabilities, and Independence

Barthel Scale or Barthel ADL Index (Maloney & Barthel, 1965)

The *Barthel Scale* is an ordinal scale used to measure performance in activities of daily living. There are 10 performance items

Table 6–2. Measures of Neurologic Status, Disabilities and Independence

Test Name	Measurements
Barthel Scale/Barthel ADL Index (Maloney & Barthel, 1965)	Measures performance in activities of daily living (ADLs) using a 10-item rating on ADLs and mobility. Used to predict independence following hospital discharge.
Canadian Neurological Scale (CNS; Côté et al., 1986)	Measures consciousness, orientation, motor function, and facial weakness using an 8-item scale. Can be accessed online.
Frenchay Activities Index (FAI; Holbrook & Skilbeck, 1983)	Measures daily living activities in stroke survivors in domestic work, leisure/work, and outdoor activities. Rates the frequency with which activity has been undertaken over the past 3–6 months. Can be accessed online.
Modified Rankin Scale (mRS; van Swieten, Koudstaal, Visser, Schouten, & van Gijn, 1988)	Measures degree of disability or dependence in daily activities because of neurological disability, using a 6-item scale. Can be accessed online.
National Institutes of Health Stroke Scale (NIHSS; Brott et al., 1989)	Documents neurological status in acute stroke patients using a 15-item scale to evaluate effect of acute cerebral infarction on consciousness, language, dysarthria, motor strength, ataxia, sensory loss, visual-field loss, and extraocular trained observer rates the patient to perform in these areas. Can be accessed online.

and each performance item is rated on this scale with a given number of points assigned to each level or ranking. It uses 10 variables describing activities of daily living and mobility. A higher number is associated with a greater likelihood of being able to live at home with a degree of independence following discharge from hospital.

Canadian Neurological Scale (CNS; Côté, Hachinski, Shurvell, Norris, & Wolfson, 1986)

The CNS is an 8-item scale that measures consciousness, orientation, motor function, and facial weakness. It is accessible at http://www.gbhn.ca/ebc/documents/CanadianNeurologicalScaleAug2007.pdf

Frenchay Activities Index (FAI; Holbrook & Skilbeck, 1983)

The FAI assesses a broad range of activities of daily living in patients recovering from stroke. The items included can be separated into three factors: domestic work, leisure/work, and outdoor activities. The frequency with which each item or activity is undertaken over the past 3 to 6 months is assigned a score of 1 to 4, where a score of 1 is indicative of the lowest level of activity. The FAI can be accessed from http://www.rehabmeasures.org/PDF%20Library/Frenchay%20Activities%20Index.pdf

Modified Rankin Scale (mRS; van Swieten, Koudstaal, Visser, Schouten, & van Gijn, 1988; Banks & Marotta, 2007)

The mRS is a commonly used scale for measuring the degree of disability or dependence in the daily activities of people who have suffered a stroke or other causes of neurological disability. It is a 6-level outcome scale used to assess level of function in neurological disease. The scale runs from 0 to 6, running from perfect health without symptoms to death and can be accessed at http://www.strokecenter.org/wp-content/uploads/2011/08/modified_rankin.pdf

National Institutes of Health Stroke Scale (NIHSS; Brott et al., 1989)

The NIHSS can be used as a clinical stroke assessment tool to evaluate and document neurological status in acute stroke patients. The stroke scale is valid for predicting lesion size and can serve as a measure of stroke severity. The NIHSS has been shown to be a predictor of both short and long-term outcome of stroke patients. The NIHSS is a 15-item neurologic examination stroke scale used to evaluate the effect of acute cerebral infarction on the levels of consciousness, language, neglect, visual-field loss, extraocular movement, motor strength, ataxia, dysarthria, and sensory loss. A trained observer rates the patient's ability to answer questions and perform activities. The NIHSS may be accessed at http://www.ninds.nih.gov/doctors/NIH_Stroke_Scale.pdf

Discussion of the modified NIHSS is described by Meyer, Hemmer, Jackson & Lyden (2002).

Aphasia Batteries

A list of suggested aphasia batteries and assessments related to language function may be found in Table 6–3.

Table 6–3. Suggested Aphasia Batteries

Test Name	Measurement
Aphasia Diagnostic Profiles (ADP; Helm-Estabrooks, 1992)	Nine subtests yield composite scores and profiles of patient's performance. Provides information on type and severity of aphasia, means of expression, social-emotional state during testing. and the nature of the errors.
Aphasia-Language Performance Scales (ALPS; Keenan & Brassell, 1975)	Uses four 1-item scales to measure listening, talking, reading, and writing. Test is available in English and Spanish.
Boston Diagnostic Aphasia Examination–3 (BDAE-3; Goodglass, Kaplan, & Barresi, 2000)	Determines disorders of language function and aphasic syndromes. The ***Boston Naming Test*** assesses visual confrontation naming ability. A short form is available for rapid assessment. Entire test measures perceptual modalities, processing functions, and response modalities.
Comprehensive Aphasia Test (CAT; Swinburn, Porter, & Howard, 2004)	Measures cognition, language, and disability using a cognitive screen, a language battery, and a disability questionnaire.
Discourse Comprehension Test, Second Edition (Brookshire & Nicholas, 1997)	Appropriate for aphasia, right-hemisphere brain damage or TBI. Assesses listening and reading comprehension and retention of stated and implied ideas using stories.
Examining for Aphasia; Assessment of Aphasia and Related Impairments–Fourth Edition (EFA-4; LaPointe & Eisenson, 2008)	Assesses aphasia and impact of aphasia on the patient's quality of life.
Multilingual Aphasia Examination, Third Edition (MAE-3; Benton, Hamsher, & Sivan, 1994)	Uses 11 tests and rating scales to assess visual naming, repetition, fluency, spelling, articulation, aural comprehension, reading, and writing.
Multilingual Aphasia Examination, Spanish Version (MAE-S; Rey, Sivan, & Benton, 1994)	For use with Spanish/English bilingual populations. Measures visual naming, repetition, fluency, articulation, spelling, aural comprehension, and reading and writing in 11 tests and rating scales.
Object and Action Naming Battery (Druks & Masterson, 2000)	Assesses verb knowledge of persons with aphasia.
Philadelphia Naming Test (PNT; Roach, Schwartz, Martin, Grewal, & Brecher, 1996)	Measures anomia using 175 words and pictures.

continues

Table 6–3. *continued*

Test Name	Measurement
Porch Index of Communicative Ability–Revised (PICA-R; Porch, 2001)	Measures communicative ability using a battery of 18 subtests for gestural, verbal, and graphic abilities at varying levels of difficulty.
Quantitative Production Analysis (QPA; Berndt, Wayland, Rochon, Saffran, & Schwartz, 2000)	Measures sentence production through a storytelling format.
Revised Token Test (RTT; McNeill & Prescott, 1978)	Measures auditory processing through a series of increasingly complex directions.
The Reporter's Test (DeRenzi & Ferrari, 1978)	Patient is asked to verbally report what the examiner is doing with an array of token. Patient is scored on accurately producing a connected sequence of words.
Western Aphasia Battery–Revised (WAB-R; Kertesz, 2006)	Measures linguistic skills most often affected by aphasia in addition to key nonlinguistic skills. Provides differential diagnosis information. The WAB-R is a widely used clinical assessment tool.

Aphasia Diagnostic Profiles (ADP; Helm-Estabrooks, 1992)

The ADP assesses patients with aphasia using nine subtests that create composite scores and a series of complementary profiles of the patient's performance: Aphasia Severity Profile, Alternative Communication Profile, Classification Profile, Behavioral Profile, and Error Profile. This test provides information on the type and severity of aphasia, the means of expression (gestural and linguistic), overall social-emotional state during testing, and whether errors were communicative, noncommunicative, or nonaphasic.

Aphasia-Language Performance Scales (ALPS; Keenan & Brassell, 1975)

The ALPS obtains information needed to measure language impairment, predict language prognosis, plan treatment, identify recovery levels, and write comprehensive reports. Four 10-item scales measure listening, talking, reading, and writing with right/wrong/partial scoring. This test is available in both English and Spanish.

Boston Diagnostic Aphasia Examination–3 (BDAE-3; Goodglass, Kaplan, & Barresi, 2000)

This comprehensive assessment determines and distinguishes disorders of language function and neurologically recognized aphasic syndromes. The BDAE-3 includes the Boston Naming Test to assess visual confrontation naming abilities and a short form for rapid diagnostic classification and quantitative assessment. The BDAE-3 evaluates perceptual modalities (auditory, visual, and gestural), processing functions (comprehension, analysis, problem solving), and response modalities (writing, articulation, and manipulation).

Comprehensive Aphasia Test (CAT; Swinburn, Porter, & Howard, 2004)

The CAT assesses people who have acquired aphasia. The battery contains a cognitive screen, a language battery, and a disability questionnaire.

Discourse Comprehension Test, Second Edition (Brookshire & Nicholas, 1997)

This instrument provides data for adults with aphasia, right-hemisphere brain damage, or TBI by assessing listening and reading comprehension and retention of stated and implied ideas conveyed through test stories. The test stories are controlled for length, grammatical complexity, listening difficulty, and reading level.

Examining for Aphasia: Assessment of Aphasia and Related Impairments–Fourth Edition (EFA-4; LaPointe & Eisenson, 2008)

The EFA-4 has subtests that measure the cognitive, personality, and linguistic modifications that accompany acquired aphasia. This test includes a personal history form and assesses visual, auditory and tactile recognition; auditory and reading comprehension in words, sentences and paragraphs; and expressive/productive skills in mathematical computation, automatic language and other expressive areas that parallel receptive skills assessed. Persons from diverse ethnic groups are included in the revised normative data.

Multilingual Aphasia Examination, Spanish Version (MAE-S; Rey, Sivan, & Benton, 1994)

A standardized assessment for use with Spanish/English bilingual populations, the MAE-S examines visual naming, repetition, fluency articulation, spelling, aural comprehension, reading, and writing; it has 11 tests and rating scales.

Multilingual Aphasia Examination, Third Edition (MAE; Benton, Hamsher, & Sivan, 1994)

The MAE assesses visual naming, repetition, fluency, articulation, spelling, aural comprehension, reading, and writing; it has 11 tests and rating scales.

Object and Action Naming Battery (Druks & Masterson, 2000)

This battery provides a thorough assessment of verb knowledge in patients with aphasia.

Philadelphia Naming Test (PNT; Roach, Schwartz, Martin, Grewal, & Brecher, 1996)

The PNT measures anomia through 175 words and pictures.

Porch Index of Communicative Ability–Revised (PICA-R; Porch, 2001)

The PICA-R measures communicative ability of brain injured adults using a battery of 18 subtests that measure gestural, verbal, and graphic abilities at different levels of difficulty. The multidimensional scoring system describes accuracy, responsiveness, completeness, promptness, and efficiency of response.

Quantitative Production Analysis (QPA; Berndt, Wayland, Rochon, Saffran, & Schwartz, 2000)

The QPA characterizes aspects of aphasic sentence production. The analysis system is carried out on samples of narrative speech elicited from aphasic patients in a storytelling format. Irrelevant and/or non-propositional content is omitted according to stated criteria, and the resulting sample is analyzed on the basis of a number of structural and morphological indices.

The Reporter's Test (DeRenzi & Ferrari, 1978)

The Reporter's Test requires the patient to verbally report to a hypothetical third person what the examiner is doing with an array of tokens. The patient is scored on whether he or she has accurately produced a connected sequence of words.

Revised Token Test (RTT; McNeil & Prescott, 1978)

The RTT tests for auditory processing inefficiencies and disorders associated with brain damage, aphasia, and certain language learning disabilities.

Western Aphasia Battery–Revised (WAB-R; Kertesz, 2006)

The WAB-R is an individually administered assessment for adults with acquired neurological disorders (e.g., as a result of stroke, head injury, dementia). Like the previous edition, WAB-R assesses the linguistic skills most frequently affected by aphasia, in addition to key nonlinguistic skills, and provides differential diagnosis information.

Bedside Measures

Table 6–4 gives suggested bedside measurements. Bedside measures include those that can be given in 30 minutes or less.

Bedside Evaluation Screening Test–Second Edition (BEST-2; West, Sands, & Ross-Swain, 1998)

The BEST-2 assesses and quantifies language disorders in adults resulting from aphasia. Test results give sufficient clinical information to set treatment goals and objectives. Administration time is 20 minutes.

Bedside Form, Western Aphasia Battery–Revised (WAB-R; Kertesz, 2006)

Administration time is 15 minutes.

Boston Assessment of Severe Aphasia (BASA; Helm-Estabrooks, Ramsberger, Morgan & Nicholas, 1989)

The BASA identifies and quantifies preserved skills in patients with severe or global aphasia and is appropriate for early bedside poststroke administration. Gestural and verbal responses are scored, as are refusals, affective responses, and perseverative responses. Tasks and modalities measured include auditory comprehension, buccofacial or limb praxis, gesture recognition, oral and gestural expression, reading comprehension, writing, and visual-spatial tasks. Administration time is 20 to 30 minutes.

Boston Naming Test, Boston Diagnostic Examination for Aphasia–3 (BDAE-3; Goodglass, Kaplan, & Barresi, 2000)

Administration time is 15 minutes.

Table 6–4. Suggested Bedside Assessments for Adults with Aphasia

Test Name	Administration Time in Minutes	Measurement
Bedside Evaluation Screening Test–Second Edition (BEST-2; West, Sands, & Ross-Swain, 1998)	20	Measures language disorders in adults with aphasia. Allows for setting treatment goals and objectives.
Bedside Form, Western Aphasia Battery–Revised (WAB-R; Kertesz, 2006)	15	See Table 6–3
Boston Assessment of Severe Aphasia (BASA; Helm-Estabrooks, Ramsberger, Morgan, & Nicholas, 1989)	20–30	Measures preserved skills in patients with severe or global aphasia. Gestural and verbal responses are scored. A full range of abilities are assessed.
Burns Brief Inventory of Communication and Cognition (Burns Inventory; Burns, 1997)	30/each inventory	Measures deficits in inventories for the right and left hemisphere and for complex neuropathology.
Quick Assessment for Aphasia (Tanner & Culbertson, 1999)	10–15	Basic skills: verbal labeling, answering question, giving basic information, and general conversation.
Scales of Cognitive and Communicative Ability for Neurorehabilitation (SCCAN; Milman & Holland, 2012)	30	Assesses cognitive-communication skills and and functional ability in patients in rehabilitation hospitals, clinics, and skilled nursing facilities.
Short Form, Boston Diagnostic Examination for Aphasia–3 (BDAE-3; Goodglass, Kaplan, & Barresi, 2000)	20–30	See Table 6–3
Short-Form, Philadelphia Naming Test (PNT30; Walker & Schwartz, 2012)	15	See Table 6–3

Burns Brief Inventory of Communication and Cognition (Burns Inventory; Burns, 1997)

The Burns Inventory helps evaluate individuals with communication or cognitive deficits resulting from neurological injury and assists in selecting appropriate treatment targets and functional treatment goals. This test includes three inventories: Right Hemisphere, Left Hemisphere, and Complex Neuropathology.

Administration time for each inventory is 30 minutes.

Quick Assessment for Aphasia (Tanner & Culbertson, 1999)

The *Quick Assessment* for Aphasia measures basic skills such as verbal labeling, answering questions, giving basic information, and general conversation. Administration time is 10 to 15 minutes.

Scales of Cognitive and Communicative Ability for Neurorehabilitation (SCCAN; Milman & Holland, 2012)

The SCCAN assesses cognitive-communicative deficits and functional ability in patients in rehabilitation hospitals, clinics, and skilled nursing facilities. Administration time is 30 minutes.

Short Form, Boston Diagnostic Examination for Aphasia–3 (BDAE-3; Goodglass, Kaplan, & Barresi, 2000)

Administration time is 20 to 30 minutes.

Short-Form Philadelphia Naming Test (PNT30; Walker & Schwartz, 2012)

Measures anomia through 30 words and pictures. Administration time is 15 minutes.

Functional Communication Assessments

Table 6–5 gives a list of suggested functional communication assessments.

Assessment of Language-Related Functional Activities (ALFA; Baines, Heeringa, & Martin, 1999)

The ALFA is designed to assess a person's ability to perform 10 language-related functional tasks—for example, using the telephone, counting money, and reading instructions.

Communication Abilities in Daily Living Test–2 (CADL-2; Holland, Frattali, & Fromm, 1999)

The CADL-2 is a supplemental aphasia tool that assesses the functional communication skills of adults with aphasia, mental retardation, hearing impairment, Alzheimer's disease, or traumatic brain injury.

Functional Assessment of Communication Skills in Adults (ASHA-FACS; Frattali, Holland, Thompson, Wohl, & Ferketic, 1995)

The ASHA-FACS assists in measuring and recording the functional communication of adults with speech, language, and cognitive communication disorders. This instrument assesses social communication; communication of basic needs; reading, writing, and number concepts; and daily planning.

Functional Communication Profile Revised (FCPR; Kleinman, 2003)

The FCPR has 10 subtests that assess sensory-motor skills, attentiveness, receptive language, expressive language, pragmatic and social language, speech, voice, oral fluency, and non-oral communication.

Table 6–5. Suggested Functional Communication Assessments for Adults with Aphasia

Test Name	Measurement
Assessment of Language-Related Functional Activities (ALFA; Baines, Heeringa, & Martin, 1999)	Assesses ability in 10 language-related daily living tasks.
Communication Abilities in Daily Living Test–2 (CADL-2; Holland, Fratteli, & Fromm, 1999)	Measures functional communication skills in adults with neurological disorders.
Functional Assessment of Communication Skills in Adults (ASHA-FACS; Frattali, Holland, Thompson, Wohl, & Freketic, 1995)	Assesses social communication, communication of basic needs, reading, writing, number concepts, and daily planning.
Functional Communication Profile Revised (FCPR; Kleinman, 2003)	Uses 10 subtests to measure sensory-motor skills, attentiveness, receptive and expressive language, pragmatic and social language, speech, voice, oral fluency, and non-oral communication.
Informal Pragmatic Protocol (Prutting & Kirchner, 1987)	Rates 30 features of verbal and nonverbal conversation.
Inpatient Functional Communication Interview (IFCI; O'Halloran, Toffolo, Worrall, Code, & Hickson, 2004)	Measures how well in patients who are in acute care are able to communicate in hospital situations.

Informal Pragmatic Protocol (Prutting & Kirchner, 1987)

This measure addresses 30 features of conversation and provides ratings (appropriate, inappropriate, not observed) for verbal (for example, topic selection and initiation, turn-taking behaviors) and nonverbal (for example, gesture, posture, proximity) behaviors in conversation.

Inpatient Functional Communication Interview (IFCI; O'Halloran, Worrall, Toffolo, Code & Hickson, 2004)

The IFCI measures how well in-patients who have communication disorders and who are in acute care are able to communicate in relevant hospital situations.

Related Assessments

Table 6–6 shows suggested related assessments for use with persons with aphasia.

Auditory Discrimination: Goldman-Fristoe-Woodcock Test of Auditory Discrimination (G-F-W TAD; Goldman, Fristoe, & Woodcock, 1970).

The G-F-W TAD evaluates the patient's ability to discriminate speech sounds in quiet and noise.

Table 6–6. Suggested Related Assessments for Adults with Aphasia

Test Name	Measurements
Assessment of Nonverbal Communication (Duffy & Duffy, 1984)	Measures ability in pantomime recognition and production.
Geriatric Depression Scale (GDS; Yesavage et al., 2008)	Measures depression in a self-rating scale of 30 items in a yes/no format. Available online.
Goldman-Fristoe-Woodcock Test of Auditory Discrimination (G-F-W TAD; Goldman, Fristoe, & Woodcock, 1970)	Evaluates the patient's ability to discriminate speech sounds in quiet and noise.
McMaster Family Assessment Device (Epstein, Baldwin, & Bishop, 1983)	Assesses family relationships through a 60-item self-reporting instrument. Scores on six dimensions: problem solving, communication, roles, affective responsiveness and involvement, and behavioral control. Available online.
Measures of Skill in Supported Conversation/ Measures of Level of Participation in Conversation (for partners with aphasia) (MSC/MPC; Kagan et al., 2004)	Two measures: MSC measures conversation partner's skill; MPC measures participation in conversation by person with aphasia. Available online.
Multimodal Communication Screening Test for Persons with Aphasia (MCST-A; Garrett & Lasker, 2005)	Allows for differentiation of those who would benefit from partner-dependent communication strategies and patients who could learn to use AAC systems.
Swanson Cognitive Processing Test (SCPT; Swanson, 1996)	Measures cognitive functioning in semantic association and categorization, auditory digit span, nonverbal and picture sequencing, phrase recall, story retelling, rhyming, spatial organization, directions, and mapping skills.

Cognition: Swanson Cognitive Processing Test (SCPT; Swanson, 1996).

The SCPT measures semantic association and categorization; auditory digit, nonverbal, and picture sequencing; phrase recall, story retelling, rhyming; spatial organization, directions, and mapping skills. More

assessments of cognitive functioning may be found in Chapter 4.

Depression: Geriatric Depression Scale (GDS; Yesavage et al., 1982–1983)

The GDS is a self-rating scale with 30 items in a yes/no format. The GDS is accessible from http://en.wikipedia.org/wiki/Geriatric_Depression_Scale. A 15-item short form of the GDS is available at http://www.chcr.brown.edu/GDS_SHORT_FORM.PDF. Instructions for scoring the short form may be accessed at http://geriatrics.uthscsa.edu/tools/GDS%20short%20form.pdf

Family Relationships: McMaster Family Assessment Device (MFAD; Epstein, Baldwin, & Bishop, 1983)

The MFAD is a 60-item self-reporting instrument intended to evaluate a number of aspects of family relationships. Items are phrased to denote both effective and affective domains. The MFAD generates scores on six dimensions: problem solving, communication, roles, affective responsiveness, affective involvement, and behavioral control. This test may be accessed at http://web.up.ac.za/User Files/FAD.pdf

Nonverbal Communication: Assessment of Nonverbal Communication (Duffy & Duffy, 1984)

This assessment measures a patient's ability in pantomime recognition and production.

Selection of Augmentative and Alternative Communication Devices: Multimodal Communication Screening Test for Persons with Aphasia (MCST-A; Garrett & Lasker, 2005)

The MCST-A enables clinicians to differentiate those individuals who would benefit most from partner-dependent communication strategies (e.g., written choice conversation, partner-presented symbol choices, tagged yes/no questions) and

those who could learn to use augmentative and alternative communication (AAC) systems (e.g., digitized speech devices that store complete messages; multilevel devices with stored messages and spelling capabilities) to communicate independently.

Supported Conversation: Measures of Skill in Supported Conversation/ Measures of Level of Participation in Conversation (for Partners With Aphasia) (MSC/ MPC; Kagan et al., 2004)

The MSC and MPC are two complementary measures designed to capture elements of conversation between adults with aphasia and their speaking conversation partners. The MSC provides an index of the conversation partner's skill in providing conversational support. The MPC provides an index of the level of participation in conversation by the person with aphasia. Available online at http://www.aphasia.ca/wp content/uploads/2012/03/ mscpc.pdf

INTERVENTION FOR APHASIC DISORDERS

The World Health Organization (2001) emphasizes that the ultimate goal of rehabilitation should be to return the individual to the activities and life participation typical for the person's social role. Efficacious intervention for aphasia refers to improvements in language that exceed what can be expected from spontaneous recovery. The focus should be on retraining the person with aphasia to regain as much pre-stroke language ability as possible. The policy of the American Speech-Language-Hearing Association (ASHA)

(2004b) policy on intervention for adults with language disorders is:

> Adults receive intervention and/or consultation services when their ability to communicate effectively and participate in social, educational, or vocational activities is impaired because of a language disorder and when there is a reasonable expectation of benefit to the individual in body structure/function and/or activity/participation. Interventions that enhance activity and participation through implementation of strategies or modification of contextual factors may be warranted even if the prognosis for improved body structure/function is limited.

There is no timeline for intervention. Patients can show improvement immediately after a neurological episode and may continue to benefit from therapy for months and years after a stroke. ASHA (2008a) goes further to state: "Clinicians and researchers now understand that positive changes can also occur long after the stroke that produced aphasia, dispelling the notion that language rehabilitation undertaken very soon after stroke made the biggest difference."

Timing and Frequency of Therapy

Assessment and a program of treatment can begin as soon as the patient is alert and conscious. Aphasia treatment should begin as early as possible and as soon as the patient can tolerate therapy. Spontaneous recovery does account for the revitalization of language skills, but, according to Laska and colleagues (2001), 43% of persons with a diagnosis of aphasia at onset were found to have significant aphasia after 18 months. Therefore, clinicians

should expect that treatment is an ongoing process that requires periodic assessments as long as there are clear objectives and measurable progress. Taylor-Goh (2005), for example, found that individuals with persistent aphasia at 6 months poststroke should be considered for further speech and language treatment either within a group or in one-on-one individual settings.

In general, there is support for more intensive treatment over less intensive treatment, particularly for chronic aphasia. Although there are few definitive data on the effects of treatment intensity on quality of life for persons with aphasia, evidence suggests that aphasia treatment is effective in improving functional communication and receptive/expressive language skills (Brady, Kelly, Godwin & Enderby, 2012; Cherney, Patterson, & Raymer, 2011).

Models of Intervention

Tippett (2012) describes two models of intervention for persons with aphasia. One is a therapist-directed model in which the clinician establishes objective, measurable goals that target impairment in specific domains, such as auditory comprehension at a sentence level. This approach is followed by a medical model that emphasizes impairment of function. This model has been the standard for intervention; however, it does not take into consideration the patient's family preferences, the social/communication/physical context in which the patient is functioning, or the environmental and personal barriers that impede recovery.

In the second model, the patient-centered model, the clinician encourages patients and families to identify goals that are important to them. Within the patient-centered model is the construct of context. Contextual factors for disability are considered to act as barriers or facilitators of the disability. Both environmental factors, or those factors external to the person, and personal factors, such as internal premorbid factors such as age, health status, gender, and coping style, are considered to affect the level of disability and therefore recovery (Tippett, 2012; Worrall, Papathanasiou, & Sherratt, 2013).

Within the framework of the patient-centered model, patient perceptions of the impact of communication disability should be assessed. This information enables the clinician to understand the patient's response to disability. An assessment that can be used, for example, is the Burden of Stroke Scale (BOSS; Doyle, McNeil, Hula, & Mikolic, 2003), which is a health-status assessment instrument designed to measure patient-reported difficulty in multiple domains of functioning, psychological distress associated with specific functional limitations, and general well-being. This assessment can be used to complement formal assessment of aphasia and related areas. The clinician should observe the patient in the daily living setting to determine the contextual needs of the patient (for example, number and availability of communication partners, level of family support, communicative needs within the living context).The final step should be negotiation between the patients and speech-language pathologist to define a treatment plan.

It is important to understand that both the therapist-directed and the patient-centered models have their place in aphasia rehabilitation. The International Classification of Functioning, Disability and Health adopts a biosocial approach that combines both the medical

and the social approaches. According to Worrall and colleagues (2013), this combined or holistic approach is "well suited to aphasia rehabilitation because historically both the medical and social models have been considered as separate and distinct approaches to aphasia rehabilitation" (p. 94).

Therapist-Directed Approaches

Persons with aphasia are heterogeneous in their clinical presentations because of difference in health status, coping strategies to disability, severity of aphasia, number and extent of related disorders (for example, word-finding difficulty, visual disturbances, cognitive impairments), age, personality, and lesion site and size. Intervention should, therefore, be individualized for the patient's needs. In planning a rehabilitation program, from the perspective of the medical model, there are patients whose aphasia diagnosis warrants therapist-direct intervention, as in the case of a patient who needs to decrease stereotyped vocalizations in order to regain control of voluntary utterances. There may also be those who need direct stimulation in specific language areas, such as auditory comprehension deficits or agrammatism. When treating an impairment, the clinician helps the patient by modifying or supplementing a stimulus, or by providing informative feedback (Davis, 2000). There are specific theory-driven approaches that address areas within aphasia that are theory driven. A number of influential therapy techniques are appropriate under the therapist-directed model. These are the stimulation approach, Melodic Intonation Therapy (MIT), Visual Action Therapy (VAT), Voluntary Control of Involuntary Utterances (VCIU), mapping therapy, chaining and verb network strengthening, and naming facilitation.

Stimulation Approach. Credited to Schuell (1969), this approach is one of the most widely used in aphasia therapy, and the approach is synonymous with traditional therapy. The stimulation approach corresponds with Lubinski's (1988) Skills Approach, in which standardized tests are used to determine areas of deficit. The clinician builds a therapeutic regimen around repairing these deficits. Drill and activities in the stimulation approach tend to be noncontextual; however, consistent and repetitious work in targeted problem areas is effective for some patients. In this approach: (1) the clinician initiates or demonstrates the desired response, (2) the patient imitates the clinician's demonstration or modeling, and (3) the clinician reinforces the patient's response.

Melodic Intonation Therapy (MIT). The American Academy of Neurology determined that Melodic Intonation Therapy (Albert, Sparks, & Helm, 1973; Helm-Estabrooks & Albert, 2004) holds promise for treating aphasia. This is perhaps the first aphasia therapy to receive this commendation (Holland, Fromm, DeRuyter, & Stein, 1996). This approach seeks to reestablish some speech in patients through reorganization of speech production processes using melodic intonation, a right-hemisphere function. In this therapy, common words and phrases are turned into melodic phrases emulating typical speech intonation and rhythmic patterns. MIT is particularly effective in treating nonfluent aphasia.

Visual Action Therapy (VAT). Visual action therapy (Helm-Estabrooks, Fitzpatrick, & Barresi, 1982) involves a patient in several steps of object manipulation to train the use of pantomime gestures. The program begins with matching tasks for perception and recognition of objects and proceeds to gesturing of functioning with the object in hand, and then without the object. Patients with Broca's aphasia may be able to use more gestures than speech, and this approach helps to facilitate their ability to: (1) communicate with others and (2) transition from gestures to meaningful speech.

Using gestures to enhance aurally presented stimuli is an important part of retraining. Records (1994) used three types of stimuli presentation: (1) visual-only, (2) auditory-only, and (3) a combination of audio and visual stimuli presentation. Listeners with aphasia were grouped as high- or low-language comprehension from their standardized tests. Gestural information significantly contributed to the responses of the lower-comprehension group.

Voluntary Control of Involuntary Utterances (VCIU). In this approach (Helm & Barresi, 1980), the clinician reads aloud an utterance and presents the printed form of the utterance to the patient. If the patient repeats the clinician's utterance as was read aloud, the utterance is considered to be volitional. If a different word was produced, a stimulus card is written for the word. No treatment is pursued for any utterance that is difficult for the patient to produce a second time. Object-picture tasks are presented in transition to naming tasks. VCIU is designed to enable clinicians to work with persons with severe aphasia, such as global aphasia, and persons with severe Wernicke's aphasia.

Mapping Therapy. Mapping therapy is designed to repair a disability in comprehension of sentence production by tapping into the mental processes that lead to formulating a grammatically intact sentence. One approach (Byng, Nickels, & Black, 1994) is to have the patient sort color-coded phrases into a sentence. The patient then describes the action using color cues. Patients who have agrammatic production and relatively intact judgment for what should be grammatically correct are possible candidates for this technique.

Chaining and Verb Network Strengthening.
Therapy strategies for agrammatic production include chaining and verb network strengthening treatment. Chaining (forward and reverse) is an approach in which sentences are elicited through modeling. Chaining breaks tasks/words/ sentences into small parts and teaches the beginning (or end) part first (Thompson & McReynolds, 1986). A verb network strengthening treatment approach is designed to improve word retrieval in simple active sentences. Verbs are trained with pairs of related nouns to improve sentence production.

Naming Facilitation.
Naming is greatly aided by the use of cuing to trigger a response. Naming abilities in persons with aphasia was studied by Freed, Marshall, and Nippold (1995). Results of their study indicated that persons diagnosed with aphasia who developed their own associations for word-symbolic pairs performed better when ready-made associations were used during training. Ability to create easily imaged cues was not related to the severity of the language impairment. An example was given to a subject who had been an artist before his stroke. His cue for "whisky" was "drunk flower," which served him well in each of the trials. The authors noted that it was the most severe subjects who seemed to be the most motivated to succeed.

Client-Centered Approaches

In the client-centered approach, the focus is less on the aphasia syndrome and type of language impairment and more on the patient in the context of a disability that is causing difficulty in communicating with others, restricting natural movement within the environment, and changing how the patient views him/herself as a disabled but valuable person. Because of the more collaborative nature of this approach, effort is taken to consider the patient and the patient's significant publics, for example, family members and/ or caregivers, and their wishes for change (Byng & Duchen, 2005). An important feature of the client-centered approach is that education and training efforts involve the client and those important to the client. The client becomes part of the decision-making process about treatment.

Several approaches are influential in affecting outcome. Those are conversational training and coaching, response elaboration training, contextualized approach to treatment of fluent or Wernicke's aphasia, reciprocal scaffolding, Supported Conversation for Adults With Aphasia, total communication, PACE, augmentative/assistive communication, effectiveness and opportunity approaches, script training, support for living with aphasia, patient participation in community aphasia groups, aphasia-friendly formatting, and patient use of aphasia organizations.

Conversational Training.
This treatment is designed to improve communication between the person with aphasia and primary communication partners. The clinician serves as the facilitator, or coach, for both partners. This is a also form of pragmatic treatment in which the clinician works to improve social communication

deficits, such as appropriate word choice, nonverbal communication, and understanding the rules of conversation.

Conversational Coaching. This is an approach in which the clinician acts as a communication strategy coach to both the person with aphasia and the communication partner (Hopper, Holland, & Rewega, 2002). First, effective communication strategies for both the communication partner and the person with aphasia are established equally; both have their set of strategies to learn and apply. A conversational situation is created, such as viewing a short video clip. One partner views the clip and communicates the information to the other, while the clinician acts as coach, scaffolding and cueing the use of effective strategies in both partners.

Response Elaboration Training (RET). Response elaboration training (Kearns, 1985, 1986; Kearns & Scher, 1989; Kearns & Yedor, 1991) is a strategy that works well with persons with aphasia. This is a form of "loose training" in which the emphasis is on patient-initiated responses and reinforcement of the content of the responses rather than the form of the response. In this procedure, the clinician or the communication partner and the patient select a conversational topic. The clinician/partner provides a series of prompts and asks the partner to add on to his or her original production. The goal is to lengthen the number of utterances produced by the patient. This approach is particularly effective with persons with nonfluent aphasia, but relies heavily on the patient's having memory and executive functioning (Hinckley, 2009).

Contextualized Approach to Treatment of Fluent or Wernicke's Aphasia. This

strategy has been described by Marshall (2001). In this approach, the ability of fluent aphasic patients to engage in turn taking is used to benefit structure discourse in a conversational setting. The focus of treatment is on identifying key words and relevant meaning units through strategy use and scaffolding.

Reciprocal Scaffolding. Reciprocal scaffolding enhances conversational coaching and training, and is a treatment approach in which communication skills are addressed in natural, relevant situations where the person with aphasia practices conversational skills by taking on the role of instructor to others during conversations about topics of interest to the person with aphasia. The conversational relationship allows both parties to demonstrate and reinforce communication strategies (asha.org).

Supported Conversation for Adults with Aphasia (SCA). Supported conversation for adults with aphasia (Kagan, Black, Duchan, Simmons-Mackie, & Square, 2001) is a program accessible through the Aphasia Institute that uses a set of techniques to encourage conversation when working with someone with aphasia through spoken and written key words, body language and gestures, hand drawings, and detailed pictographs.

SCA is designed to help people who have difficulty with expressive language be able to express their opinions and feelings in a way that makes them feel valued and heard. Through the program's techniques, conversation partners such as family members, doctors, nurses, or friends can help break down the communication barrier and help people with aphasia rejoin life's conversations. The SCA program is designed to acknowledge the communicative competence of a person with aphasia and assist the person to demonstrate that competence.

Total Communication. This approach involves use of residual speech along with expanded use of multiple modalities such as gesture, body movement, facial expression, prosody, writing, drawing (Ross, Winslow, Marchant, & Brumfitt, 2006), and gestural codes such as Amer-Ind Code and Blissymbols (Davis, 2000). In addition, relevant low-tech augmentative communication books and/or boards and remnant books (e.g., a visual record including remnants of daily activities such as movie ticket stub, receipt, invitation, photos; Ho, Weiss, Garrett, & Lloyd, 2005; Simmons-Mackie, 2009) or high-tech electronic devices are introduced within the total communication package. The aphasia literature seems to address aspects of total communication in three relatively distinct paths: training of compensatory strategies, AAC, and supported conversation. These are overlapping aspects of the total communication package and should be introduced in an integrated manner (Simmons-Mackie, 2009).

PACE. PACE is an acronym for Promoting Aphasics Communicative Effectiveness, a program designed by Davis and Wilcox (1985). PACE is a dynamic approach to treatment. The intervention encourages clinicians to incorporate the extralinguistic parameters of purpose, setting, and participants in the intervention program. The treatment goal is to improve conversational skills by allowing the person with aphasia to use any modality to communicate messages. Both the person with aphasia and the clinician take turns as message sender or receiver, promoting active participation.

Augmentative/Assistive Communication. There is consensus that with training and careful selection of appropriate devices, persons with aphasia will benefit from augmentative and assistive communication and tools (Bourgeois, Fried-Oken & Rowland, 2010). Johnson, Hough, King, Vos, and Jeffs (2008) examined abilities of three individuals with chronic nonfluent aphasia using a dynamic display AAC device to enhance communication. The device, Dialect with Speaking Dynamically Pro, was tailored to each participant's skill level using a treatment protocol adapted from Koul, Corwin, and Hayes (2005) in which the primary caregiver was the spouse. Participants with aphasia showed improvement in pre- and posttreatment measures for quality and effectiveness of communication, and two participants showed improved linguistic and cognitive functioning.

The use of computers in therapy serves the purpose of increasing frequency of therapy by allowing patients to practice specific exercises at home. Computer-assisted interactive therapy can help people with aphasia retrieve certain parts of speech, such as the use of verbs, can be used to treat reading disorders, and can be used to provide an alternative system of communication for people who have difficulty with expressive language (Aftonomas, Steele & Wertz, 1997; Katz & Wertz, 1997). Auditory discrimination software with training exercises can also help patients who have problems perceiving the difference between phonemes.

Commercially available programs like Lingraphica™ use a multimodal treatment approach. Patients are reported to increase natural and expressive language with this program (Aftonomos, Appelbaum, & Steele, 1997, 1999). Another commercially available computer software program is AphasiaMate™ (Archibald, Orange, & Jamieson, 2009), which is a comprehensive computer-based language therapy program with eight modules of learning. Archibald and her colleagues (2009) found increased improvement in language and functional communication skills, particularly for persons with moderate to severe aphasia.

Effectiveness and Opportunity Approaches. Lubinski (1988) described two strategies for language intervention for adults with aphasia, which she labeled the Effective Approach and the Opportunity Approach. Lubinski was particularly concerned about the nursing home environment, in which older residents with communication impairments have little opportunity for socialization and communication interaction (Lubinski, 1988; Lubinski, Morrison, & Rigrodsky, 1981).

Lubinski (1988) argued that the stimulation approach, or the Skills Approach, is not the most effective one for the nursing home environment. By the very definition of nursing home placement, persons with aphasia are more dependent and more likely to be more seriously impaired. The environment does not lend itself readily to repetitive drill work, which may seem childish and demeaning to the patient. The Skills Approach may be too unrealistic and frustrating for a frailer nursing home resident. Families and funding agencies may also see the patient's lack of progress as a deterrent to their willingness to continue to pay for services.

The Effectiveness Approach, therefore, is a viable alternative to the stimulation or Skills Approach. In the Effectiveness Approach, the patient is encouraged to use whatever means possible to communicate with the aid of a trusted communication partner. The patient and the partner share the burden for initiating and repairing communication. Patients may use whatever modality is successful in getting the message across, including communication boards, writing, gestures, pictures, and other similar devices.

Lubinski's Opportunity Approach to language therapy is optimally designed for older persons in less than stimulating environments. Individuals, however, must want to communicate. In many long-term care centers, both the internal and external environments may require modifications to increase opportunities for communication. The external environment needs to provide opportunities for interaction through socialization activities, such as dining in groups, and communication partners of choice (Brush & Calkins, 2008). The internal environment of the patient may need guidance in the ways in which the patient/resident is to be open to communication opportunities.

Script Training. Script training is a treatment approach in which the clinician and person with aphasia construct a monologue or dialogue that is practiced intensely so that the person with aphasia can communicate about a topic of interest to them.

Living with Aphasia. For those who live with aphasia, there are many challenges in adjustment to disabilities and self-image. The first three months post-onset are particularly challenging as patients struggle to adjust to life as a person with aphasia (Worrall, Simmons-Mackie, & Brown, 2012). In a study of 15 participants with aphasia, Grohn, Worrall, Simmons-Mackie, and Brown (2012) used semistructured interviews and self-perceived ratings to determine how successfully respondents felt they were living with aphasia. The respondents indicated that they felt a need to do things in order to be actively engaged in rehabilitation and to increase independence and life purpose. Additionally, respondents stressed the importance of social supports, the value of rehabilitation; a need to adapt and make adjustments; and a positive outlook.

Fraas and Calvert (2009) observed that persons with brain injuries need to have a means to redefine themselves in the aftermath of physical and emotional changes. They found that guided narratives or personal stories allow a narrator to talk with others in a group setting about his or her conceptualization of life and identity since brain injury. Although these researchers were investigating the effects of TBI on self-actualization (see Chapter 5), persons with aphasia also need opportunities to see themselves as persons who have survived a catastrophic health event but who have a future.

A new test, available from the Aphasia Institute, allows clinicians to assess patient information on the impact of aphasia and the factors that affect quality of life and factors that worsen or lessen disability. The test, *Assessment for Living with Aphasia* (ALA), can be ordered from the Aphasia Institute (http://www.aphasia.ca), and provides quantitative and qualitative data from the perspective of the person living with aphasia. The ALA, developed with funding from the Ontario Ministry of Health and Long-Term Care, via the Ontario Stroke Network, uses graphics and pictures suitable for persons with aphasia who have a wide range of aphasia severity.

Community Aphasia Groups. Participation-oriented aphasia groups not only foster and reinforce total communication, but also provide a group identity and develop membership in a social community. These are important goals to counter the social isolation often experienced by those with severe aphasia (Simmons-Mackie & Damico, 2009). Aphasia support groups offer patients and their families opportunities to learn more about aphasia, health and wellness steps to take to ensure quality of life, and socialization. Locations and times of community-based aphasia support groups can be accessed at local offices of the American Heart Association. The National Stroke Association (http://www.stroke.org) has a registry of stroke support groups that can accessed online.

Aphasia-Friendly Formatting. Written materials developed for patients and their families should be easy to understand. The National Stroke Association (http://www.stroke.org) has online resources, among them Stroke 101, an easy to understand fact sheet about stroke in English and Spanish.

Aphasia Organizations. There are several aphasia organizations that offer information to clinicians and researchers as well as education and support to persons with aphasia and their families/caregivers through brochures and fact sheets, online education, community programs, webinars, and other resources:

- **American Speech-Language-Hearing Association** (http://www.asha.org)
- **National Stroke Association** (http://www.stroke.org)
- **American Stroke Association/ American Heart Association** (http://www.strokeassociation.org/STROKEORG/)
- **Aphasia Institute** (http://www.aphasia.ca), a nonprofit organization in Canada.

- ◆ **Aphasia United**, represents the collective voices of organizations of people living with aphasia, aphasia service providers, and aphasia researchers through global strategic action. http://www.aphasiaunited.org/
- ◆ **Aphasia Hope Foundation**, a nonprofit foundation promoting research into the prevention and cure of aphasia and ensuring that survivors of aphasia have access to the best treatments available at http://www.aphasiahope.org/
- ◆ **Aphasia Now**, an organization created by people with aphasia for people with aphasia. http://www.aphasianow.org/ (United Kingdom)

Additional Therapy Approaches

Cognitive Rehabilitation

There is agreement that some persons with aphasia will also demonstrate disorders of cognitive functioning (Arkin, 1991; Helm-Estabrooks, 2002). Murray (2012) investigated cognitive disorders in 78 subjects and hypothesized that individuals with aphasia would display variable deficit patterns on tests of attention and other cognitive functions and that their attention deficits, particularly those of complex attention functions, are related to their language and communication status. Results showed that the group with aphasia performed significantly more poorly than the control group on the cognitive measures but displayed variability in the presence, types, and severity of their attention and other cognitive deficits.

Strategies for rehabilitation of cognitive deficits are also described in detail in Chapter 4. Both spaced retrieval training (Brush & Camp, 1998) and errorless learning are well-established techniques that work well with persons with aphasia who also have memory impairments (Fillingham, Sage, & Lambon-Ralph, 2006).

Memory aids such as memory wallets and personal digital assistants, such as iPhones, can be used to help persons with aphasia maintain schedules, telephone numbers, and other important information and hold conversations (Hoerster, Hickey, & Bourgeois, 2001; Gentry, Wallace, Kvarfordt, & Lynch, 2008). Computer-based learning programs like PSS-CogRehab use eight software modules that include 67 computerized therapy tasks, most of which can be adapted to fit the needs of the patient. The focus of the individual exercises extends from simple attention and executive skills, through multiple avenues and modalities of visuospatial and memory skills. The program also includes problem-solving skills ranging from the simple to extremely complex (Bracy, 1994).

Treatment for Reading and Writing Disorders

Most individuals with severe aphasia have concomitant impairments of spoken and written language. For individuals with reading impairments (alexia), treatment should focus on training the impaired component or incorporating strategies to compensate for impairment (e.g., semantic approach, improving speed and efficiency of letter identification) (Taylor-Goh, 2005).

Writing impairment (agraphia) can result from damage to one or more of the critical components of the cognitive processes that support written spelling. Therapy directed toward lexical semantic and nonlexical spelling processes can improve spelling abilities of individuals with acquired writing impairments or can be used efficiently to compensate for the impaired components (Papathanasiou & Cséfalvay, 2013).

Beeson and colleagues (Beeson, 1999; Beeson, Hirsch, & Rewega, 2002) describe the Copy and Recall Treatment (CART) as an exemplar of a lexical-semantic approach to intervention for agraphia. CART involves repeated copying of target words while the patient looks at pictured stimuli, followed by asking the patient to write the name of the picture in repeated trials. Originally, CART was used to structure homework but was later found to be an effective approach to be used for some persons with severe aphasia.

Beeson, Higginson, and Rising (2013) used cell phone texting as a way to implement CART for a 31-year-old patient with severe Broca's aphasia. This novel approach, called T-CART, for texting using the alphabet on the cellular telephone, was found to be an effective treatment for the patient. The patient's wife worked outside of the home, and the patient was able to communicate with her through texting. He was also able to use texting as a way to communicate with his wife in face-to-face interactions. There were, however, several caveats to this treatment. According to Beeson and his associates (2013), the patient was within the age range of adults who commonly use text messaging, he already owned a cell phone with a pull-out keyboard, and he had the motivation and desire to learn to use his phone for texting. Despite his right hemiparesis, the patient easily held the phone and pushed keys using his left hand. He could independently put the phone into the text-messaging mode, and after treatment, he routinely used text messaging to communicate with his family. There are no research reports to confirm that this approach is appropriate for older adults with aphasia, but as most persons now have cell phones and use texting, it would appear that this may be a viable complement to paper and pencil and gesturing communication for most adults.

Summary

Speech-language pathologists, as members of a comprehensive rehabilitation team, have multiple responsibilities for assessing patients with aphasia. Preassessment activities include gathering all relevant data from other professionals and family members and other significant persons in the patient's support network. Neurological examination reports provide information that will be helpful for determining a preliminary diagnosis, the patient's prognosis for recovery, and the extent and severity of the brain damage. There are significant neurological findings that can affect outcome. Altered consciousness and visual field defects as well as neurobehavioral findings of cognitive deficits and affective disorders are highly predictive of language rehabilitation prognosis. These findings should be considered when making a determination of aphasia severity.

Case history intake provides important information about a patient's poststroke ability in language and about the patient's life before stroke. Probes into the psychosocial domains can assist the clinician to understand the patient's cultural environment and coping strategies for illness and disability. Family preinter-views can assist the clinician in docu-menting family dynamics, resources, and stressors. Interview questions to the fam-ily before or during the assessment fur-ther enable clinicians to interpret how the patient and family perceive the nature of stroke and aphasia and what their expec-tations are for the patient's progress while in therapy.

Many standardized tests are appro-priate for adults with aphasia, among them instruments that evaluate overall function, comprehensive aphasia assess-ment, bedside assessments, functional assessments, and assessments that tap specialized and related areas of function-ing, such as family assessment. Results of testing are designed to assist clinicians in determining a patient's residual abilities as well as strengths and weakness in com-municative functioning.

There are two important theories about intervention. One is that therapy should be directed by the clinician who, after careful review of the diagnostic data, develops a program of intervention that is designed to rehabilitation specific areas of aphasia deficits. This approach, which is therapist directed, is effective but does not invest the patient or the patient's fam-ily in the decisions for therapy. Another school of thought is that therapy should be guided by the patient's and the patient's family in light of their under-standing of the context of the patient. This approach is client centered and takes into consideration all of the social and self-identification/esteem concerns that a per-son recovering from a major health crisis will probably experience. As each theory has its merits, clinicians should include both in individualized treatment plans to meet the needs of the patient. Several

strategies are discussed in this section that are appropriate under the therapist-directed and the client-centered models of care. Examples under therapist-directed care include MIT and VCIU, both of which are considered to be effective pro-grams for nonfluent aphasia. An example under client-centered care includes PACE and use of community aphasia groups and resources. PACE is designed to enable persons with aphasia to use and practice their skills with communication partners in a dynamic approach to treatment. Com-munity aphasia groups are considered to be an effective way to involve persons with aphasia and their families in social interaction.

II. RIGHT-HEMISPHERE DISORDERS

Perceptions of the role of the right hemi-sphere in language and cognition have evolved over the last several decades. Historically, the right hemisphere was thought to have three nonlinguistic func-tions: (1) a site of speech in left-handers, (2) the hemisphere that could take over functions after damage to the left hemi-sphere in children and some adults, and (3) the hemisphere most likely to be impli-cated in denial or neglect in hemipare-sis. Very little linguistic functioning was attributed to the right hemisphere. Little importance was given to higher executive functioning. Major findings were in the areas of constructional difficulty, impaired nonverbal perceptual functioning, spa-tial ability, constructional capability, and impaired memory for faces.

Constructional difficulty was found to be more frequent and more intense after right lesions compared with left lesions. Right-hemisphere lesions led to other difficulties in nonverbal perceptual functions, including those involving musical capacities, visual form, color, and stereoscopic vision. Lesions in the right hemisphere were observed also to disrupt functions on tasks requiring spatial judgments and perceptions. Disordered drawing, copying, and contructional capabilities, as well as impairment in face and form perception, were documented for right-hemisphere lesions (Mateer, 1989). Impairment in memory for unfamiliar faces shown in photographs and in recognition of photographs of familiar people was a consistent finding after right temporal lobe lesions (Teuber, 1975).

Three decades ago, speech-language pathologists began to report an increase in the number of patients with both focal and diffuse right-hemisphere lesion (Murdoch, 1990; Tompkins, 1995). Approximately one-half of the patients with right-hemisphere disorders (RHD) presented with communication disorders (Joanette, Goulet, & Hannequin, 1990). Those persons who had language disorders also had a greater incidence of familial left-handedness and less education than persons with RHD without language disorders. In addition, these persons were more likely to have cortical rather than subcortical lesions.

Generally, although the language components of phonology, syntax, and semantics appeared to be more intact in persons with RHD, there were demonstrated problems with communicating effectively. Patients evaluated produced impulsive answers with unnecessary detail, focused on insignificant details in conversation, had difficulty interpreting figurative language, demonstrated reduced sensitivity to emotional tone, and evidenced difficulties in comprehen-

sion and production of normal variations in intonation (Joanette et al., 1990; Myers, 1983, 1991, 1996; Ross, 1981; Tompkins, Boada, & McGarry, 1992; Tompkins et al., 1993). Hence, the more current theories on cognitive and communication disorders associated with RHD lesions suggested that language may be impaired in different ways depending on whether the damage is to the left or the right hemisphere.

According to Davis (2000), persons with nondominant or right-hemisphere strokes often were not referred to speech-language pathologists because their primary disorders were not seen to be the disorders of syntax or word-finding that are seen in persons with aphasia. Now, patients may be referred for the following reasons:

1. The patient has a swallowing problem or motor speech deficit.
2. Someone with an old right-hemisphere infarct has recently sustained a left-hemisphere stroke.
3. The patient has communicative difficulties caused by a right-hemisphere stroke.

Disorders of Language and Cognition Associated with RHD

Three major components of language and cognitive disorders associated with RHD are linguistic deficits, nonlinguistic deficits, and extralinguistic deficits.

Linguistic Deficits

As the fundamental components of language are largely mediated by the left hemisphere, the linguistic deficits observed in RHD are typically mild and have the least effect on the patient's communication disorder (Murdoch, 1990). When linguistic deficits are observed, they include:

◆ problems in auditory comprehension of complex material;

◆ difficulties with word finding, word fluency, and body part naming; and

◆ difficulty with oral sentence reading, and writing problems, such as, grapheme substitutions and omissions.

Eisenson (1962) was among the first to suggest that there were subtle language impairments that could result from damage to the right hemisphere. Later studies confirm that RHD can cause language impairments in auditory comprehension, word retrieval, discourse coherence, and pragmatics.

Auditory Comprehension Deficits. Evidence suggests that RHD can produce deficits in auditory comprehension, including comprehension of complex auditory information. Keller, Schlenker and Pigache (1995) reported that there may be a selective impairment of auditory attention in persons with vascular lesions of the right hemisphere. Keller and his colleagues used strings of auditory digits presented diotically (one digit string to both ears) and dichotically (simultaneous presentation of a different digit string to both ears). Compared with persons with CHI, the persons with stroke-induced RHD made significantly more errors on dichotic subtests independent of speed of presentation. These results suggested that the attention deficits is due to differential disruptions of the cortical network includ-

ing prefrontal, anterior cingulate, and temporoparietal structures of the right hemisphere.

Tompkins (2008) conjectures that there are multiple phases involved in language comprehension in the right hemisphere. One phase, the initial phase, also called the Construction phase (Kintsch, 1998), involves automatic and context specific processes. Incoming words trigger background knowledge and activate concepts that are independent of a broader context. In this phase, the word "car" can trigger the concepts of toy car, model car, family car or sedan, and armored car, among others.

The second phase of such accounts, termed the Integration phase (Kintsch, 1998), is context dependent. Aspects of context are brought to bear on an emerging interpretation. The processes that occur in this phase combine incoming text with prior text information and with what is known about the world. In the second phase, which is context driven, the words "speeding ticket" establish the context, which makes toy car and armored car irrelevant. This pruning and weeding of words that do not fit the context is termed suppression (Tompkins, 2008).

The intact right hemisphere is proposed to "coarsely code'" linguistic input. This means that the right-hemisphere superior temporal and inferior parietal regions (Jung-Beeman, 2005) activate extensive semantic fields of words, including distantly related, peripheral meanings and features (Coulson & Williams, 2005; Faust, Barak, & Chiarello, 2006; Faust & Lavidor, 2003) that may not be activated in the left hemisphere.

Coarse semantic coding is thought to make the right hemisphere sensitive to semantic overlap between words. The right hemisphere, therefore, may be specialized for making novel semantic connections that aid the processing of unfamiliar sentences and/or the right hemisphere may support additional processing required to make sense of distant semantic relations. These processes are considered to be important for some kinds of inferencing and nonliteral language interpretation (Blake, 2009;Tompkins, Baumgaertner, Lehman, & Fassbinder, 2000). Adults with RHD are thought to have a deficit in coarse semantic coding, which leads to difficulty in aspects of normal comprehension that are supported by coarse coding (Tompkins, Kiepousniotou, & Scott, 2013).

Word Retrieval Deficits and Discourse. Word retrieval deficits occur frequently among persons with RHD (Diggs & Basili, 1987; Myers, 1996; Tompkins, 1995; Varley, 1995). Unlike patients with left-hemisphere damage, patients with RHD have less severe and frequent problems with naming, single-word comprehension, and word definition tasks. Patients with RHD tend to make more visually based errors than patients with aphasia. For example, extension cord may be given as the name for snake (Tompkins, 1995). Patients with RHD tend also to have particular difficulty with naming categories or collective nouns (Myers & Brookshire, 1994). Patients may be able to name the individual elements belonging to a particular category, for example, apple, banana, pear, rather than assigning the name fruit.

Using a confrontation naming task of collective and single nouns, Myers and Brookshire (1994) found that their patients with RHD performed poorly on collective noun naming and concluded that there may be a relationship between severity of neglect and impairment on confrontational naming. Naming deficits may be

more related, therefore, to cognitive rather than to visual factors in that patients had more semantic and listing errors than neglect and visual confusion errors. Varley (1995) found similar evidence that RHD language disorders are the result of broad cognitive disintegration.

Patients with RHD may have particular difficulties when discourse contains ambiguous or conflicting elements that make multiple interpretations possible. In discourse production, although there is considerable variability among persons with RHD, some consistencies in diminished informational content, difficulty telling a coherent story, and excessive detail and overpersonalization have been reported (Tompkins, Klepousniotou, & Scott 2013).

Nonlinguistic Impairments

Anosognosia. A frequent symptom of right parietal lobe damage is denial of illness, or anosognosia, specifically for the existence of left hemiplegia. Denial may take the form of inference, underestimation, or denial of major disabilities. Pimenthal and Kingsbury (1989a), however, viewed anosognosia and denial as two separate entities. Anosognosia may be the more inclusive term, and denial, both explicit verbal denial and implicit denial, may be a more specific variety of anosognositic awareness. Denial, then, suggests more than unawareness; it involves active negating or refusing to accept a disability or condition.

Neglect. Despite the fact that brain-injured patients often have relatively spared speech, language, and memory abilities, their prognosis for recovery of independent function is not good (Jehkonen, Laihosalo, & Kettunen, 2006). Even global aphasia and right hemiparesis may not have as great an effect on the ability to become independent. Patients with RHD may exhibit unilateral neglect, which is the failure to attend to one side of the body or to respond to stimuli in the visual field contralateral to the site of lesion, despite normal integrity of the sensory modalities (Myers, 1996).

According to Kolb and Whishaw (1990), neglect is a perceptual disorder following right parietal lesions. Patients may have impaired use of margins and punctuation in writing, fail to attend to the left side of space, have impaired localization skills, fail to look to the left side of a page while reading, and may omit the left when drawing or copying a figure. The devastating effect of neglect on recovery may occur because it consists of a cluster of symptoms, affecting several areas of vital importance in daily life.

Patients with RHD usually have trouble with awareness of things placed to the left of their bodies (body-centered neglect), to the left of their heads (head-centered neglect), or in their left visual field (eye-centered or retinotopic neglect). Sometimes a patient will neglect the left "side" of a visual object no matter where it is placed in the environment (object-centered neglect) (Barrett, 2000). The majority of studies report neglect of the left side. However, there have been isolated reports of right-sided neglect following RHD.

Unilateral neglect may be the result of an intrahemispheric disconnection syndrome in that damage to the long-range white matter pathways connecting parietal and frontal areas within the right hemisphere may be a major cause of neglect. Hence, neglect may not result from damage to a single cortical region. Rather, neglect may be caused by a disruption of large networks made up of distant cortical regions (Bartolomeo, de Schotten, & Doricchi, 2007).

The following case history information provided by Kolb and Whishaw (1990, p. 424) illustrates the typical symptoms of neglect associated with right parietal lesions:

Mr. P., a 67-year-old man, suffered a right parietal stroke and exhibited the following symptoms: Mr. P. neglected the left side of his body and of his world. When asked to lift up his arms, he failed to lift his left arm but could do so if one took his arm and asked him to lift it. When asked to draw a clock face, he crowded all the numbers on the right side of the clock. When asked to read compound words such as ice cream of football, he read cream and ball. When he dressed, he did not attempt to put on the left side of his clothing (a form of dressing apraxia) and when he shaved, he shaved only the right side of his face. He ignored tactile sensation on the left side of his body.

Unilateral neglect has been a major focus of research because the impairment is related to many deficits in RHD. Barrett (2000) focuses on the following, related deficits:

◆ *Disordered spatial perception.* Subjects with neglect usually have disordered spatial perception. They are unable to take note of relevant, interesting, or novel events that occur on the left side of space, although their vision, hearing, and touch in that region is not usually severely impaired.

◆ *Emotional disorders.* People with neglect often have disorders of emotional perception and communication that have catastrophic consequences for their family and work relationships. Specifically, after right-hemisphere stroke, persons with RHD can have difficulty expressing emotions through the use of prosodic feature of speech (aprosodia), although some persons may recognize that their voice does not convey their emotions to others (Brookshire, 1992). Patients will lack the appropriate intonation to convey happiness, sadness, surprise, anger, or disappointment. These patients are described as having a flat affect and monotone speech, and in some cases, may appear to be clinically depressed (Ross, 1981). Contrastively, increased intonational variation or hypermelodicity has been reported (Colsher, Cooper, & Graff-Radford, 1987). Problems with comprehension of prosodic variations have been reported. Impaired interpretation of affective prosody of speech has been observed particularly in patients with temporoparietal lesions (Joanette et al., 1990).

◆ *Hypoarousal.* People with neglect after right-hemisphere stroke often appear more indifferent or apathetic than they did before the event. They may rarely move, speak, or initiate behaviors compared with their premorbid norm. When this deficit in arousal is severe, patients may demonstrate *abulia*, a profound passivity and indifference to their environment.

◆ *Motor bias.* Persons with neglect may have trouble activating a motor response, especially if a left-sided limb must be activated, or if either limb must be moved into left space. Like someone steering a shopping cart with a stuck wheel, they may have a "motor bias" or "turning tendency" toward their good, right field. This is termed *directional hypokinesia* or *hemihypokinesia* (Coslett, Bowers, Fitzpatrick, Haws, & Heilman, 1990).

◆ *Personal Neglect.* Persons with neglect may pay little attention to external items on the left, but they can neglect the left side of their bodies. These patients may fail to wash, groom, or dress the left side of their face and/or body. Some of these subjects can be observed to "forget" about their left arm even when it is capable of some movement and may let the arm drag in the wheel of their wheelchair. They may lie on the limb in a manner likely to impair circulation or joint mobility (Barrett, 2000).

Prosopagnosia. Prosopagnosia falls within the category of nonlinguistic disorders that are associated with RHD also. Prosopagnosia refers to an acquired deficit in the recognition and identification of familiar human faces. The disorder occurs with both bilateral lesions of mesial occipitotemporal areas and unilateral right-hemisphere lesions. The primary cause of this disorder appears to be a deficit in perceiving and processing contextual information (Brookshire, 1992). Patients may have difficulty identifying photographs of famous people, recognizing faces, and perceiving line-drawn faces and cartoons.

Difficulty in appropriately producing facial expression is a problem for patients with RHD (see Emotional Disorders). Although less has been written about the facial expression of emotion, some investigators (Ladavas, Umilta, & Ricci-Bitti, 1980) report that there is greater movement of the left side of the face when the patient expresses emotion.

Extralinguistic Impairments

Aprosodia. Patients may have difficulty interpreting prosodic and facial and situational cues that signal the emotional content of the message. Prosody, the aspect of language by which different emotions are conveyed through variations in intonation, rhythm, and stress, is mediated by the right hemisphere. Perceptual, global, and motor disorders have been ascribed to aprosodia (Leon & Rodriguez, 2008). Patients with RHD have difficulty expressing emotions through the use of prosodic features of speech, although some may recognize that their voice does not convey their emotions to others (Brookshire, 1992).

Deficits of Pragmatic Language. Pragmatics is the appropriate use of language and the ability to convey meaning beyond the actual words through gesture, body language, facial expression, changes in the vocal inflection, and intonation (Pimenthal & Kingsbury, 1989b). Pragmatics also refers to the context-appropriate use of language and communicative functions. Context includes the identities of the participants in verbal exchanges and their beliefs, knowledge, and intentions, as well as the temporal and spatial dimensions of the communicative event. Myers (1991) and Tompkins (1995) found that patients with RHD exhibit pragmatic disorders in:

◆ proxemics, or respecting personal space and personal and social distance (Hall, 1963)
◆ difficulty in organizing information in an efficient, meaningful way
◆ a tendency to produce impulsive answers that are tangential and related
◆ difficulty distinguishing between what is important and what is not
◆ a tendency to over personalize external events
◆ a reduced sensitivity to the communicative situation or to the pragmatic aspects of communication
◆ difficulty understanding and producing indirect requests ("Can you pass the salt?")
◆ a decreased sensitivity to listener needs and situations

Others (Prutting & Kitchner, 1987) observed that patients with RHD have problems with proxemics, gesture, question formulation, topic change, appropriate topic selection and maintenance, and repairing misunderstandings through turn taking. Tompkins (1995) also found that many individuals with RHD are impulsive, talk excessively, interject irrelevant and inappropriate comments, and generate impulsive responses. They may have problems with observing turn-taking rules, staying on topic, and maintaining eye contact with the listener.

Difficulties with Abstract Meanings. Patients with RHD have a tendency to lend a literal interpretation to figurative language and to have difficulty grasping figurative and implied meanings in narratives, humor, and in conversation, particularly with interpretation of idioms, metaphors, and figures of speech (Tompkins et al., 1992). Individuals with RHD tend to respond only to the literal interpretation of what they see or hear.

Patients may also have difficulty with answering questions about the relationships among characters or events in a story, difficulty matching a metaphor to its pictured representation, or even problems selecting the appropriate punchline to a joke. Patients have problems with distinguishing the literal from the implied meaning in instructions. For example, when asked to give the days of the week, a patient may respond, "Monday, Tuesday, Wednesday, Thursday, Friday." When cued to continue, the patient may reply, "You didn't say the weekend."

In general, patients with RHD tend to focus on irrelevant or insignificant details and fail to synthesize information in discourse, whether in narrative or conversation. For extensive reviews of discourse and related problems, the reader is referred to Cherney and Canter (1993), Joanette and colleagues (1990), Myers (1996), and Tompkins (1995).

To account for the impairment in the interpretation of figurative and implied meanings in patients with RHD, Myers (1991) proposed that inference failure, which refers to faulty inferencing, can occur at all levels of cognitive and perceptual processing. Inferencing involves recognizing relationships between key elements of meaning and other contextual cues. Impaired comprehension of facial and prosodic features and difficulty with interpreting nonliteral expressions are indicative of inference failure.

Myers and Brookshire (1994) provided further evidence for an underlying inference deficit in a study of the effects of visual and inferential complexity on the picture description of patients with no brain damage (NBD) and patients with RHD. Both groups of subjects mentioned essentially the same number of major concepts in response to visually simple and complex pictures. However, the patients with RHD tended to generate fewer major concepts in all conditions compared with the NBD subjects. The impaired ability of patients with RHD to describe more detailed picture scenes is more related to the inferential than to the visual complexity of pictured stimuli.

The ability to appreciate, understand, or produce humor has not been well documented. Clinically, some adults with RHD react to cartoons with unrestrained hilarity; this is more likely with frontal lobe damage. Humor production has been observed clinically to be, at times, disinhibited, crude, suggestive, or otherwise inappropriate in some adults with RHD (Tompkins et al., 2013). Impaired ability to understand humor or sarcasm is a hallmark of right-hemisphere damage. However, not all elements of humor may be lost. In a study of elements of humor, Brownell, Michel, Powelson, and Gardner (1987) noted that persons with right-hemisphere deficits exhibited a selective attraction to humorous story endings that contained an element of surprise but were not otherwise coherent with the body of the joke.

Disorders of Visual Processing. Pimenthal and Kingsbury (1989a, 1989b) categorized components of right-hemisphere syndromes linked to specific underlying disorders of visual processing. These include disorders of gaze stability, which incorporates visual scanning deficits; disorders of visuoverbal processing; and disorders of visuosymbolic processing. Disorders of gaze stability produce problems with the ability to focus on and track reading material. Disorders of visuoverbal processing disrupt reading comprehension or decoding and produce alexia. The alexia may be the result of neglect or due to deficits in visual recognition and scanning. Writing deficits, or agraphia, are demonstrated in the patient's inability to write and is the consequence or errors in visuoverbal encoding. Disorders of visuosymbolic processing may interrupt the ability to perform arithmetical processes, or acalculia. Acalculia may occur from lesions anywhere in either the right or left hemispheres and it is postulated that there may be a general reduction in cerebral activation after a right hemisphere infarct (Coslett, Bowers, & Heilman, 1987; Pimenthal & Kingsbury, 1989a). These visual processing disorders are significant for language expression and comprehen-

sion, and are shown in Table 6–7 with the suspected sites of lesions.

Disorders of Orientation. Patients with RHD are often disoriented to place and time, but are generally more oriented to person (Pimenthal, 1985, 1986). Patients with disorientation to place may be able to include both a correct and an incorrect place. For example, a patient who lives in Washington DC and who is in the Providence Hospital may respond that he is in his house, which is called Providence Hospital. Patients may also misname the place or give an erroneous description, such as: "This is the nursing motel." Patients with disorientation to time may produce errors in the time of day, the name of the day, month, or years and may show confusion on the seasons.

Disorders of Attention and Memory. Adults with stroke-induced RHD may

Table 6–7. Classification of Selected Right Hemisphere Visual Syndromes That Impair Language Functions

Disorders of Visual Processing	Relationship to Language	Site of Lesion
Disorders of gaze stability	Causes problems in reading	Frontal lobe eye fields
Disorders of visuospatial processing	Alexia	Hemialexia can result from lesions to the splenium of the corpus callosum. Visuospatial alexia can occur from lesions in the right occipital cortex or from subcortical disconnections.
	Agraphia	Visuospatial agraphia results from lesions to the frontoparietal or temporoparieto-occipital areas.
Disorders of visuosymbolic processing	Acalculia	Left or right hemispheres, anywhere

Source: Adapted from Pimenthal, P. A., & Kingbury, N. A. (1989b). *Mini inventory of right brain injury.* Austin, TX: Pro-Ed.

have difficulty in dividing and switching attention, which portends limitations to social activities and performance of family roles (Lehman & Tompkins, 2000). Many adults with RHD have deficits in estimated verbal working memory capacity for language. Good working memory capacity for language is associated with higher level cognitive performance, such as resolving inconsistencies in narratives and revising inferences in tasks with relatively high processing demands. Impaired spatial working memory can co-occur with and complicate the neglect syndrome (Marsh & Hillis, 2008).

Deficits in Executive Functioning. Patients with RHD can have deficits with aspects of executive functioning, such as planning, organization, reasoning, and problem solving. Difficulties have been documented in record-keeping, adhering to checklists, organizing schedules, keeping of belongings, and managing time (Klonoff, Sheperd, O'Brien, Chiapello, & Hodak, 1990).

ASSESSMENT OF RHD

Assessment of the adult patient with RHD should include measures of linguistic, nonlinguistic, and extralinguistic functioning. Traditional tests of aphasia have not been found to be adequate for this purpose; however, subtests designed to assess auditory comprehension and word finding will be helpful in the assessment of language, detailed earlier in this chapter. A variety of measures, both formal and informal, should be used to diagnose language and related disorders. Extralinguistic behaviors such as conversational style, interpretation, and production of discourse and pragmatic skills are shaped by cultural influences and experiences. The clinician should use sensitivity when designating language behaviors as deficient or abnormal (Tompkins, 1995). Cultural sensitivity has been covered in depth in Chapter 2.

CLINICAL ASSESSMENT

Standardized Testing

There are several tests that will help the clinician assess the unique and often subtle communicative difficulties associated with RHD. These are:

Aprosodia Battery (Ross, Thompson, & Yenkosky, 1997)

This battery, described by Ross (1997), is a bedside assessment for prosody. The test consists of a variety of tasks assessing repetition of affective prosody, identification of affective prosody, and discrimination between two sentences spoken in differing affective prosodic tones. It also assesses ability to understand gestures associated with emotional states.

Mini Inventory of Right Brain Injury-2 (MIRBI-2; Pimenthal & Knight, 2000)

The MIRBI-2 is a 27-item screening measure with ratings for affective language, primary impairments, and pragmatic language, such as humor and metaphor. This instrument is brief enough to be used at bedside.

Prosody-Voice Screening Profile (PVSP; Shriberg, Kwaitkowski, & Rasmussen, 1990)

Expressive prosodic deficits can be measured using the PVSP, which collects spontaneous speech in order to assess the prosodic and vocal characteristics of the speaker. Phrasing, rate, stress, pitch loudness, and vocal quality are transcribed and judged for appropriateness.

Rehabilitation Institute of Chicago Evaluation of Communication Problems in Right Hemisphere Dysfunction–3 (RICE-3; Halper, Cherney, & Burns, 2010)

This evaluation assesses general behavior patterns, visual scanning and tracking, writing, pragmatic communication, and metaphoric language. General behavior tasks include orientation examined in an interview. Visual scanning and tracking is measured through writing tasks. Pragmatic communication is profiled with general rating scales for intonation, gesture, conversational skills, and narrative abilities. Metaphoric language is examined by asking a patient to explain proverbs and idioms.

Right Hemisphere Language Battery (RHLB; Bryan, 1989)

The RHLB has seven subtests that measure lexical-semantic comprehension, metaphor appreciation in listening and reading, verbal humor appreciation, comprehension of inferred meaning, production of emphatic stress, and conversational discourse. The MIRBI-2 includes a revised Right-Left Differential Scale with an updated cutoff score for right-brain impairment.

Ross Information Processing Assessment, Second Edition (RIPA-2; Ross-Swain, 1996)

RIPA assesses auditory processing and retention, immediate and recent memory,

temporal orientation (recent and remote), information recall, environmental orientation, organization, spatial orientation, problem solving, and reasoning skills.

Table 6–8 provides a summary of suggested assessments appropriate for use with adults with RHD. Other suggested assessments include function communication, discourse, and cognitive assessments, which are described earlier in this chapter.

Informal Measures

Responses to situation or action pictures, interview questions, or open-ended questions and responses in general conversation can be analyzed for appropriateness or verbal production (Morganstein & Smith, 1993). Other measures include observing the patient's communication with family, nursing staff, and other rehabilitation specialists to assess pragmatic skills (Tompkins, 1995).

PATIENT MANAGEMENT

Patients with RHD cognitive-language disorders are heterogeneous and varied in their symptoms. Intervention programs should be comprehensive yet highly individualized (Boone & Plante, 1993). The primary area of language impairment in patients with RHD involves linguistic and extralinguistic deficits. Specifically, right-hemisphere lesions might affect four different components of verbal communication: prosody, discourse, semantics, and pragmatics. Treatment for these deficits and those of nonlinguistic deficits such as neglect are appropriate and efficacious, using a client-centered model of service delivery. The American Speech-Language-Hearing Association's (2008) Treatment

Table 6–8. Suggested Assessments for Adults with Right Hemisphere Damage

Test Name	Measurement
Aprosodia Battery (Ross, Thompson, & Yenkowsky, 1997)	Bedside assessment of repetition of affective prosody, understanding gestures associated with emotional states, and identification and discrimination of affective prosody.
Mini-Inventory of Right Brain Injury–2 (MIRBI-2; Pimenthal & Knight, 2000)	A 27-item screening measure with ratings for affective language, primary impairments, and pragmatic, such as humor and metaphor. This tool can be used at bedside.
Prosody-Voice Screening Profile (PVSP; Shriberg, Kwaitkowski, & Rasmussen, 1990)	Assesses prosodic and vocal characteristics of the speaker. Measures vocal quality, pitch, loudness, phrasing, and rate.
Rehabilitation Institute of Chicago Evaluation of Communication Problems in Right Hemisphere Dysfunction–3 (RICE-3; Halper, Cherney, & Burns, 2010)	Assesses general behavior, visual scanning and tracking, writing, pragmatic communication, and metaphoric language.
Right Hemisphere Language Battery (RHLB; Bryan, 1989)	Uses 7 subtests to measure lexical-semantic comprehension, metaphor appreciation, verbal humor appreciation, comprehension of inferred meaning, emphatic stress production, and conversational discourse.
Ross Information Processing Assessment, Second Edition (RIPA-2; Ross-Swain, 1996)	Assesses auditory processing and retention, immediate and recent memory, temporal orientation, information recall, environmental orientation, organization, spatial orientation, problem solving, and reasoning skills.

Efficacy Summary on Cognitive-Communication Disorders Resulting from Right Hemisphere Brain Damage reports:

> [D]ata from ASHA's National Outcomes Measurement System (NOMS) show that for patients with right hemisphere cerebrovascular disease who received speech-language pathology services, 73%improved in problem solving, 80% increased attention, 74% improved memory, and 77% improved in pragmatics. Treatments for visuospatial neglect have been shown to be effective primarily when they are intensive, encourage active scanning or internal cueing (as opposed to clinician-driven cues, such as "look to the left"), or involve left limb movement combined with scanning tasks.

As persons with RHD have historically not been seen by speech-language pathologists routinely, there are few research studies about approaches to treatment. However, treatment can be either theoretically motivated or based on deficits as shown through assessments.

Considering the paucity of evidence in the field of practice, clinicians can look to treatment from other populations, specifically, treatments for persons with dementia and TBI. After the assessment phase, it is important to develop an intervention program that will address the communication and functional needs of the individual. The patient and his family should therefore choose the intervention goals together with the clinician in order to set a collaborative base. As underlined by Tompkins (1995), the goals should target the most prejudicial deficits in everyday communication activities. The family has to be involved all along the therapy to obtain a better generalization to different contexts (Ferré, Ska, Lajoie, Bleau, & Joanette, 2011).

Even though more research needs to be done to develop efficacy studies based on evidence-based practices, some clinical guidelines are useful for clinicians to develop an appropriate intervention program for their patients with RHD. Myers (1996) suggested that treatment address the following areas:

♦ Aspects of general and spatial attention, including arousal, selective attentive, vigilance, and maintenance of attention
♦ Inferences, including the detection of stimuli, awareness of stimulus significance, integration of information, and association with prior experiences
♦ Verbal efficiency in topic maintenance and reduction of verbal irrelevancies
♦ Level of informative content with particular emphasis on increasing specificity and number of concepts

♦ Capacity to generate alternate meanings, humor, and intended meanings and ability to accommodate new information
♦ Pragmatic aspects of communication, rules of conversation, and awareness of situational context.

Although there is great variability of profiles among RHD adults, three guidelines offered by Ferré and his associates (2011) seem relevant:

1. Raise the awareness of the deficits. Clinicians can also suggest real-life examples and analogies, through a pictographic symbol illustrating the maladapted situation of communication (e.g., a highway illustrating the main theme, exit roads suggesting the diverging commentaries). Symbols can be used during therapy and progressively replaced by verbal signals or gestures to diminish feedback and to abide by the second guideline.

2. Organize tasks into a hierarchy of increasing difficulty. It is possible to vary the level of difficulty by modifying the perceptibility of stimuli (visual versus verbal presentation, unimodal versus multimodal, font, size, background, etc.), by changing their internal characteristics (frequency, imageability, organization in space, etc.), or by multiplying the contexts (structured to various complex natural settings).

3. Take into account the basic cognitive impairments (e.g., memory, attention, mental flexibility). Offer a facilitative context appropriate for each type of deficit that can be withdrawn in order to adopt a more realistic and complex context of communication. Each facilitator should be adapted to the specific

disorder (e.g., by controlling the presentation of the stimuli in the visual space for hemi-neglect patients).

Treatment for neglect and related disorders represents a challenge for clinicians. Readers are encouraged to read the review article on treatment for unilateral neglect by Barrett (2000). Although treatment should be individualized, it may be beneficial for all patients with RHD to work initially on improving attention and orientation. The following tasks proposed by Swindell and colleagues (1994) have been used successfully for patients with RHD and can be incorporated in therapy where appropriate:

◆ Sequencing tasks for helping patients with organization of verbal materials
◆ Tasks that focus on the comprehension and production of emotional tone
◆ Tasks that require the selection of critical items of a pictures or a story
◆ Tasks that emphasize visuospatial perception to assist reading and writing abilities
◆ Tasks requiring limits on speaking time to help patients avoid digression and perseveration
◆ Tasks requiring patients to watch for cues to assist with eye contact, topic maintenance, and turn taking during conversation.

Myers (1996) and Tompkins (1995) recommended the inclusion of two main types of tasks to achieve treatment efficacy: (1) compensatory tasks and (2) facilitation tasks. Compensatory tasks are used to teach the patient new strategies and to focus on using intact skills to compensate for areas of deficit. Facilitation tasks are used to stimulate the recovery of deficits and focus on theory of impaired processes.

Very few training programs have been published for use with adults with RHD. One such program that is available and has been found to be effective with this population is *Lessons for the Right Brain* (Anderson & Crowe-Miller, 1982). This set of five 64-page workbooks, published by Pro-Ed, helps the individual learn and retrieve such skills as writing notes, telling time, reading street maps, and finding phone numbers. Workbooks are included for memory, reading and writing, visual perception and attention, thought organization, and self-perception/organizing functional information. A memory workbook is available from http://www.thera pro.com/Lessons-for-the-Right-Brain-Memory-Workbook-P6521.aspx

Summary

The right hemisphere also plays an important role in language and cognitive skills. Historically, the right hemisphere was considered to be silent during language. It is now widely accepted that lesions in the right hemisphere can cause denial of illness and unilateral neglect, and impair auditory comprehension of complex information, orientation, inferencing, prosody, memory, attention, visuospatial ability, reading, and writing due to visuosymbolic disorders, word fluency, discourse, pragmatics, executive functioning, and ability to understand and produce abstract language in three broad categories: linguistic, nonlinguistic, and extralinguistic disorders. In particular, nonlinguistic disorders such as unilateral neglect, a major characteristic of RHD, are associated with many other disorders that impair language. There is evidence to support that rehabilitation of unilateral neglect, usually left-side unilateral neglect, has favorable outcomes for cognition and language.

Comprehensive batteries are available for speech-language pathologists to examine both linguistic and extralinguisic behaviors, such as discourse and pragmatics, and some nonlinguistic areas, like unilateral neglect. Additionally, a protocol to examine prosody is available. Including testing for functional communication and cognitive functioning, selected subtests from aphasia batteries and informal assessments will provide clinicians with a holistic view of the person with RHD.

There is a need for more research on RHD to establish the efficacy of treatment approaches and the best evidence-based therapies. At present, it is accepted that rehabilitation should focus on both cognitive and language disorders. Therefore, guidelines and tasks to assist the clinician should be useful for developing an appropriate and individualized plan of treatment.

EDUCATION AND COUNSELING FOR FAMILIES OF PATIENTS WITH APHASIA AND RIGHT-HEMISPHERE DISORDERS

The vast majority of persons with aphasia are stroke survivors. Adjusting to the functional and communication impairments that are frequently associated with stroke recovery presents major challenges for both the survivor and the family. Coping with caregiving for a person with aphasia is often difficult and stressful (Draper et al., 2007). Clark (1991) outlined several sources of stress related to caregiving for a person after stroke: lack of community and family support, lack of information about resources, guilt from decisions to institutionalize a stroke survivor, and the emotional and physical toll of caregiving.

Flasher and Fogle (2012) define counseling in the context of speech-language services for families as an interactive process for information gathering in which the professional uses listening, rapport-building, and emphatic skills to understand the uniqueness of the patient and the patient's family. At times, counseling also means helping the family to adjust to the long-term consequences of a neurological disorder that has changed the person they knew significantly.

Fox (2013) recommends involving the family in every aspect of the treatment process in a collaborative partnership, using the Self-Anchored Rating Scale as an approach to involve families of persons with aphasia in treatment goal setting. This approach minimizes the family's frustration, emphasizes the family strengths, and focuses on identifying solutions and reasonable treatment goals. Family members are given assignments that build upon their successes in ways that invest the family in the intervention process.

Brochures, while useful, are insufficient sources of information to families. This type of information should be used as part of an ongoing program of family education and counseling (Family Caregiver Alliance, n.d.; Wahrborg, 1991). For families who speak a language other than English, bilingual reading materials should be used to assist them in comprehending the effects of stroke on language.

Families also need help in identifying materials appropriate for their persons with aphasia to use at home. The recommended materials should be age appropriate, easily understood, and written in a font size that is easy to read. The American Speech-Language-Hearing Association has printed materials and videos on aphasia. Information about these materials can be accessed at http://www.asha .org. In addition to communication boards and other low-tech devices, commercially available software, like Parrot and Lingraphica, can be used at home and in the clinical setting.

Support groups and Web-based resources are also sources of information and support for families. Please refer to the section in this chapter on Client-Centered Therapy for information about accessing a directory of support groups and websites that will be helpful to families.

Family members and/or caregivers of adults with RHD will need special support and counseling. Unlike persons with aphasia, language skills of patients with RHD may appear to the family to relatively intact. The family may act with dismay when told that their patient needs speech-language therapy and may become defensive or angry. The role of the speech-language pathologist is to educate the family about critical areas of language, visuospatial processing, pragmatics, higher cognitive impairments, and other behaviors that can disrupt the patient's ability to return to previous roles at home and in society. The patient's motivation is a critical factor in recovery.

Before planning an educational program, however, it will be important to find out what is already known by the family as a point of departure. Suggested questions are found earlier in this chapter and family responses can be used to develop verbal and written information that is appropriate and easy to understand.

Educational materials should be in the family's primary language. Patients with RHD and their families may find it difficult to accept that intervention is needed because the patient may appear to be behaving and speaking normally. Denial of illness and disability that frequently accompanies RHD may be misinterpreted by the family as the patient's good adjustment to the change in health status. Professionals may encounter defensiveness and anger from the family when advised that the patient has problems with judgment, planning, memory, or pragmatics. Family members may view these problems as symptomatic of the patient's being stubborn or, worse, old and foolish. Education and counseling will be important to inform families about RHD and its possible effects on critical areas of functioning that can impair family relationships, social interactions, reentry to work or other productive endeavors, and quality of life.

STUDY QUESTIONS

1. What are the major types of cerebrovascular accidents? How are they different?

2. What is aphasia?

3. What diseases or conditions can cause aphasia?

4. What are the differences between mild, moderate, and severe aphasia?

5. What is meant by nonfluent and fluent aphasia?

6. What are the transcortical aphasias? How are they different?

7. What is a pure aphasia?

8. What are the types of aphasia considered to be nonfluent and fluent?

9. What are the naming disorders associated with aphasia?

10. In what ways can altered consciousness portend recovery from aphasia?

11. What types of language disturbances occur with lesions to the basal ganglia and thalamus?

12. What factors need to be considered in establishing a prognosis?

13. Why are bedside tests advisable in an acute care setting?

14. What role does cognition play in aphasia?

15. What assessments for cognitive function are suggested?

16. What assessments for aphasia are suggested?

17. What are the related assessments that are suggested?

18. Distinguish between therapist-directed and client-centered therapy.

19. Which approaches are most appropriate for therapist-directed therapy?

20. Which strategies are most appropriate for client-centered therapy?

21. What kinds of linguistic deficits occur in some persons with RHD?

22. What kinds of nonlinguistic and extralinguistic deficits occur in some persons with RHD?

23. How is unilateral neglect associated with other disorders in RHD?

24. What are the guidelines for rehabilitation of RHD disorders?

25. What is a visuosymbolic disorder and how is it related to agraphia?

26. What tests are available to assess cognitive-communication disorders in persons with RHD?

27. What are some specific therapy techniques to consider for an adult with RHD?

28. Why might families of patients with RHD become defensive about therapy?

29. Why is it important for persons with RHD to receive speech-language pathology services?

30. What resources, programs, and websites are helpful for families and patients with left- and/or right-hemisphere damage?

REFERENCES

Adair, J. C., Nadeau, S. E., Conway, T. W., Gonzalez-Rothi, L. J., Heilman, P. C., Green, I. A., & Heilman, K. M. (2000). Alterations in the functional anatomy of reading induced by rehabilitation of an alexic patient. *Neuropsychiatry, Neuropsychology, and Behavioral Neurology, 13,* 303–311.

Aftonomos, L. B., Appelbaum J. S., & Steele, R. D. (1999) Improving outcomes for persons with aphasia in advanced community-based treatment programs. *Stroke, 30,* 1370–1379.

Aftonomos, L. B., Steele R. D., & Wertz, R. T. (1997) Promoting recovery in chronic aphasia with an interactive technology. *Archives of Physical Medicine and Rehabilitation, 78,* 841–846.

Aggarwal, N. T., Schneider, J. A., Wilson, R. S., Beck, T. L., Evans, D. A., & De Carli, C. (2012). Characteristics of MR infarcts associated with dementia and cognitive function in the elderly. *Neuroepidemiology, 38,* 41–47.

Albert, M. L., Sparks, R. W., & Helm, N. A. (1973). Melodic intonation therapy for aphasia. *Archives of Neurology, 2,* 130–131.

American Speech-Language-Hearing Association. (2004a). *Communication facts: Special populations: Stroke—2004 edition.* Retrieved from http://www.asha.org/research/reports/stroke/

American Speech-Language-Hearing Association. (2004b). *Preferred practice patterns for the profession of speech-language pathology* [Preferred practice patterns]. Retrieved from http://www.asha.org/policy

American Speech-Language-Hearing Association. (2008a). *Treatment efficacy summary on aphasia from left hemisphere stroke*. Retrieved from http://www.asha.org/uploadedFiles/public/TreatmentEfficacySummaries2008.pdf#search =%22American%22

American Speech-Language-Hearing Association. (2008b). *Treatment efficacy summary on cognitive-communication disorders resulting from right hemisphere brain damage*. Retrieved from http://www.asha.org/uploadedFiles/public/TreatmentEfficacySummaries2008.pdf#search=%22American%22

Anderson, K., & Crowe-Miller, P. (1982). *Lessons for the right brain series*. Austin, TX: Pro-Ed.

Archibald, L. M. D., Orange, J. B., & Jamieson, D. J. (2009). Implementation of computer-based language therapy in aphasia. *Therapeutic Advances in Neurological Disorders, 2*, 299–311.

Arkin, S. (1991). Memory training in early Alzheimer's disease: An optimistic look at the field. *American Journal of Alzheimer's Care and Related Disorders and Research, 7*, 17–25.

Baillieux, H., De Smet, H. J., Dobbeleir, A., Paquier, P., De Deyn, P., & Mariën, P. (2010). Cognitive and affective disturbances following focal cerebellar damage in adults: A neuropsychological and SPECT study. *Cortex, 46*, 869–879.

Baillieux, H., De Smet, H. J., Lesage, G. Paquier, P., De Deyn, P. P., & Mariën, P. (2006). Neurobehavioral alterations in an adolescent following posterior fossa tumor resection. *Cerebellum, 5*, 289-295.

Baillieux, H., De Smet, H., Paquier, P., De Deyn, P., & Mariën, P. (2008). Cerebellar neurocognition: Insights into the bottom of the brain. *Clinical Neurology and Neurosurgery, 110*, 763–773.

Baines, K. A., Heeringa, H. M., & Martin, A. W. (1999). *Assessment of Language-Related Functional Activities*. Austin, TX: Pro-Ed.

Bakar, M., Kirshner, H. S., & Wertz, R. T. (1996) Crossed aphasia. Functional brain imaging with PET or SPECT. *Archives of Neurology, 53*, 1026–1032.

Banks, J. L., & Marotta, C. A. (2007). Outcomes validity and reliability of the modified Rankin scale: Implications for stroke clinical trials: A literature review and synthesis. *Stroke, 3*, 1091–1096.

Barrett, A. M. (2000). Treatment of unilateral neglect in patients with right hemisphere brain damage. *Perspectives on Neurophysiology and Neurogenic Speech and Language Disorders, 10*, 18–26.

Bartolomeo, P., de Schotten, M. T., & Doricchi, F. (2007). Left unilateral neglect as a disconnection syndrome. *Cerebral Cortex, 17*, 2479–2490.

Beeson, P. M. (1999). Treating acquired writing impairments: Strengthening graphemic representations. *Aphasiology, 13*, 767–785.

Beeson, P. M., Bayles, K. A., Rubens, A. B., & Kaszniak, A. W. (1993). Memory impairment and executive control in individuals with stroke-induced aphasia. *Brain and Language, 45*, 253–275.

Beeson, P. M., Higginson, K., & Rising, K. (2013). Writing treatment for aphasia: A texting approach. *Journal of Speech, Language, and Hearing Research, 56*, 945–955.

Beeson, P. M., Hirsch, F., & Rewega, M. A. (2002). Successful single-word writing treatment: Experimental analysis of four cases. *Aphasiology, 16*, 473–491.

Belay, E. D., & Schoenberger, L. B. (2005). The public health impact of prion diseases. *Annual Reviews of Public Health, 26*, 191–212. doi:10.1146/annurev.publhealth.26.021304.144536

Benjamin, L. A., Bryer, A., Emsley, H. C., Khoo, S., Solomon, T., & Connor, M. D. (2012). HIV infection and stroke: Current perspectives and future directions. *Lancet Neurology, 11*(10), 878–890. doi:10.1016/S1474-4422(12)70205-3

Benson, D. R. (1979). Neurologic correlates of anomia. In H. Whitaker & H. A. Whitaker (Eds.), *Studies in neurolinguistics* (Vol. 4, pp. 293–328). New York, NY: Academic Press.

Benton, A. L., Hamsher, D. S., & Sivan, A. B. (1994). *Multilingual Aphasia Examination–Third edition*. Lutz, FL: Psychological Assessment Resources.

Berndt, R. S., Wayland, S., Rochon, E., Saffran, E., & Schwartz, M. (2000). *Quantitative Production Analysis (QPA)*. New York, NY: Psychology Press.

Blake, M. L. (2009). Inferencing processes after right hemisphere brain damage: Maintenance of inferences. *Journal of Speech, Language, and Hearing Research, 52*, 359–372.

Boone, D. T., & Plante, E. (1993). *Human communication and its disorders* (2nd ed.). Englewood Cliffs, NJ: Prentice-Hall.

Bourgeois, M., Fried-Oken, M., & Rowland, C. (2010, March 16). *AAC strategies and tools for persons with dementia.* Retrieved from http://www.asha.org/Publications/leader/2010/100316/AACStrategies.htm

Bracy, O. L. (1994). *PSSCogRehab* [Computer Software]. Indianapolis, IN: Psychological Software Services.

Brady, M. C., Kelly, H., Godwin, J., & Enderby, P. (2012). Speech and language therapy for aphasia following stroke. *Cochrane Database of Systematic Reviews, 5:* CD000425. doi:10.1002/14651858.CD000425.pub3

Bryan, K. (1989). *Right hemisphere language battery.* London, UK: Whurr.

Brookshire, R. H. (1992). *An introduction to communication disorders* (4th ed.). St. Louis, MO: Mosby-Year Book.

Brookshire, R. H., & Nicholas, L. E. (1997). *Discourse Comprehension Test* (2nd ed.). Albuquerque, NM: PICA Programs.

Brott, T., Adams, H. P., Olinger, C. P., Marler, J. R., Barsan, W. G., Biller, J., . . . Walker, M. (1989). Measurements of acute cerebral infarction: A clinical examination scale. *Stroke, 20,* 864–870.

Brownell, H. H., Michel, D., Powelson, J., & Gardner, H. (1993). Surprise but not coherence: Sensitivity to verbal humor in right-hemisphere patients. *Brain and Language, 18,* 20–27.

Brush, J. A., & Calkins, M. P. (2008, June 17). Environmental interventions and dementia: Enhancing mealtimes in group dining rooms. *The ASHA Leader,* pp. 24–25.

Brush, J. A., & Camp, C. J. (1998). Using spaced retrieval as an intervention during speech-language therapy. *Clinical Gerontologist, 19,* 51–64.

Burke, H. L., Yeo, R. A., Delaney, H. D., & Conner, L. (1993). CT scan cerebral hemispheric asymmetries: Predictors of recovery from aphasia. *Journal of Clinical and Experimental Neuropsychology, 15,* 191–204.

Burns, M. S. (1997). *Burns Brief Inventory of Communication and Cognition (Burns Inventory).* San Antonio, TX: Pearson.

Butzkueven, H., Evans, A. H., Pitman, A., Leopold, C., Jolley, D. J., Kaye, A. H., . . . Davis, S. M. (2000). Onset seizures independently predict poor outcome after subarachnoid hemorrhage. *Neurology, 56,* 1423–1424.

Byng, S., & Duchan, J. (2005). Social model philosophies and principles: Their applications to therapies for aphasia. *Aphasiology, 19*(10/11), 906–922.

Byng, S., Nickels, L., & Black, M. (1994). Replicating therapy for mapping deficits in agrammatism: Remapping the deficit? *Aphasiology, 8,* 315–341.

Cappa, S. F., Perani, D., Bressi, S., Paulesu, E., Franceschi, M., & Fazio, F. (1993). Crossed aphasia: A PET follow-up study of two cases. *Journal of Neurology, Neurosurgery and Psychiatry, 56,* 665–671.

Cappa, S. F., Perani D., Grassi, F., Bressi S., Alberoni, M., Franceschi M., . . . Fazio, F. (1997). A PET follow-up study of recovery after stroke in acute aphasics. *Brain and Language, 56,* 55–67.

Centers for Disease Control and Prevention. (2012). *About prion disease.* Retrieved from http://www.cdc.gov/ncidod/dvrd/prions/

Cherney, L. R., & Canter, G. J. (1993). Informational content in the discourse of patients with probable Alzheimer's disease and patients with right brain damage. *Clinical Aphasiology, 21,* 123–134.

Cherney, L. R., Patterson, J. P., & Raymer, A. S. (2011). Intensity of aphasia therapy: Evidence and efficacy. *Current Neurology and Neuroscience Reports, 11,* 560–569.

Clark, L W., (1991). Caregiver stress and communication management in Alzheimer's disease. In D. N. Ripich (Ed.), *Handbook of geriatric communication disorders* (pp. 127–141). Austin, TX: Pro-Ed.

Colsher, P. L., Cooper, W. E., & Graff-Radford, N. (1987). Intonational variability in the speech of right-hemisphere damaged patients. *Brain and Language, 32,* 379–383.

Conner, L. T., Brady, T. S., Snyder, A. Z., Lewis, C., Blasi, V., & Corbetta, M. (2006). Cerebellar activity switches hemispheres with cerebral recovery in aphasia. *Neuropsychologia, 44,* 171–177.

Cornelissen, K., Laine, M., Tarkiainen, A., Jarvensivu, T., Martin, N., & Salmelin, R. (2003). Adult brain plasticity elicited by anomia treatment. *Journal of Cognitive Neuroscience, 15,* 444–461.

Coslett, B., Bowers, D., & Heilman, K. (1987) Reduction in cerebral activation after right hemisphere stroke. *Neurology, 37,* 957–962.

Côté, R., Hachinski, V. C., Shurvell, B. L., Norris, J. W., & Wolfson, C. (1986). The Canadian Neurological Scale: A preliminary study in acute stroke. *Stroke, 17*, 731–737.

Coulson, S., & Williams, R. F. (2005). Hemispheric differences and joke comprehension. *Neuropsychologia, 43*, 128–141.

Crosson, B., Moore, A., McGregor, K. M., Chang, Y. L., Benjamin, M., Gopinath, K., . . . White, K. D. (2009). Regional changes in word-production laterality after a naming treatment designed to produce a rightward shift in frontal activity. *Brain and Language, 111*, 73–85.

Cummings, J. L., & Mega, M. S. (2003). *Neuropsychiatry and behavioral neuroscience*. New York, NY: Oxford University Press.

Damasio, A. R., Damasio, H., Rizzo, M., Varney, N., & Gersh, F. (1982). Aphasia with nonhaemorrhagic lesions in the basal ganglia and internal capsule. *Archives of Neurology, 39*, 15–20.

Damasio, A., & Geschwind, N. (1984). The neural basis of language. *Annual Review of Neuroscience, 7*, 127–147.

Damasio, H., & Damasio, A. (1980). The anatomical bases of conduction aphasia. *Brain, 103*, 337–353.

Davie, G. L., Hutcheson, K. A, Barringer, D. A., Weinberg, J. S., & Lewin, J. S. (2009). Aphasia in patients after brain tumour resection. *Aphasiology, 23*, 1196–1206.

Davis, G. A. (2000). *Aphasiology: Disorders and clinical practice*. Needham Heights, MA: Allyn & Bacon.

Davis, G. A., & Wilcox, M. J. (1985). *Adult aphasia rehabilitation: Applied pragmatics*. San Diego, CA: College-Hill Press.

DeRenzi, E., & Ferrari, C. (1978). The reporter's test: A sensitive test to detect expressive disturbances in aphasics. *Cortex, 14*, 278–293.

De Reuck, J., De Clerck, M., & Van Maele, G. (2006). Vascular cognitive impairment in patients with late-onset seizures after an ischemic stroke. *Clinical Neurology and Neurosurgery, 108*, 632–637.

D'Esposito, M., & Alexander, M. P. (1995). Subcortical aphasia: Distinct profiles following left putaminal hemorrhage. *Neurology, 45*, 38–41.

Diggs, C., & Basili, A. (1987). Verbal expression of right cerebrovascular accident patients: Convergent and divergent language. *Brain and Language, 30*, 130–146.

Doyle, P., McNeil, M., Hula, W., & Mikolic, J. (2003). The Burden of Stroke Scale (BOSS): Validating patient-reported communication difficulty and associated psychological distress in stroke survivors. *Aphasiology, 14*, 291–304.

Draper, B., Bowring, G., Thompson, C., Van Heyst, J., Conray, P., & Thompson, J. (2007). Stress in caregivers of aphasic stroke patients: A randomized controlled trial. *Clinical Rehabilitation, 21*, 122–130.

Druks, J., & Marshall, J. C. (1995). When passives are easier than actives: Two case studies of aphasic comprehension. *Cognition, 55*, 311–331.

Druks, J., & Masterson, J. (2000). *Object and Action Naming Battery*. New York, NY: Psychology Press.

Duffy, R. J., & Duffy, J. R. (1984). *Assessment of nonverbal communication*. Tigard, OR: C. C. Publications.

Eisenson, J. (1962). Language and intellectual modifications associated with right cerebral damage. *Language and Speech, 5*, 49–53.

El, S., Annegers, J. F., Hauser, W. A., O'Brien, P. C., & Whisnant, J. P. (1996). Population-based study of seizure disorders after cerebral infarction. *Neurology, 46*, 350–355.

Engelter, S. T., Gostynski, M., Papa, S., Frei, M., Born, C., Ajadacic-Gross, V., . . . Lyrer, P. A. (2006). Epidemiology of aphasia attributable to first ischemic stroke. *Stroke, 37*, 1379–1394. doi:10.1161/01.STR.0000221815.64093.8c

Epstein, N. B., Baldwin, L. M., & Bishop, D. S. (1983). The McMaster family assessment device. *Journal of Marital and Family Therapy, 9*, 171–180.

Fabbro, F., Moretti, R., & Bava, A. (2000). Language impairments in patients with cerebellar lesions. *Journal of Neurolinguistics, 13*, 173–188.

Family Caregiver Alliance. (n.d.) *The stresses of caregiving*. Retrieved from http://www.caregiver.org/caregiver/jsp/content_node.jsp?nodeid=891

Faust, M., Barak, O., & Chiarello, C. (2006). The effects of multiple script priming on word recognition by the two cerebral hemispheres: Implications for discourse processing. *Brain and Language, 99*, 247–257.

Faust, M., & Lavidor, M. (2003). Semantically convergent and semantically divergent priming in the cerebral hemispheres: Lexical decision and semantic judgment. *Cognitive Brain Research, 17*, 585–597.

Ferré, P., Ska, B., Lajoie, C., Bleau, A., & Joanette, Y. (2011). Clinical focus on prosodic, discursive and pragmatic treatment for right hemisphere damaged adults: What's right? *Rehabilitation Research and Practice, 2011*, 1–10.

Fiez, J. A., Petersen, S. E., Cheney, M. K., & Raichle, M. E. (1992). Impaired nonmotor learning and error detection associated with cerebellar damage: A single-case study. *Brain, 115*, 155–178.

Fillingham, J. K., Sage, K., & Lambon Ralph, M. (2005).The treatment of anomia using errorless learning. *Neuropsychological Rehabilitation, 16*, 129–154.

Flasher, L. V., & Fogle, P. T. (2012). *Counseling skills for speech-language pathologists and audiologists.* Clifton Park, NY: Delmar Cengage Learning.

Fox, L. (2013). *SIGnatures: Family friendly.* Retrieved from http://www.asha.org/Publications/leader/2013/13091/SIGnatures-Family-Friendly.htm

Fraas, M. R., & Calvert, M. (2009). The use of narratives to identify characteristics leading to a productive life following acquired brain injury. *American Journal of Speech-Language Pathology, 18*, 315–328. doi:10.1044/1058–0360(2009/08–0008)

Frattali, C. M., Holland, A. L., Thompson, C. K., Wohl, C., & Ferketic, M. (1995). *Functional Assessment of Communication Skills in Adults* (ASHA–FACS). Rockville, MD: American Speech-Language-Hearing Association.

Freed, D. B., Marshall, R. C., & Nippold, M. A. (1995). Comparison of personalized cueing and provided cueing on the facilitation of verbal labeling by aphasic subjects. *Journal of Speech and Hearing Research, 38*, 1081–1090.

Fridriksson, J., Baker, J. M., & Richardson, J. D. (2010, July 06). What can neuroimaging tell us about aphasia? *The ASHA Leader.*

Garrett, K. C., & Lasker, J. P. (2005). AAC for adults with aphasia. In D. Beukelman & P. Mirenda (Eds.), *Augmentative and alternative communication: Supporting children and adults with complex communication needs.* Baltimore, MD: Paul H. Brookes.

Gasparini, M., Di Piero, V., Ciccarelli, O., Cacioppo, M. M., Panatano, P., & Kebzum, G. L. (1999). Linguistic impairment after right cerebellar stroke: A case report. *European Journal of Neurology, 6*, 353–356.

Gebreyohanns, M., & Adams, R. J. (2004). Sickle cell disease: Primary stroke prevention. *CNS Spectrum, 9*, 445–449.

Gentry, T., Wallace, J., Kvarfordt, C., & Lynch, K. (2008). Personal digital assistants as cognitive aids for individuals with severe traumatic brain injury: A community-based trial. *Brain Injury, 22*, 19–24.

Geschwind, N. (1967). The varieties of naming errors. *Cortex, 3*, 97–112.

Goldenberg, G., & Spatt, J. (1994). Influence of size and site of cerebral lesions on spontaneous recovery of aphasia and on success of language therapy. *Brain and Language, 47*, 684–698.

Goldman, R., Fristoe, M., & Woodcock, R. W. (1970). *Goldman-Fristoe-Woodcock Test of Auditory Discrimination* (G-F-W TAD). San Antonio, TX: Pearson.

Goodglass, H., & Geschwind, N. (1976) Language disorders (aphasia). In E. C. Carterette & M. Friedman (Eds.), *Handbook of perception* (Vol. 7, pp. 389–428). New York, NY: Academic Press.

Goodglass, H., & Kaplan, E. (1983). *Assessment of aphasia and related disorders* (2nd ed.). Philadelphia, PA: Lea and Febiger.

Goodglass, H., Kaplan, E., & Barresi, B. (2000). *Boston Diagnostic Aphasia Examination–3 (BDAE-3).* Austin, TX: Pro-Ed.

Gresham, G. E., Duncan, P. W., Stason, W. B., Adams, H. P., Adelman, A. M., Alexander, D. N., . . . Trombly, C. A. (1995). *Post-stroke rehabilitation. Clinical practice guidelines, No. 16,* Public Health Service, Agency for Health Care Policy and research. (AHCPR Publication No. 95-62). Rockville, MD: U.S. Department of Health and Human Services.

Groher, M. (1977). Language and memory disorders following closed head trauma. *Journal of Speech and Hearing Research, 20*, 212–223.

Grohn, B., Worrall, L. E., Simmons-Mackie, N., & Brown, K. (2012). The first 3-months post-stroke:What facilitates successfully living with aphasia? *International Journal of Speech-Language Pathology, 4*, 390–400.

Haartman, H. J., & Kolk, H. H. (1994). On-line sensitivity to subject-verb agreement violations in Broca's aphasics: The role of syntactic complexity and time. *Brain and Language, 46*, 493–516.

Hall, E. T. (1963). A system for the notation of proxemic behavior. *American Anthropologist, 65*, 1003–1026.

Halper, A. S., Cherney, L. R., & Burns, M. S. (2010). *Rehabilitation Institute of Chicago evaluation of communication problems in right hemisphere dysfunction.* Chicago, IL: Author.

Hebb, A. O., & Ojemann, G. A. (2013). The thalamus and language revisited. *Brain and Language, 126,* 99–108. doi:10.1016/j.bandl.2012.06.010.

Helm, N., & Barresi, B. (1980). Voluntary control of involuntary utterances: A treatment approach for severe aphasia. In R. Brookshire (Ed.), *Clinical Aphasiology Conference Proceedings.* Minneapolis, MN: BRK.

Helm-Estabrooks, N. (1984). Severe aphasia. In A. L. Holland (Ed.), *Language disorders in adults* (pp. 159–176). San Diego, CA: College-Hill Press.

Helm-Estabrooks, N. (1992). Overview of treatment of aphasia. In J. Cooper (Ed.), *Aphasia treatment: Current approaches and research opportunities* (pp. 1–6). U.S. Department of Health and Human Services, Public Health Services, National Institutes of Health, NIH Publication No. 93-3424.

Helm-Estabrooks, N. (2002). Cognition and aphasia: A discussion and a study. *Journal of Communication Disorders, 35,* 171–186.

Helm-Estabrooks, N., & Albert, M. L. (2004). Melodic intonation therapy. In *Manual of aphasia and aphasia therapy* (2nd ed., pp. 221–233). Austin, TX: Pro-Ed.

Helm-Estabrooks, N., & Barresi, B. (1980). Voluntary control of involuntary utterances: A treatment approach for severe aphasia. In R. Brookshire (Ed.), *Clinical aphasiology conference proceedings.* Minneapolis, MN: BRK.

Helm-Estabrooks, N., Fitzpatrick, P. M., & Barresi, B. (1982). Visual action therapy for global aphasia. *Journal of Speech and Hearing Disorders, 47,* 385–389.

Helm-Estabrooks, N., Ramsberger, G., Morgan A. R., & Nicholas, M. (1989). *Boston Assessment of Severe Aphasia.* Austin, TX: Pro-Ed.

Henics, T. ,& Wheatley, D. N. (1999). Cytoplasmic vacuolation, adaptation and cell death: A view on new perspectives and features. *Biology of the Cell, 91,* 485–498.

Herrman, M., Bartels, C., & Wallesch, C. W. (1993). Depression in acute and chronic aphasic: Symptoms, pathoanatomical-clinical correlations and functional implications. *Journal of Neurology, Neurosurgery, and Psychiatry, 56,* 672–778.

Hier, D. B., Yoon, W. B., Mohr, J. P., Price, T. R., & Wolf, P. A. (1994). Gender and aphasia in the stroke data bank. *Brain and Language, 47,* 155–167.

Highnam, C. L., & Bleile, K. M. (2011). Language in the cerebellum. *American Journal of Speech-Language Pathology, 20,* 337–347. doi:10.1044/1058–0360(2011/10–0096)

Hinckley, J. (2009). Clinical decision-making for stroke and aphasia in the older adult. *Perspectives on Gerontology, 14,* 4–11. doi:10.1044/gero 14.1.4

Ho, K., Weiss, S., Garrett, K., & Lloyd, L. *(2005).* The effect of remnant and pictographic books on the communicative interaction of individuals with global aphasia. *Augmentative and Alternative Communication, 21,* 218–232.

Hoerster, L., Hickey, E. M., & Bourgeois, M. S. (2001). Effects of memory aids on conversations between nursing home residents with dementia and nursing assistants. *Neuropsychological Rehabilitation, 11,* 399–427.

Holbrook, M., & Skilbeck, C. E. (1983). An activities index for use with stroke patients. *Age and Ageing, 12,* 166–170.

Holland, A. L., Fratteli, C., & Fromm, D. (1999). *Communication Abilities of Daily Living* (2nd ed.). Austin, TX: Pro-Ed.

Holland, A. L., Fromm, D. S., DeRuyter, F., & Stein, M. (1996). Treatment efficacy: Aphasia. *Journal of Speech and Hearing Research, 39,* S27–S36.

Horner, J. (1984). Moderate aphasia. In A. L. Holland (Ed.), *Language disorders in adults* (pp. 133–158). San Diego, CA: College-Hill Press.

Hopper, T., Holland, A., & Rewega, M. *(2002).* Conversational coaching: Treatment outcomes and future directions. *Aphasiology, 16,* 745–761.

Horner, S., Ni, X. S., Buft, M., & Lechner, H. (1995). EEG, CT and neurosonographic findings in patients with postischemic seizures. *Neurological Science, 132,* 57–60.

Jehkonen, M., Laihosalo, M., & Kettunen, J. (2006). Anosognosia after stroke: Assessment, occurrence, subtypes and impact on functional outcome reviewed. *Acta Neurologica Scandinavia, 114,* 293–306.

Joanette, Y., Goulet, P., & Hannequin, D. (1990). *Right hemisphere and verbal communication.* New York, NY: Springer-Verlag.

Johnson, R. K., Hough, M. S., King, K. A., Vos, P., & Jeffs, T. (2008). Functional communication in individuals with chronic severe aphasia using augmentative communication. *Augmentative and Alternative Communication, 24,* 269–280. doi:10.1080/07434610802463957

Jung-Beeman, M. (2005). Bilateral brain processes for comprehending natural language. *Trends in Cognitive Sciences, 9,* 512–518.

Kagan, A., Black, S. E., Duchan, J. F., Simmons-Mackie, N., & Square, P. (2001). Training volunteers as conversation partners using "Supported conversation for adults with aphasia" (SCA): A controlled trial. *Journal of Speech, Language, and Hearing Research, 44,* 624–638.

Kagan, A., Winckel, J., Black, S., Duchan, J. F., Simmons-Mackie, N., & Square, P. (2004). A set of observational measures for rating support and participation in conversation between adults with aphasia and their conversation partners. *Topics in Stroke Rehabilitation, 11,* 67–83.

Kang, E. K., Sohn, H. M., Han, M. K., Kim, W., Han, T. R., & Paik, N. J. (2010). Severity of post-stroke aphasia according to aphasia type and lesion location in Koreans. *Journal of Korean Medical Science, 25,* 123–127.

Katz, R .C., & Wertz, R. T. (1997) The efficacy of computer-provided reading treatment for chronic aphasic adults. *Journal of Speech-Language-Hearing Research, 40,* 493–507.

Kauhanen, M. L., Korpelainen, J. T., Hiltunen, P., Määtta, R., Mononen, H., Brusin, E., . . . Myllvlä, V. V. (2000). Aphasia, depression, and non–verbal cognitive impairment in ischaemic stroke. *Cerebrovascular Diseases (Basel, Switzerland), 6,* 455–461.

Kavanagh, D. O., Lynam, C., Düerk, T., Casey, M., & Eustace, P. W. (2010).Variations in the presentation of aphasia in patients with closed head injuries. *Case Reports in Medicine.* doi:10.1155/2010/678060

Kearns, K. P. (1985). Response elaboration training of patient initiated utterances. In R. H. Brookshire (Ed.), *Clinical aphasiology* (Vol. 15, pp. 196–204). Minneapolis, MN: BRK.

Kearns, K. P. (1986). Systematic programming of verbal elaboration skills in chronic Broca's aphasia. In R. C. Marshall (Ed.), *Case studies in aphasia rehabilitation* (pp. 225–244). Austin, TX: Pro-Ed.

Kearns, K. P., & Scher, G. P. (1989). The generalization of response elaboration training effects. *Clinical Aphasiology, 18,* 223–245. Minneapolis, MN: BRK.

Kearns, K. P., & Yedor, K. (1991). An alternating treatments comparison of loose training and a convergent treatment strategy. *Clinical Aphasiology, 20,* 223–238. Minneapolis, MN: BRK.

Keenan, J. S., & Brassell, E. G. (1975). *Aphasia-Language Performance Scales* (ALPS). St. Louis, MO: Pinnacle Press.

Keller, I., Schlenker, A., & Pigache, R. M. (1995). Selective impairment of auditory attention following closed head injuries or right cerebrovascular accidents. *Cognitive Brain Research, 3,* 9–15.

Kennedy, M., & Murdoch, B. E. (1993). Chronic aphasia subsequent to striatocapsular and thalamic lesions in the left hemisphere. *Brain and Language, 44,* 284–295.

Kertesz, A. (1982). *Western Aphasia Battery.* New York, NY: Grune & Stratton.

Kertesz, A. (2006). *Western Aphasia Battery–Revised* (WAB-R). San Antonio, TX: Pearson.

Kertesz, A., Lau, W. K., & Polk, M. (1993). The structural determinants of recovery in Wernicke's aphasia. *Brain and Language, 44,* 153–164.

Kintsch, W. (1998). *Comprehension: A paradigm for cognition (xvi).* New York, NY: Cambridge University Press.

Kirshner, H. S., Tanridag, O., Thurman, L., & Whetsell, W. O. (1987). Progressive aphasia without dementia: Two cases with focal spongiform degeneration. *Annals of Neurology, 22,* 527–532. doi:10.1002/ana.4102204 13

Kleinman, L. I. (2003). *Functional Communication Profile, Revised* (FCPR). East Moline, IL: Linguisystems.

Klonoff, P. S., Sheperd, J. C., O'Brien, K. P., Chiapello, D. A., & Hodak, J. A. (1990). Rehabilitation and outcome of right-hemisphere stroke patients: Challenges to traditional diagnostic and treatment methods. *Neuropsychology, 4,* 147–163.

Kolb, B., & Whishaw, I. Q. (1990). *Fundamentals of neuropsychology.* New York, NY: W. H. Freeman.

Koul, R. K., Corwin, M., & Hayes, S. (2005). Production of graphic symbol sentences by individuals with aphasia: Efficacy of a computer-based augmentative and alternative communication intervention. *Brain and Language, 92,* 58–77.

Ladavas, E., Umilta, C., & Ricci-Bitti, P. (1980). Evidence of sex difference in right hemisphere dominance for emotion. *Neuropsychologia, 18,* 361–366.

LaPointe, L. L., & Eisenson, E. (2008). *Examining for Aphasia: Assessment of aphasic and related impairments-fourth edition* (EFA–4). Austin, TX: Pro-Ed.

Laska, A. C., Hellblom, A., Murray, V., Kahan, T., & Von Arbin, M. (2001). Aphasia in acute stroke and relation to outcome. *Journal of Internal Medicine, 249,* 413–422.

Legar, A., Demonet, J.-F., Ruff, S., Aithamon, B., Touyeras, B., Puel, M., . . . Cardebat, D. (2002). Neural substrates of spoken language rehabilitation in an aphasic patient: An fMRI study. *NeuroImage, 17,* 174–183.

Lehman, M. T., & Tompkins, C. (2000). Inferencing in adults with right hemisphere brain damage: An analysis of conflicting results. *Aphasiology, 14,* 485–499.

Leon, S. A., & Rodriguez, A. D. (2008). Aprosodia and Its Treatment. *Perspectives on Neurophysiology and Neurogenic Speech and Language Disorders, 18,* 66–72.

Linebaugh, C. W. (1984). Mild aphasia. In A. L. Holland (Ed.), *Language disorders in adults* (pp. 113–132). San Diego. CA: College-Hill Press.

Lingraphica. (n.d.). *Who gets aphasia?* Retrieved from http://www.aphasia.com/about-apha sia/who-gets-aphasia

Lloyd-Jones, D., Adams, R., Carnethon, M., De Simone, G., Ferguson, B., Flegal, K., . . . Hong, Y. (2009). Heart disease and stroke statistics—2009 update. A report from the American Heart Association Statistics Committee and Stroke Statistics Subcommittee. *Circulation, 119,* e21–e181.

Lubinski, R. (1988). A model for intervention: Communication skills, effectiveness, and opportunity. In B. B. Shadden (Ed.), *Communication behavior and aging: A sourcebook for clinicians* (pp. 294–308). Baltimore, MD: Williams & Wilkins.

Lubinski, R., Morrison, E., & Rigrodsky, S. (1981). Perception of spoken communication by elderly chronically ill patients in an institutional setting. *Journal of Speech and Hearing Disorders, 46,* 405–412.

Mahoney, F. L., & Barthel, D. (1965). Functional evaluation: The Barthel index. *Maryland State Medical Journal, 14,* 56–61.

Marien, P., Baillieux, H., De Smet, H. J., Engelborghs, S., Wilssens, I., & Paquier, P. (2009). Cognitive, linguistic and affective disturbances following a right superior cerebellar artery infarction: A case study. *Cortex, 45,* 527–536.

Marien, P., Saerens, J., Nanhoe, R., Moens, E., Nagels, G., Pickut, B. A., & De Deyn, P. P. (1996). Cerebellar induced aphasia: Case report of cerebellar induced prefrontal aphasic language phenomena supported by SPECT findings. *Journal of Neurological Sciences, 144,* 34–44.

Marsh, E. B., Hillis, A. E. (2008) Dissociation between egocentric and allocentric visuospatial and tactile neglect in acute stroke. *Cortex, 44,* 1215–1220.

Marshall, R. C. (2001). Management of Wernicke's aphasia: A context-based approach. In R. Chapey (Ed.), *Language intervention strategies in aphasia and related neurogenic communication disorders* (4th ed., pp.435-456). Baltimore: Lippincott Williams & Williams.

Mateer, C. A. (1989). Neural correlates of language function. In D. P. Kuehn, M. L. Lemme, & J. M. Baumgartner (Eds.), *Neural bases of speech, hearing and language* (pp. 259–291). Boston, MA: College-Hill Press.

Mayer, J. F. (2008). Brain tumors frequently encountered by speech-language pathologists: A review and tutorial. *Perspectives on Neurophysiology and Neurogenic Speech and Language Disorders, 18,* 4129–4136. doi:10.1044/nnsld18.4

McNeill, M. E., & Prescott, R. W. (1978). *Revised Token Test.* Austin, TX: Pro-Ed.

Mega, M. S., & Alexander, M. P. (1994). Subcortical aphasia: The core profile of capsulostriatal infarction. *Neurology, 44,* 1824–1829.

Meyer, B. C., Hemmen, T. M., Jackson, C. M., & Lynden, P. D. (2002). Modified National Institutes of Health Stroke Scale for use in stroke clinical trials. *Stroke, 33,* 1261–1266.

Milman, L. H., & Holland, A. L. (2012). *SCCAN Scales of Cognitive and Communicative Ability for Neurorehabilitation.* East Moline, IL: Linguisystems.

Morgenstein, S., & Smith, M. (1993). Aphasia and right-hemisphere disorders. In W. A. Gordon (Ed.), *Advances in stroke rehabilitation.* Boston, MA: Andover Medical.

Morris, P. L., Robinson, R. G., & Raphael, B.(1993). Emotional lability after stroke. *Australian and New Zealand Journal of Psychiatry, 27,* 601–605.

Murdoch, B. E. (1990). *Acquired speech and language disorders: A neuroanatomical and functional neurological approach.* Baltimore, MD: Paul H. Brookes.

Murray, L. L. (2012). Attention and other cognitive deficits in aphasia: Presence and relation to language and communication measures. *American Journal of Speech-Language Pathology, 21,* 551–564.

Myers, P. S. (1983). Treatment of right hemisphere communication disorders. In W. H. Perkins (Ed.), *Current therapy in communication disorders* (Vol. 3, pp. 57–67). New York, NY: Thieme-Stratton.

Myers, P. S. (1991). Inference failure: The underlying impairment in right-hemisphere communication disorders. *Clinical Aphasiology, 20,* 167–180.

Myers, P. S. (1996, March). *Neglect, attention, and right hemisphere communication disorders.* Paper presented at the Maryland Speech-Language-Hearing Association Annual Convention, Bowie.

Myers, P. S., & Brookshire, R. H. (1994). The effects of visual and inferential complexity on the picture descriptions of non-brain-damaged and right-hemisphere-damaged adults. *Clinical Aphasiology, 22,* 25–34.

Naesar, M. A., & Palumbo, C. L. (1994). Neuroimaging and language recovery in stroke. *Journal of Clinical Neurophysiology, 11,* 150–174.

Narushima, K., Chan, K. L., Kosler, J. T., & Robinson, R. G. (2003). Does cognitive recovery after treatment of poststroke depression last? A 2-year follow-up of cognitive function associated with poststroke depression. *American Journal of Psychiatry, 160,* 1157–1162.

National Aphasia Association. (2011). http://www.aphasia.org

National Institute of Deafness and Other Communication Disorders. (n.d.). *Aphasia.* Retrieved from http://www.nidcd.nih.gov/health/voice/pages/aphasia.aspx

National Stroke Association. (2008). http://www.stroke.org

National Stroke Association. (2012). *Aphasia.* http://www.stroke.org

Nicholas, L. E., & Brookshire, R. H. (1993). A system for scoring main concepts in the connected speech of non-brain-damaged and aphasic speakers. *Clinical Aphasiology, 21,* 87–99.

Nishio, S., Takemura, N., Ikai, Y., & T. Baba, T (2004). Sensory aphasia after closed head injury. *Journal of Clinical Neuroscience, 11,* 442–444.

Oczna, K. (2012). Homonymous hemianopsia. *Klinika Oczna, 114,* 226–229.

O'Halloran, R., Worrall, L., Toffolo, D., Code, C., & Hickson, L. (2004). *Inpatient Functional Communication Interview (IFCI).* Oxon, UK: Speechmark.

Ojemann, G. A. (1979). Subcortical language mechanisms. In H. Whitaker & H. A. Whitaker (Eds.), *Studies in neurolinguistics* (Vol. 1, pp. 103–138). New York, NY: Academic Press.

Okuda, B., Tanaka, H., Tachibana, H., Kawabata, K., & Sugita, M. (1994). Cerebral blood flow in subcortical global aphasia: Perisylvanian cortical hypoperfusion as a crucial role. *Stroke, 25,* 1495–1499.

Ortiz, G., Koch, S., Romano, J. G., Forteza, A. M., & Rabinstein, A. A. (2007). Mechanisms of ischemic stroke in HIV-infected patients. *Neurology, 68,* 1257–1261. doi:10.1212/01.wnl.0000259515.45579.1e

Ozeren, A., Sarica, Y., & Efe, R. (1994). Thalamic aphasic syndrome. *Acta Neurologica Belgium, 94,* 205–208.

Papathanasiou, I., & Cséfalvay, Z. (2013). Written language and its impairments. In I. Papathanasiou, P. Coppen, & C. Potagas (Eds.), *Aphasia and related neurogenic communication disorders* (pp. 173–196). Burlington, MA: Jones & Bartlett Learning.

Paratz, E. D. (2011). The significance of aphasia in neurological cancers. *Australian Medical Student Journal, 2,* 15–18.

Pataraia, E., Billingsley-Marshall, R. L., Castillo, E. M., Billingsley-Marshall, R. L., McGregor, A. L., Breier, J. I., . . . Papanicolaou, A. C. (2005). Organization of receptive language-specific cortex before and after left temporal lobectomy. *Neurology, 64,* 481–487.

Patel, M., Coshall, C., Rudd, A. G., & Wolfe, C. D. (2003). Natural history of cognitive impairment after stroke and factors associated with its recovery. *Clinical Rehabilitation, 17,* 158–166.

Paulus, K. S., Magnano, I., Conti, M., Galistu, P., D'Onofrio, M., & Satta, W. (2004). Pure post stroke cerebellar affective syndrome: A case report. *Neurological Sciences, 25,* 220–224.

Pedersen, P. M., Jorgensen, H. S., Nakayama, H., Raaschou, H. O., & Olsen, T. S. (1994). Aphasia in acute stroke: Incidence, determinants, and recovery. *Annals of Neurology, 38,* 659–666.

Pimenthal, P. A. (1985). *A guide to right brain injury: Communication suggestions for persons with right hemisphere injury and the right hemisphere deficit checklist.* Chicago, IL: Neurotest Associates.

Pimenthal, P. A. (1986). Alterations in communication: Biopsychosocial aspects of aphasia, dysarthria, and right hemisphere syndromes in the stroke patient. *Nursing Clinics of North America, 21,* 321–337.

Pimenthal, P. A., & Kingsbury, N. A. (1989a). *Neuropsychological aspects of right brain injury.* Austin, TX: Pro-Ed.

Pimenthal, P. A., & Kingsbury, N. A. (1989b). *Mini Inventory of Right Brain Injury.* Austin, TX: Pro-Ed.

Pimenthal, P. A., & Knight, J. (2000). *Mini Inventory of Right Brain Injury–2.* Austin, TX: Pro-Ed.

Porch, B. E. (2001). *Porch Index of Communicative Ability–Revised* (PICA-R). Albuquerque, NM: PICA Programs.

Potagas, C., Kasselimis, D. S., & Evdokimidis, J. (2013). Elements of neurology essential for understanding the aphasia. In I. Papathanasiou, P. Coppens, & C. Potagas (Eds.), *Aphasia and related neurogenic communication disorders* (pp. 23–48). Burlington, MA: Jones & Bartlett Learning.

Price, C. J., & Crinion, J. (2005). The latest on functional imaging studies of aphasic stroke. *Current Opinion in Neurology, 18,* 429–434.

Prutting, C. A., & Kirchner, D. M. (1987). A clinical appraisal of the pragmatic aspects of language. *Journal of Speech and Hearing Disorders, 52,* 105–119.

Pulvermüller, F., Hauk, O., Zohsel, K., Neininger, B., & Mohr, B. (2005). Therapy-related reorganization of language in both hemispheres of patients with chronic aphasia. *Neuroimage, 28,* 481–491.

Pulvermüller, F., & Schonle, P. W. (1993). Behavioral and neuronal changes during treatment of mixed transcortical aphasia: A case study. *Cognition, 48,* 139–161.

Records, N. J. (1994). A measure of the contribution of a gesture to the perception of speech in listeners with aphasia. *Journal of Speech and Hearing Research, 37,* 1086–1099.

Rey, G. J., Sivan, A. B., & Benton, A. L. (1994). *Multilingual Aphasia Examination, Spanish version.* Lutz, FL: Psychological Assessment Resources.

Roach, A., Schwartz, M.F., Martin, N., Grewal, R. S., & Brecher, A. (1996). The Philadelphia Naming Test: Scoring and rationale. *Clinical Aphasiology, 24,* 121–133.

Robin, D. A., & Schienberg, S. (1990). Subcortical lesions and aphasia. *Journal of Speech and Hearing Disorders, 55,* 90–100.

Rosen, H. J., Petersen, S. E., Linenweber, M. R., Snyder, A. Z., White, D. A., Chapman, L., . . . Corbetta, M. (2000). Neural correlates of recovery from aphasia after damage to left inferior frontal cortex. *Neurology, 55,* 1883–1894.

Ross, E. (1981). The aprosodias: Functional-anatomical organization of the affective components of language in the right hemisphere. *Archives of Neurology, 38,* 561–569.

Ross, E. D. (1997). Right hemisphere syndromes and the neurology of emotions. In S. C. Schacter & O. Devinsky, O. (Eds.), *Behavioral neurology and the legacy of Norman Geschwind* (pp. 183–191). Philadelphia, PA: Lippincott-Raven.

Ross, E., Thompson, R., & Yenkosky, J. (1997). Lateralization of affective prosody in brain and the collosal integration of hemispheric language functions. *Brain and Language, 56,* 27–54.

Ross, A., Winslow, I., Marchant, P., & Brumfitt, S. (2006). Evaluation of communication, life participation and psychological well-being in chronic aphasia: The influence of group intervention. *Aphasiology, 20,* 427–448.

Ross-Swain, D. (1996). *Ross Information Processing Test, Second edition* (RIPA-2). Austin, TX: Pro–Ed.

Rubens, A. B. (1979). Transcortical motor aphasia. In H. Whitaker & H. A. Whitaker (Eds.), *Studies in Neurolinguistics* (Vol. 1, pp. 293–303). New York, NY: Academic Press.

Schmahmann, J. D. (2003). Vascular syndromes of the thalamus. *Stroke, 34,* 2264–2278.

Schmahmann, J. D., & Sherman, J. C. (1998). The cerebellar cognitive affective syndrome. *Brain, 121,* 567–579.

Schmahmann, J. D., Weilburg, J., & Sherman, J. (2007). The neuropsychiatry of the cerebellum—insights from the clinic. *Cerebellum, 6,* 254–267.

Schuell, H. (1969). *The Minnesota Test for Differential Diagnosis of Aphasia.* Minneapolis: University of Minnesota Press.

Seddoh, S. A. K., Robin, D. M., Sim, H-S., Hageman, C., Moon, J. B., & Folkins, J. W. (1996). Speech timing in apraxia of speech versus conduction aphasia. *Journal of Speech and Hearing Research, 39,* 590–603.

Serrano, S., Domingo, J., Rodriguez-Garcia, E., Castro, M. D., & del Ser, T. (2007). Frequency of cognitive impairment without dementia in patients with stroke: A two-year follow-up study. *Stroke, 38,* 105–110.

Servan, J., Verstichel, P., Catala, M., Yakovleff, A., & Rancurel, G. (1995). Aphasia and infarction of the posterior cerebral artery territory. *Journal of Neurology, 242*, 87–92.

Shafi, N., & Carozza, L. (2012, July 31). *Treating cancer-related aphasia.* http://www.asha.org/Publications/leader/2012/120731/Treating-Cancer-Related-Aphasia.htm

Shriberg, L. D., Kwiatkowski, J., & Rasmussen, C. (1990). *The Prosody-Voice Screening Profile.* Tucson, AZ: Communication Skill Builders.

Silveri, M. C., Leggio, M. G., & Molinari, M. (1994). The cerebellum contributes to linguistic production: A case of agrammatic speech following a right cerebellar lesion. *Brain, 121*, 2175–2187.

Simmons-Macke, N., (2009).Thinking beyond language: Intervention for severe aphasia. *Perspectives on Neurophysiology and Neurogenic Speech and Language Disorders, 19*, 15–22. doi:10.1044/nnsld19.1.15

Simmons-Mackie, N., & Damico, J. S. (2009). Engagement in group therapy for aphasia. *Seminars in Speech and Language, 30*, 18–26.

Stoodley, C. J., & Schmahmann, J. D. (2009). The cerebellum and language: Evidence from patients with cerebellar degeneration. *Brain and Language, 110*, 149–153.

Swanson, H. L. (1996). *Swanson Cognitive Processing Test* (SCPT). Austin, TX: Pro-Ed.

Swinburn, K., Porter, G., & Howard, D. (2004). *Comprehensive Aphasia Test* (CAT). New York, NY: Psychology Press.

Swindell, C. S., & Hammons, J. (1991). Poststroke depression: Neurologic, physiologic, diagnostic, and treatment implications. *Journal of Speech and Hearing Research, 34*, 325–333.

Tanner, D., & Culbertson, W. (1999). *Quick Assessment for Aphasia.* Oceanside, CA: Academic Communication Associates.

Taylor-Goh, S. (Ed.). (2005). *Royal College of Speech and Language Therapists Clinical Guidelines: 5.12 Aphasia.* Bicester, UK: Speechmark.

Teuber, H-L. (1975). Effects of focal brain injury on human behavior. In D. B. Tower (Ed.), *The nervous system Vol. 2: The clinical neurosciences* (pp. 457–480). New York, NY: Raven.

Thompson, C. K. (2000). Neuroplasticity: Evidence from aphasia. *Journal of Communication Disorders, 33*, 357–366.

Thompson, C. K. (2004). Neuroimaging: Applications for studying aphasia. In L. L. LaPointe (Ed.), *Aphasia and related disorders* (pp. 19–38). New York, NY, NY: Thieme.

Thompson, C. K., & McReynolds, L. V. (1986). *Wh*-interrogative productive in agrammatic aphasia: An experimental analysis of auditory-visual stimulation and direct-production treatment. *Journal of Speech and Hearing Research, 29*, 193–206.

Tippett, D. C. (2012).Current concepts in treatment planning: patient centered and evidence-based practice in speech-language pathology. *Perspectives on Gerontology, 17*, 27–33. doi:10.1044/gero17.1.27

Tompkins, C. A. (1995). *Right hemisphere communication disorders: Theory and management.* San Diego, CA: Singular.

Tompkins, C. A. (2008). Theoretical considerations for understanding "understanding" by adults with right hemisphere brain damage. *Perspectives on neurophysiology and Neurogenic Speech and Language Disorders, 18*, 45–54.

Tompkins, C. A., Baumgaertner, A., Lehman, M. T., & Fassbinder, W. (2000). Mechanisms of discourse comprehension impairment after right hemisphere brain damage: Suppression in lexical ambiguity resolution. *Journal of Speech, Language, and Hearing Research, 43*, 62–78.

Tompkins, C. A., Boada, R., & McGarry, K. (1992). The access and processing of familiar idioms by brain-damaged and normally aging adults. *Journal of Speech and Hearing Research, 35*, 626–637.

Tompkins, C. A., Boada, R., McGarry, K., Jones, J., Rahn, A. E., & Rainer, S. (1993). Connected speech characteristics of right-hemisphere-damaged adults: A re-examination. *Clinical Aphasiology, 21*, 113–122.

Tompkins, C., Klepousniotou, E., & Scott, G. (2013). Treatment of right hemisphere disorders. In I. Papathanasiou, P. Coppens, & C. Potagas (Eds.), *Aphasia and related neurogenic communication disorders* (pp. 345–364). Sudbury, MA: Jones & Bartlett.

Torvik, A. (1984). The pathogenesis of watershed infarcts in the brain. *Stroke, 15*, 221–223.

Tzeng, B. C., Chen, C. Y., Lee, C. C., Chen, F. H., Chou, T. Y., & Zimmerman, R. A. (1997). Rapid spongiform degeneration of the cerebrum and cerebellum in Creutzfeldt–Jakob encephalitis: Serial MR findings. *American Journal of Neuroradiology, 18*, 583–586.

van Swieten, J. C., Koudstaal, P. J., Visser, M. C., Schouten, H. J. A., & van Gijn, J. (1988).

Interobserver agreement for the assessment of handicap in stroke patients. *Stroke, 19,* 604–607.

Varley, R. (1995). Lexical-semantic deficits following right-hemisphere damage: Evidence from verbal fluency tasks. *European Journal of Disordered Communication, 30,* 362–371.

Verduzco, L. A., & Nathan, D. G. (2009). Sickle cell disease and stroke. *Blood, 114,* 5117–5125.

Vignolo, L. A. (1988). The anatomical and pathological basis of aphasia. In F. C. Ross, R. Whurr, & M. A. Wyke (Eds.), *Aphasia* (pp. 227–249). London, UK: Whurr.

Vindiola, M., & Rapp, B. (2005). The neural consequences of behavioral intervention in dysgraphia. *Brain and Language, 95,* 237–238.

Vukovic, M., Vuksanovic, J., & Vukovic, I. (2008). Comparison of the recovery patterns of language and cognitive functions in patients with post-traumatic language processing deficits and in patients with aphasia following a stroke. *Journal of Communication Disorders, 41,* 531–552.

Wahrborg, P. (1991). *Assessment and management of emotional and psychosocial reactions to brain damage and aphasia.* San Diego, CA: Singular.

Walker, G. M., & Schwartz, M.F. (2012). Short-Form Philadelphia Naming Test: Rationale and empirical evaluation. *American Journal of Speech-Language Pathology, 21,* S140–S153.

Walker-Batson, D., Wendt, J. S., Devous, M. D., Barton, M. M., & Frederick, J. (1988). A long-term follow-up case study of crossed aphasia assessed by single-photon emission tomography (SPECT), language, and neuropsychological testing. *Brain and Language, 33,* 311–322.

Weiller, C., Isensee, C., Rijntjes, M., Huber, W., Muller, S., Bier, D., . . . Diener, H. C. (1995). Recovery from Wernicke's aphasia: A positron emission tomographic study. *Annals of Neurology, 37,* 723–732.

Wells, E. M., Walsh, K. S., Khademian, Z. P., Keating, R. F., & Packer, R. S. (2008). The cerebellar mutism syndrome and its relation to cerebellar cognitive function and cerebellar cognitive affective behavior. *Developmental Disabilities Research and Review, 14,* 221–228.

West, J. F., Sands, E. S., & Ross-Swain, D. (1998). *Bedside Evaluation Screening Test–Second Edition* (BEST-2). Austin, TX: Pro-Ed.

Whatley, B. R., Li, L., & Chin, L-S. (2008). The ubiquitin-proteasome system in spongiform degenerative disorders. *Biochimica et Biophysica Acta (BBA)—Molecular Basis of Disease, 1782,* 700–712.

Wierenga, C. E., Maher, L. M., Moore, A. B., Swearengin, J., Soltysik, D. A., Peck, K., . . . Crosson, B. (2006). Neural substrates of syntactic mapping treatment: An fMRI study of two cases. *Journal of the International Neuropsychological Society, 12,* 132–146.

World Health Organization. (n.d.). *Stroke, Cerebrovascular Accident.* Retrieved from http://www.who.int/topics/cerebrovascular_accident/en/

World Health Organization. (2001). *International Classification of Functioning.* Geneva, Switzerland: Author.

Worrall, L., Papathanasiou, H., & Sherratt, S, (2013). Therapy approaches to aphasia. In I. Papathanasiou, P. Coppen, & C. Potagas (Eds.), *Aphasia and related neurogenic communication disorders* (pp. 93–112). Burlington, MA: Jones & Bartlett Learning.

Worrall, G. B., Simmons-Mackie, N., & Brown, K. (2012). The first 3-months post-stroke: What facilitates successfully living with aphasia? *International Journal of Speech-Language Pathology, 14,* 390–400. doi:10.3109/17549507.2012.692813

Yesavage, J. A., Brink, T. L., Rose, T. L., Lum, O., Huang, V., Adey, M., & Leirer, V. O. (2008). Development and validation of a geriatric depression screening scale: A preliminary report. *Journal of Psychiatric Research, 17,* 37–49.

Glossary

Abstract langusage. Words or expressions that take on meaning other than the literal translation—for example, "a rolling stone gathers no moss."

Abulia. A disorder of lack of will or initiative.

Acalculia. The inability to perform simple arithmetic functions because of brain damage.

Acetylcholine (Ach). Neurotransmitter in the peripheral and central nervous system. Ach is a neurotransmitter at the neuromuscular junction and in autonomic ganglia.

Acetylcholinesterase (ACHE). An enzyme that hydrolyzes or breaks up the neurotransmitter acetylcholine at neuromuscular junctions and brain cholinergic synapses, and thus terminates signal transmission.

Acquired immune deficiency syndrome (AIDS). The final stage of HIV disease, which causes severe damage to the immune system.

Activities of daily living (ADLs). Mobility and self-care functions such as dressing, bathing, feeding, toileting, grooming, and transfers, such as chair to bed and in and out of bath, that a person must be to perform to be independent.

Acute stage of recovery. The initial stage of recovery following an illness or head injury when the symptoms are most severe prior to recovery. Usually the first 4 days following the injury.

Adrenergic. Activated by or capable of releasing epinephrine or an epinephrine-like substance, especially in the sympathetic nervous system.

Agnosia. Loss of the ability, due to brain damage, to recognize and differentiate sensory the sensory stimuli, although the sensory mechanisms are intact.

Agraphia. Loss of the ability to use the written symbols of language because of brain damage.

Alar lamina. The alar plate (or alar lamina) is a neural structure in the embryonic nervous system, part of the dorsal side of neural tube, that involves the communication of general somatic and general visceral sensory impulses.

Alcohol abuse. Intake of large quantities of alcohol to the extent that reversible or irreversible neurotoxic and nutritional deficiencies result.

Alexia. Loss of the ability to comprehend written language because of brain damage.

Alpha-synuclein. A synuclein protein of unknown function primarily found in neural tissue, making up as much as 1% of all proteins in the cytosol. It is predominantly expressed in the neocortex, hippocampus, substantia nigra, thalamus, and cerebellum. Alpha-synuclein aggregates to form insoluble fibrils in pathological conditions characterized by Lewy bodies, such as Parkinson's disease, dementia with Lewy bodies and multiple system atrophy such as Alzheimer's disease.

Alzheimer's disease (AD). A degenerative neurological disorder characterized by progressive deterioration of memory, cognition, personality, and language because of changes in neurochemistry and abnormal histopathological findings, such as neuritic plaques, neurofibrillary tangles, and granulovascuolar degeneration.

Amnesia. Inability to make enduring new memories due to lesions in the lateral thalamus, medial temporal lobe, lateral thalamus, or the basal nucleus of Meynert. Also, a condition characterized by the loss of memories, such as of facts, information, and experiences. Two types associated with head injury are anterograde and retrograde amnesias.

Anemia. A condition resulting from an insufficient number of healthy red blood cells to carry adequate oxygen to body tissues.

Aneurysm. A sac formed by the widening of the wall of an artery.

Anomia. A language impairment characterized by word-finding difficulties due to brain damage. May occur with or without aphasia.

Anomic aphasia. This term is applied to persons who are left with a persistent inability to supply the words for the very things they want to talk about—particularly the significant nouns and verbs. As a result their speech, while fluent in grammatical form and output is full of vague circumlocutions and expressions of frustration. They understand speech well, and in most cases, read adequately. Difficulty finding words is as evident in writing as in speech (National Aphasia Association).

Anosmia. Loss of smell.

Anosodiaphoria. A somatosensory agnosia or a sign of neglect syndrome an acknowledgment of the problem, but lack of concern (i.e., patient seems indifferent to the existence of their handicap), specifically with regard to indifference to paralysis.

Anosognosia. Denial of illness, e.g., hemiparesis. Unawareness of an important loss of body function.

Anoxia. Absence of oxygen supply to tissue despite an adequate perfusion of blood in the tissue.

Anterograde amnesia (AGA). A type of posttraumatic amnesia characterized by difficulty creating new memories following the head injury.

Aphasia. Loss of language and communication function due to central nervous system damage.

APOE gene (Apolipoprotein E). The *APOE* gene provides instructions for making a protein called apolipoprotein E. This protein combines with fats (lipids) in the body to form molecules called lipoproteins. Lipoproteins are responsible for packaging cholesterol and other fats and carrying them through the bloodstream.

Apraxia of speech. Loss of the ability to execute motor sequences because of loss of motor planning. Apraxia is not due to paralysis or paresis but occurs from lesions in the left parietal and frontal lobes.

Aprosodia. Inability to produce the melodic contour, pausal phenomena, and stress of spoken language. Also, the inability to display affect.

Arcuate fasciculus. The bundle of axons connecting Wernicke's area to Broca's area.

Arterial hypotension. Low arterial blood pressure.

Arterial hypoxemia. Reduction of oxygen to the most severely injured parts of the brain.

Arteriosclerosis. A group of diseases characterized by thickening and loss of elasticity of arterial walls.

Astereognosis. The inability to identify objects if placed in the affected hand.

Atresia. Closure of a normal body opening as in an artery due to vascular pathology such as thrombosis or embolism.

Auditory agnosia. A relatively rare condition that typically occurs in conjunction with other auditory processing disorders, is due to difficulty distinguishing environmental and nonverbal auditory cues including difficulty distinguishing speech from nonspeech sounds even though hearing is usually normal.

Augmentative and alternative communication (AAC). Augmentative and alternative communication, also known as AAC, is a term that is used to describe various methods of communication that can help people who are unable to use verbal speech to communicate. AAC can benefit a wide range of individuals, from a beginning communicator to a more sophisticated communicator who generates his own messages (http://www .prentrom.com/what-is-augmentative-and-alternative-communication).

Autosomal. Refers to any of the 22 paired chromosomes in humans.

Axon. Single process that extends from the cell body of the neuron and conducts impulses away from the cell body.

Axonal shearing. Refers to the stretching and tearing of axon fibers during an acceleration-deceleration head injury.

Basal ganglia. Masses of gray matter situated in the cerebral hemisphere and upper brainstem. Usually included are the caudate nucleus, putamen, and globus pallidus. The substantia nigra is often included as part of the basal ganglia.

Basal lamina. One of the pair of longitudinal zones of the embryonic neural tube, from which develop the ventral gray columns of the spinal cord and the motor centers of the brain.

Basal nucleus of Meynert. Also referred to as the nucleus basalis of Meynert, abbreviated NBM and also known as the nucleus basalis, is a group of neurons in the substantia innominata of the basal forebrain that has wide projections to the neocortex and is rich in acetylcholine and choline acetyltransferase. In Parkinson's and Alzheimer's diseases the nucleus undergoes degeneration. A decrease in acetylcholine production is seen in Alzheimer's disease, Lewy body dementia, and some Parkinson's disease patients showing abnormal brain function, leading to a general decrease of mental capacity and learning.

Binswanger's disease. A rare form of infarction that affects the white matter more than the gray and occurs predominantly in the temporal and occipital lobes. Believed to be due to arteriosclerosis of the penetrating arteries in these areas and to result in dementia with a typically rapid progression.

Blast injury. A complex type of physical trauma resulting from direct or indirect exposure to an explosion. Blast injuries occur with the detonation of high-order explosives as well as the deflagration of low order explosives.

Blood–brain barrier. Formed by tight junctions of the endothelial cells of the capillaries in the brain, which protect the central nervous system from undesirable substances and gross variations in the bodily environment.

Blood pressure. Pressure of the blood on the walls of the arteries that is dependent on the action of the heart, the elasticity of the walls of the arteries, and the volume and viscosity of the arterial walls. Systolic blood pressure, also called maximum blood pressure, occurs near the end of the stroke output of the left ventricle of the heart. Diastolic pressure, also called minimum pressure, occurs during the first and second heart sound, or diastole, during which the heart ventricle dilates. Normal blood pressure is 120 mm Hg systolic and 80 mm Hg diastolic.

Bradykinesia. Abnormal slowness of movement, sluggishness, or physical and mental responses.

Brain abscess. A collection of pus, immune cells, and other material in the brain.

Brain herniation. A condition in which parts of the brain are squeezed and exit past structures in the skull while still functioning adequately.

Brain reserve. The brain's resilience, its ability to cope with increasing damage.

Broca's aphasia. Named for neurologist Paul Broca, who, in 1864, described a syndrome of impaired expressive language after damage to the third frontal convolution (area 44). A nonfluent aphasia characterized by diminished speech, phonemic paraphasias, agrammatism, and omission of function words, with relative sparing of comprehension.

Brodmann areas. Brodmann areas were originally defined and numbered by the German anatomist Korbinian Brodmann based on the cytoarchitectural organization of neurons he observed in the cerebral cortex using the Nissl stain. Brodmann published his maps of cortical areas in humans, monkeys, and other species in 1909. A Brodmann area is a region of the human cerebral cortex defined based on its cytoarchitectonics, or the structure and organization of cells.

CADASIL (cerebral autosomal dominant arteriopathy with subcortical infarcts and leukoencephalopathy). An inherited form of cerebrovascular disease that occurs when the thickening of blood vessel walls blocks the flow of blood to the brain. The disease primarily affects small blood vessels in the white matter of the brain. A mutation in the Notch3 gene alters the muscular walls in these small arteries. CADASIL is characterized by migraine headaches and multiple strokes progressing to dementia. Other symptoms include cognitive deterioration, seizures, vision problems, and psychiatric problems such as severe depression and changes in behavior and personality. Individuals may also be at higher risk of heart attack.

Carotid bruit. Abnormal sound or murmur in the carotid artery.

cART. Combination antiretroviral therapy, or combinations of three or more antiretroviral drugs to suppress production of HIV replications.

Catastrophic reaction. Overwhelming feelings of sadness and anxiety in a person who has suffered brain damage.

Caudal. A synonym for the term "posterior."

Caudate nucleus. An elongated gray mass that lies adjacent to the inferior border of the anterior horn of the lateral ventricle.

Cavernous malformation. A vascular disease of the brain characterized by headaches, seizures, and cerebral hemorrhage.

Central nervous system (CNS). The CNS is composed of the brain and spinal cord and serves as the main processing and control center for the entire nervous system.

Cerebellum. Also called the little brain, the cerebellum is a structure that is located at the back of the brain, underlying the occipital and temporal lobes of the cerebral cortex.

Cerebral achromatopsia. Also known as color blindness, resulting in difficulty with recognition and categorization of colors. The individual typically sees only black, white, and shades of gray.

Cerebral atrophy. Shrinkage of brain tissue. This condition may occur with a condition known as ventricular enlargement, which is an enlargement of the ventricular system. Also, decrease in the size of neurons and neural tissue.

Cerebral edema. Diffuse posttraumatic brain swelling.

Cerebral laceration. A cut or tear in the brain tissue observed following a skull fracture, bullet, or stab wound to the head in penetrating brain injury.

Cerebrovascular accident (CVA) or stroke. An interruption or severe reduction of blood flow to the brain depriving brain tissue of oxygen, which can lead to necrosis or death of brain cells.

Cerebrum. The superiormost region of the vertebrate central nervous system and the largest and best-developed of the five major divisions of the brain. The cerebrum is the newest structure in the phylogenetic sense, with mammals having the largest and best-developed among all species.

Cholinergic. Nerve fibers that release acetylcholine at a synapse.

Choroid plexus. The choroid plexus (CP) consists of many capillaries, separated from the ventricles by choroid epithelial cells. Fluid filters through these cells from blood to become cerebrospinal fluid. Choroid plexi are present in all components of the ventricular system except for the cerebral aqueduct, frontal horn of the lateral ventricle, and occipital horn of the lateral ventricle.

Chronic traumatic encephalopathy. A form of encephalopathy that is a progressive degenerative disease, which can be definitively diagnosed only postmortem in individuals with a history of multiple concussions and other forms of head injury. CTE has been most commonly found in professional athletes participating in American football, ice hockey, professional wrestling, and other contact sports who have experienced repetitive brain trauma. It has also been found in soldiers exposed to a blast or a concussive injury, in both cases resulting in characteristic degeneration of brain tissue and the accumulation of tau protein. Individuals with CTE may show symptoms of dementia, such as memory loss, aggression, confusion, and depression, which generally appear years or many decades after the trauma.

CLAS Standards. A set of guidelines that are a comprehensive series that inform, guide, and facilitate practices related to culturally and linguistically appropriate health services. The Standards establish a blueprint for individuals as well as health and health care organizations.

Closed or nonpenetrating head injury. An injury to the head in which the integrity of the cranium is not compromised and no bone fragments or other objects penetrate the skull and dura mater. Thus even in the case of a skull fracture, the underlying dura mater and brain remain intact.

Cocaine. A mood-altering drug derived from the coca plant. May be snorted in powder form or injected. Crack cocaine is a cheaper, more accessible derivative of cocaine and is sold in rock form.

Cognition. A group of mental processes that include attention, memory, reasoning, and problem solving.

Cognitive-communication disorder. A broad term that describes a wide range of communication problems that can result from damage to regions of the brain that control thinking or cognition. This dam-age can impair the ability to transform thoughts into meaningful speech, writing, or gestures.

Cognitive impairment. A disorder affecting cognition.

Cognitive reserve. The mind's resistance to damage of the brain.

Coherence. In discourse, the logical ordering of parts.

Coma. Depression of the functions of the central nervous system.

Communication. Linguistic or nonlinguistic sharing of information by means of a symbol system.

Computerized tomography (CT). A radiographic imaging technique using a beam, which is absorbed by tissue and reconstructed to produce an image.

Concussion. A minor or mild traumatic brain injury (mTBI) that is a short loss of consciousness due to temporary loss of brain function in response to a head injury. It is the least severe and the most common type of TBI associated with a closed head injury and is classified as mTBI. Concussion results from diffuse versus focal brain injury. It is considered to be a milder form of diffuse axonal injury because the stretching of axons is less extensive. A concussion causes a variety of physical, cognitive, and emotional symptoms, which may go undetected if subtle.

Conduction aphasia. Aphasia syndrome in which patients use wrong words but are generally able to convey their thoughts and ideas well. Repetition of spoken language is poor but there is some retention of auditory comprehension.

Confabulation. Recitation of imaginary experiences to fill gaps in the memory.

Contrecoup injury. Damage resulting to an area of the brain opposite the site of the initial impact during a head injury.

Contusion. A bruise caused when blood vessels are damaged or broken due to a blow to the head.

Corpus callosum. A wide, flat bundle of neural fibers beneath the cortex at the longitudinal fissure. It connects the left and right cerebral hemispheres and facilitates interhemispheric communication. It is the largest white matter structure in the brain, consisting of 200 to 250 million contralateral axonal projections.

Corpus striatum. Includes the caudate nucleus, the putamen, and the globus pallidus.

Cortex. Also called neocortex. Superficial coat of gray matter in the cerebral hemispheres and cerebellum.

Cortical blindness. Inability to perceive visual stimuli, despite the intact vision.

Cortical deafness. Inability to perceive any auditory stimuli, despite the presence of normal hearing.

Coup injury. Damage to the brain at the exact point of impact during a head injury.

Crossed aphasia. Aphasia in a right-handed person due to a solely right cerebral lesion. Occurs in 1% to 2% of all aphasias, and characterized by confusion, memory and attention defects, and personality change (in addition to the usual language deficits). Agrammatism is common, but comprehension and naming tend to be preserved.

Cruetzfeldt–Jakob disease. A rapidly progressive disease of neuronal degeneration with viral etiology. Characterized by cortical atrophy of the frontal lobes and profound loss of neurons in the cerebral cortex, basal ganglia, thalamus, brain, and, often, the spinal cord.

Cryotococcal. Yeastlike organisms of the family Cryptococaceae.

Cultural competence. The ability to interact effectively with people of different cultures and socioeconomic backgrounds, particularly in the context of organizations whose employees work with persons from different cultural/ethnic backgrounds. Cultural competence comprises four components: (a) awareness of one's own cultural worldview, (b) attitudes toward cultural differences, (c) knowledge of different cultural practices and worldviews, and (d) cross-cultural skills. Developing cultural competence results in an ability to understand, communicate with, and effectively interact with people across cultures.

Culture. Shared meaning, including beliefs, values, and symbols, which give meaning to behavior.

Cytomegalovirus. One of a group of highly host-specific herpes viruses that infect humans, monkeys, and rodents and produces large cells with intranuclear inclusions. The virus specific to humans causes cytomegalic inclusion disease.

Deductive reasoning. A subcategory of reasoning that involves forming a specific conclusion based on general premises or the ability to go from the more general to the more specific. Also known as the "top-down" approach to reasoning, because it involves starting with a very broad statement of information then narrowing it down to a specific conclusion.

Delirium. A short-term syndrome of altered state of consciousness, cognitive change, language and memory disorders, and delusions.

Dementia. An organic syndrome characterized by decline memory and other intellectual functions in comparison with the individual's previous level of functioning.

Dementia with Lewy bodies. Progressive cognitive decline, combined with three additional defining features: (1) pronounced "fluctuations" in alertness and attention, such as frequent drowsiness, lethargy, lengthy periods of time spent staring into space, or disorganized speech, (2) recurrent visual hallucinations, and (3) Parkinsonian motor symptoms, such as rigidity and the loss of spontaneous movement. The symptoms of DLB are caused by the buildup of Lewy bodies—accumulated bits of alpha-synuclein protein—inside the nuclei of neurons in areas of the brain that control particular aspects of memory and motor control.

Dendrites. Extensions from the cell body of the neuron, which receive information from axons of neighboring cells through neurotransmitter activity at synapses.

Depression. A psychiatric syndrome characterized by dejected mood, psychomotor retardation, insomnia, and weight loss, sometimes associated with guilt feelings and somatic preoccupations, often of delusional proportions. May also be a decrease in functional activity associated with an adverse reaction to a life event.

Diabetes mellitus. A metabolic disorder in which faulty pancreatic activity impairs the ability to oxidize carbohydrates.

Diachisis. A sudden loss of function in a portion of the brain connected to a distant, but damaged, brain area. The site of the originally damaged area and of the diaschisis are connected to each other by neurons. The loss of the damaged structure disrupts the function of the remaining intact systems and causes a physiological imbalance. The injury is produced by an acute focal disturbance in an area of the brain.

Diencephalon. Formed from three swellings in the lateral wall of the third ventricle and includes the third ventricle, the thalamus, the epithalamus, and the hypothalamus.

Diffuse axonal injury (DAI). Injury caused by shearing of the axons during cranial rotation from rapid acceleration and deceleration of the brain during blunt impact head injury.

Dopamine. A neurotransmitter of the central nervous system located in the basal ganglia. Formed in the body by the decarboxylation removal of carbon dioxide of the amino acid dopa and is involved in controlling movement and posture.

Drug abuse. Overuse of any of the following: prescription drugs, nicotine, alcohol, cocaine, marijuana, heroin, and other consciousness-altering substances.

Drug toxicity. Adverse reaction to a pharmacological agent.

Dysarthria. A group of speech disorders resulting from disturbances in muscular control of the speech mechanisms caused by damage to the central or peripheral nervous system or both.

Dysphagia. Difficulty in swallowing due to dysfunction of the lips, mouth, tongue, palate, pharynx, larynx, or proximal esophagus.

Dysrhythmia. An irregularity in a rhythm, especially of heartbeats or brain waves.

Edema. Swelling of a tissue. Abnormally large amounts of fluid in the intracellular tissue spaces of the body.

Elder abuse. Doing something or failing to do something that results in harm to an elderly person or puts a helpless older person at risk of harm.

Emotional lability. See *Pseudobulbar affect*.

Encephalitis. An inflammation of cerebral tissue.

Epidemiology. A branch of medical science that deals with the incidence, distribution, and control of disease in a population.

Epstein–Barr virus. Epstein–Barr virus, frequently referred to as EBV, is a member of the herpesvirus family and one of the most common human viruses. Symptoms of infectious mononucleosis are fever, sore throat, and swollen lymph glands. Sometimes a swollen spleen or liver involvement may develop. Heart problems or involvement of the central nervous system occurs only rarely, and infectious mononucleosis is almost never fatal.

Ethics. Moral principles that govern a person's or group's behavior.

Ethnic group. A socially defined category based on common cultural heritage, shared ancestry, history, homeland, language or dialect, and possibly other aspects such as religion, mythology and ritual, cuisine, dressing style, and physical appearance.

Executive functions. Higher level cognitions such as the ability to self-regulate, metacognitive skills, comprehension of abstract ideas, and other higher level language functions.

Fictive kin. Nonblood-related persons whose relationship is as close as that of a relative.

Fluent aphasia. Impaired language with a near normal amount of speech output, but where the speech is jargon although speech is effortless, with impaired comprehension.

Frontal lobe. An area in the brain of mammals, located at the front of each cerebral hemisphere and positioned anterior to (in front of) the parietal lobe and superior and anterior to the temporal lobes. The frontal lobes are of paramount significance in determining daily capabilities, motor planning, personality manifestations, social interactions, judgments, and decisions.

Frontotemporal dementia (FTD). Describes a clinical syndrome associated with shrinking of the frontal and temporal anterior lobes of the brain. The current designation of the syndrome groups together Pick's disease, primary progressive aphasia, and semantic dementia as FTD. The symptoms of FTD fall into two clinical patterns that involve either: (1) changes in behavior or (2) problems with language. A third clinical pattern involves FTD movement disorders that affect certain involuntary, automatic muscle functions. These disorders also may impair language and behavior.

Functional assessment. A measure of a person's ability to function independently in the environment despite limitations of disease, disability, or social deprivation.

Functional MRI (fMRI). Functional magnetic resonance imaging or functional MRI (fMRI) is an MRI procedure that measures brain activity by detecting associated changes in blood flow. This technique relies on the fact that cerebral blood flow and neuronal activation are coupled. When an area of the brain is in use, blood flow to that region increases.

Gamma aminobutyric acid (GABA). The major inhibitory neurotransmitter in the brain. GABA is very widely distributed in the neurons of the cortex and contributes to motor control, vision, and many other cortical functions.

Genu. In Latin, "knee," referring to structures like the genu of the corpus callosum or the internal capsule.

Glaucoma. A group of ocular diseases that result in optic nerve damage and may cause a loss of vision. A common cause is intraocular pressure, an abnormally high pressure inside the eye.

Gliding contusion. A bruise on the surface of the cortex.

Global aphasia. Severe inability to produce, process, and understand language because of extensive damage to the left cerebral hemisphere, including the frontal and temporal lobes or the temporal lobe and the deep basal gray and subcortical white matter. The parietal lobe is often involved.

Globus pallidus. The smaller and more medial part of the lentiform nucleus of the brain, separated from the putamen by the lateral medullary lamina and subdivided by the medial medullary lamina into internal and external parts.

Glutamate. Glutamate is generally acknowledged to be the most important transmitter for normal brain function. Nearly all excitatory neurons in the central nervous system are glutamatergic, and it is estimated that over half of all brain synapses release this agent. Glutamate plays an especially important role in clinical neurology because elevated concentrations of extracellular glutamate, released as a result of neural injury, are toxic to neurons. Glutamate is a nonessential amino acid that does not cross the blood–brain barrier and must be synthesized in neurons from local precursors. The most prevalent glutamate precursor in synaptic terminals is glutamine. Glutamine is released by glial cells and, once within presynaptic terminals, is metabolized to glutamate by the mitochondrial enzyme glutaminase.

Granulovacuolar degeneration. Accumulation of fluid-filled vacuoles (small cavities) and granular debris with a cell.

Health disparities. Health disparities refer to differences between groups of people. These differences can affect how frequently a disease affects a group, how many people get sick, or how often the disease causes death. Many different populations are affected by disparities. These include racial and ethnic minorities, residents of rural areas, women, children, the elderly, and persons with disabilities.

Hematoma. A localized semisolid collection of blood outside a blood vessel. When associated with a TBI it may be found within or surrounding the brain. There are three types: epidural, subdural, and intracerebral.

Hemiachromatopsia. A loss of color perception.

Hemianopsia. Impaired vision or blindness in half of the visual field from brain damage.

Hemiparesis. Weakness on one side of the body due to brain damage.

Hemiplegia. Paralysis on one side of the body due to brain damage.

Hemispatial neglect. Inability to recognize, respond, or orient to meaningful or novel stimuli presented on the side of the body opposite to the lesion site due to faulty integration of both sensory and motor inattention.

Hemorrhage. Bleeding resulting from a tear or cut of a blood vessel, as seen in primary damage associated with head trauma.

Heroin. A highly addictive drug derived from morphine, which is obtained from the opium poppy. It is a "downer" or depressant that affects the brain's pleasure systems and interferes with the brain's ability to perceive pain (drugfree .org).

Highly active antiretroviral therapy (HAART). Antiretroviral therapy (ART) is treatment of people infected with human immunodeficiency virus (HIV) using anti-HIV drugs. The standard treatment consists of a combination of at least three drugs (often called highly active antiretroviral therapy, or HAART) that suppress HIV replication. Three drugs are used in order to reduce the likelihood of the virus developing resistance. ART has the potential both to reduce mortality and morbidity rates among HIV-infected people and to improve their quality of life.

Hippocampus. Located in the temporal lobe and considered to be a component of the limbic system that is involved in learning and auditory memory.

Human immunodeficiency virus (HIV). A virus or germ that enters the body and attacks and kills certain cells within the body, especially those that protect the body from disease. HIV infection is a condition caused by HIV. The condition gradually destroys the immune system, which makes it harder for the body to fight infections.

Huntington's disease. A rare, autosomal dominant disease that causes progressive deterioration of the brain, usually beginning with cell loss in the caudate nucleus and putamen of the basal ganglia.

Hypercapnia. Excessive carbon dioxide levels in the blood.

Hypertension. Also termed high blood pressure. A chronic medical condition in which the blood pressure in the arteries is elevated, requiring the heart to work harder than normal to circulate blood through the blood vessels. See also *Blood pressure.*

Hyponatremia. A condition resulting from sodium depletion in the body.

Hypothalamus. A portion of the diencephalon that forms the floor and a portion of the wall of the third ventricle. Involved in the activation and integration of peripheral autonomic function, endocrine regulation, and many somatic functions.

Incontinence. The inability to control bladder and/or bowel functions.

Increased intracranial pressure (ICP). Increased pressure within the skull due to the buildup of fluids from edema, hematomas, and contusions, which in severe cases may lead to brain herniation.

Inductive reasoning (or bottom-up approach). A subcategory of reasoning that involves forming a generalized conclusion from particular facts or going from the specific to more general.

Infarction. Death of tissue due to insufficient vascular circulation.

Internal capsule. Broad band of white tissue separating the lenticular nucleus from the medial caudate nucleus and thalamus.

Ischemia. Reduction in blood supply to a part of the body resulting from partial or total blockage of an artery.

Judgment. The ability to form sound opinions and make sensible decisions or reliable guesses. A higher cognitive function that is often impaired following a head injury or right-hemisphere stroke.

Korsakoff's disease. Also called chronic alcohol delirium. A neurologic syndrome resulting from chronic alcohol abuse that causes disturbances of orientation, affective lability, amnesia, confabulation, and memory loss.

Lacunar state. Syndrome of vascular dementia due to a number of lacunar infarcts.

Lacunes. Small cavities of infarcted tissue commonly observed in individuals with vascular dementia.

Lentiform nucleus. Composed of the putamen and the globus pallidus.

Lesion. A pathological or traumatic discontinuity of tissue or loss of function of a part.

Leukoencephalopathy. Any of a group of diseases affecting the white substance of the brain. The progressive multifocal leukoencephalopathy (PML) is a rare disorder that damages the material (myelin) that covers and protects nerves in the white matter of the brain. Symptoms of PML include aphasia and memory loss.

Levadopa. A precursor of the neurotransmitter dopamine that is used to treat Parkinson's disease.

Lewy bodies. Round bodies found in the vacuoles (small cavities) of cell cytoplasm in some neurons of the midbrain and seen in Parkinson's disease.

Lewy body dementia (LBD). LBD is an umbrella term for two related diagnoses. LBD refers to both Parkinson's disease dementia and dementia with Lewy bodies. See *Dementia with Lewy bodies*.

Limbic system. A collection of brain structures responsible for autonomic functions, olfaction, emotions, and memory. Includes the amygdala, hippocampus, cingulate gyrus, and septal areas.

Locus coeruleus. Also nucleus locus coeruleus (nLC). A ganglion located on the floor of the fourth ventricle of the brain.

Macrophages. Large, mononuclear, phagocytic cells in the wall of blood vessels that have a small, oval, sometimes indented nucleus and inconspicuous nucleoli. Phagocytes ingest either other small organisms or cells and foreign particles.

Magnetic resonance imaging (MRI). A high-resolution imaging technique in which photon behavior in tissue is subjected to a magnetic field that is measured and reconstructed to form an image.

Marijuana. The most often used illegal drug in this country, is a product of the hemp plant, Cannabis sativa. The main active chemical in marijuana, also present in other forms of cannabis, is THC (delta-9-tetrahydrocannabinol). Of the roughly 400 chemicals found in the cannabis plant, THC affects the brain the most (drugfree.org).

Medicaid. A United States federal reimbursement program for health care costs for families and individuals with low income and resources. Medicaid recipients must be U.S. citizens or legal permanent residents and may include low-income adults, their children, and people with certain disabilities.

Medicare. The U.S. government's health insurance program for people age 65 or older. Certain people under age 65 can qualify for Medicare too, including those with disabilities, permanent kidney failure, or amyotrophic lateral sclerosis.

Memory. The ability to encode, store, and recall information. The three main processes involved in human memory are encoding, storage, and recall.

Meninges. The meninges are the system of membranes that envelope the central nervous system. In mammals, the meninges consist of three layers: the dura mater, the arachnoid mater, and the pia mater. The primary function of the meninges and the cerebrospinal fluid is to protect the central nervous system.

Meningitis. An inflammation of the meninges.

Mesencephalon. The midbrain portion of the CNS associated with vision, hearing, motor control, sleep/wake, arousal (alertness), and temperature regulation.

Methamphetamine. An addictive stimulant that strongly activates certain systems in the brain. Also, a crystal-like powdered substance that sometimes comes in large rocklike chunks. It can be injected, smoked, snorted, or taken orally (drugfree.org.).

Metencephalon. Composed of the pons and the cerebellum; contains a portion of the fourth ventricle; and the trigeminal nerve (CN V), abducens nerve (CN VI), facial nerve (CN VII), and a portion of the vestibulocochlear nerve (CN VIII).

Microglia. Small non-neural interstitial cells that form part of the supporting structure of the CNS. These cells act as phagocytes to waste products of nervous tissue.

Mixed transcortical aphasia. Characterized by severe speaking and comprehension impairment, but with preserved repetition. The most frequent etiology of mixed transcortical aphasia is stenosis (narrowing) of the internal carotid artery.

Multiple sclerosis. A disease that involves an immune system attack against the central nervous system (brain, spinal cord, and optic nerves). As part of the immune attack on the central nervous system, myelin (the fatty substance that surrounds and protects the nerve fibers in the CNS) is damaged, as well as the nerve fibers themselves (National Multiple Sclerosis Society).

Myencephalon. Neural tube derivative that becomes the medulla oblongata.

Myocardial infarct (MI) or heart attack. Typically occurs when a blood clot blocks the flow of blood through a coronary artery (a blood vessel that feeds blood to a part of the heart muscle). The interrupted blood flow occurring during a heart attack can damage or destroy a part of the heart muscle.

Necrosis. Death of brain cells due to oxygen deprivation.

Neglect. Refers to a person's lack of awareness of a specific part of the body or external environment.

Neologism. Nonsense word generated by a person with brain damage because of deteriorated semantic and comprehension abilities.

Neural progenitor cells. Embryonic neural cells that differentiate and become neurons.

Neural tube. In an embryo, a hollow structure from which the brain and spinal cord form.

Neuritic plaques. An aggregation of neuronal debris with an amyloid core and an outer ring of granular filamentous material. Neurotic plaques are present to a great extent in the brains of persons with Alzheimer's disease.

Neurofibillary tangles. Twisted intraneuronal fibers of pairs of helically wound filaments with the cytoplasm of the neuronal cell body, which is present in the brain of patients with Alzheimer's disease.

Neurogenic language disorder. Any of the language impairments arising from damage to the CNS.

Neuron. Specialized cell body in the nervous system that receives, conducts, and transmits nervous impulses.

Neuropil. Any area in the nervous system composed of mostly unmyelinated axons, dendrites, and glial cell processes that forms a synaptically dense region containing a relatively low number of cell bodies. The most prevalent anatomical region of neuropil is the brain.

Neurotransmitter. A substance that is released from the axon terminal of an excited presynaptic neuron and travels across the synaptic cleft to either excite or inhibit the target cell. Provides communication between neurons.

Nonpenetrating head injury. See *Closed head injury*.

Norepinephrine. A neurotransmitter that, when activated, exerts effects on large areas of the brain. The effects are alertness and arousal, and it influences on the reward system. Areas of the body that produce or are affected by norepinephrine are described as noradrenergic. Noradrenergic neurons in the brain form a neurotransmitter system.

Notch3 gene. Provides instructions for producing the Notch3 receptor protein. This receptor protein is located on the surface of the muscle cells that surround blood vessels (vascular smooth muscle cells).

Occipital lobe. The visual processing center of the mammalian brain containing most of the anatomical region of the visual cortex.

Open or penetrating head injury. Occurs when the skull is fractured or penetrated, from, for example, a bullet, shrapnel, or other missile injury.

Orientation. The awareness of self in relation to one's surroundings. The subcategories are orientation to person, place, time, and situation.

Orthostatic hypotension or postural hypotension. A form of low blood pressure that occurs when standing from a seated or lying position. Symptoms are dizziness and lightheadedness that may even cause the individual to faint.

Osteoarthritis (OA) or degenerative arthritis. The most common type of arthritis caused by a joint disease resulting in cartilage loss in a joint.

Osteoporosis. A condition associated with a decrease in bone density, decreasing its strength and resulting in fragile bones. Osteoporosis literally leads to abnormally porous bone that is compressible, like a sponge.

Paraphasia. Linguistic errors that are related in meaning or type to the intended word.

Parietal lobe. A part of the brain positioned above (superior to) the occipital lobe and behind (posterior to) the frontal lobe. The parietal lobe integrates sensory information from different modalities, particularly determining spatial sense and navigation.

Parkinson's disease. A neurologic syndrome resulting from disruption of dopaminergic activity in the subcortex.

Patient Protection and Affordable Care Act (PPACA). Also known as the Affordable Care Act (ACA). Signed into law in 2010 by President Obama, the act is aimed at increasing the affordability and rate of health insurance coverage for Americans and reducing the overall costs of health care (for individuals and the government). It provides a number of mechanisms—including mandates, subsidies, and tax credits—to employers and individuals to increase the coverage rate and health insurance affordability.

Perception. The active processing of incoming sensations. It is a very complex process involving numerous aspects of brain functioning.

Perseveration. Inappropriate repetition of a response after the stimulus has faded.

Petechial hemorrhage. A form of mild hemorrhage that causes distinctive markings known as petechiae. These markings take the form of small red to purple spots, which can vary in size and distribution from a few tiny markings to an array that may look like a rash or abrasion. The most common form in the eyes is trauma.

Pick bodies. Also called Pick cells. Found in Pick's disease in the outer three layers of the cortex; characterized by argentophilic (silver and chromium) inclusions.

Pick's disease. A rare type of dementing disease characterized by marked symmetrical atrophy of the frontal and temporal lobes; Pick bodies within the neurons and inflated, swollen neurons.

Polypharmacy. The use of usually four or more medications.

Polytrauma. A medical term describing the condition of a person who has been subjected to multiple traumatic injuries.

Positron emission tomography (PET). An imaging technique using positron-emitting isotopes that are introduced into tissue. The collision of gamma rays resulting from the collision of positrons and electrons are recorded by a computer that produces a tomogram.

Positron emission tomography amyloid imaging. Method of detection of amyloid plaques in persons suspected of having Alzheimer's disease. Developed about 10 years ago, the first successful Aβ plaque-specific positron emission tomography (PET) imaging study was conducted in a living human subject clinically diagnosed with probable AD using the (11)C-labeled radiopharmaceutical Pittsburgh compound B (PiB).

Postural hypotension. See *Orthostatic hypotension.*

Posttraumatic amnesia (PTA). A state of confusion or memory loss that occurs immediately following the injury. Individuals with PTA are unable to remember events that occur after the injury. Some patients may also experience problems retaining information from one day to the next.

Posttraumatic ventricular enlargement. An enlargement of the ventricles that occurs when cerebrospinal fluid (CSF) accumulates in the brain, resulting in

dilation of the cerebral ventricles and an increase in intracranial pressure (ICP).

Pragmatics. Use of language to establish a relationship with the context of the communicative event. The context includes the identities of the participants in verbal exchanges and their beliefs, knowledge, and intentions, as well as the temporal and spatial dimensions of the communicative event.

Praxis. The doing or performance of action.

Precursor. A substance from which another, more mature or active substance is formed.

Presenile dementia. A form of dementia, of unknown cause, starting before a person is old.

Primary brain damage. Known also as primary insult or mechanical damage, primary brain damage occurs at the moment of impact and can range from large to microscopic brain lesions. Primary damage includes contusion, skull fracture, damage to blood vessels, and axonal shearing.

Primary progressive aphasia (PPA). Slowly developing aphasia with relative sparing of activities of daily living, judgment, insight, and social behavior. Cognitive problems may not appear for years after this aphasia is observed.

Prion disease. Prion diseases, or transmissible spongiform encephalopathies (TSEs), are a family of rare progressive neurodegenerative disorders that affect both humans and animals. They are distinguished by long incubation periods, characteristic spongiform changes associated with neuronal loss, and a failure to induce inflammatory response (Centers for Disease Control and Prevention).

Progressive supranuclear palsy (PSP). A neurologic syndrome of unknown etiology characterized by ventricular enlargement, loss of pigment in the substantia nigra, and marked changes in subcortical structures, as well as chronic progressive dementia and disturbances of vertical eye movements.

Prosopagnosia. An impairment in the ability to recognize familiar faces.

Proxemics. Interrelated observations and theories of man's use of space.

Pseudobulbar affect (PBA). A neurologic disorder characterized by involuntary crying or uncontrollable episodes of crying and/or laughing, or other emotional displays.

Pure aphasia. Loss of language ability in a specific modality, like reading.

Putamen. Larger and more lateral part of the lentiform nucleus, separated from the global pallidus by the lateral medullary lamina, or sheet of tissue.

Rarefaction. Diminution in density and weight, but not in volume.

Reasoning. Considered to be a higher level cognitive function often affected following a head injury and right-hemisphere damage. Two subcategories are deductive and inductive reasoning.

Regional blood flow (rBF). Measurement of the metabolic factors that control blood flow.

Reticular formation. A specialized group of nerve fibers and cells in the medulla and pons that extend upward through the midbrain and thalamus. Considered responsible for arousal from sleep, wakefulness, alerting or focusing attention, and perceptual association.

Retrograde amnesia (RGA). A form of posttraumatic amnesia in which individuals experience loss of memories that were formed shortly before the injury, particularly where there is damage to the frontal or anterior temporal regions.

Rhomencephalon. Also called the hindbrain. Includes the medulla, pons, and cerebellum.

Right-hemisphere disorders. An acquired disorder of linguistic, nonlinguistic, and extralinguistic processes resulting from damage to the right hemisphere.

Rostral. Situated or occurring near the front end of the body, especially in the region of the nose and mouth.

Secondary brain damage. Also known as secondary insult or delayed nonmechanical damage and represents a series of pathological processes initiated at the moment of injury as a direct consequence of the primary damage with subsequent clinical features. Some examples include infection, increased intracranial pressure, and hematoma.

Seizure. Occurs when the electrical system of the brain malfunctions. Instead of discharging electrical energy in a controlled manner, the brain cells keep firing. The result may be a surge of energy through the brain, causing unconsciousness and contractions of the muscles (Epilepsy Foundation).

Sensorineural hearing loss. A type of hearing loss in which the root cause lies in the vestibulocochlear nerve (cranial nerve VIII), the inner ear, or central processing centers of the brain. Sensorineural hearing loss can be mild, moderate, or severe, including total deafness.

Seropositivity. A positive reaction to a test of blood serum for a disease.

Skull fracture. A break in the skull following a head injury. There are four types: simple, linear, depressed, and compound fractures.

Single photon emission computerized tomography (SPECT). See also positron emission tomography. This measurement uses a single photon for measurement in brain tissue.

Spongiosis. Intercellular edema of the spongy layer of the skin.

Stratum pyramidale. Contains the cell bodies of the pyramidal neurons, which are the principal excitatory neurons of the hippocampus.

Stroke. Also termed cerebrovascular accident. Sudden and severe attack caused by an acute vascular brain lesion, such as hemorrhage, embolism, thrombosis, or a rupturing aneurysm.

Subacute stage of recovery. Stage that occurs between the 4th and the 21st day after an injury.

Subarachnoid hemorrhage. An intracerebral leakage of blood into the subarachnoid space.

Substantia innominata. A stratum in the human brain consisting partly of gray and partly of white substance, which lies below the anterior part of the thalamus and lentiform nucleus.

Substantia nigra. Considered one of the basal ganglia. This is a midbrain structure that has a dorsal zone of melanin-containing cells and a ventral zone that lacks melanin (dark pigment). Neurons in the substantia nigra produce dopamine.

Superior longitudinal fasciculus. A pair of long bidirectional bundles of neurons connecting the front and the back of the cerebrum.

Support network. Friends, family, coworkers, and others who provide care during a person's lifetime, but particularly when illness strikes.

Sylvian fissure. A deep fold in the cerebral cortex that runs anterior to posterior and divides the temporal and frontal lobes of the brain.

Synapse. A structure that permits a neuron to pass an electrical or chemical signal to another cell.

Synaptic transmission. The passage of a neural impulse across a synapse from one nerve fiber to another by means of a neurotransmitter.

Syncope. Loss of consciousness resulting from insufficient bloodflow to the brain.

Tactile agnosia. Inability to recognize or identify objects by touch, although normal cutaneous and proprioceptive hand sensation exists.

Talk and die or deteriorate (TADD). Called the second impact syndrome. Patient begins as mildly involved and lucid, then proceeds to coma and death or to survival with severe head injuries and disabilities within a relatively short period of time.

Tau proteins. Proteins that stabilize microtubules. Microtubules hold the cell shape and structure. Tau proteins are abundant in neurons of the central nervous system. When tau proteins are defective and no longer stabilize microtubules properly, they can result in dementias such as Alzheimer's disease.

Tegmentum. A general area within the brainstem located between the ventricular system and distinctive basal or ventral structures at each level. It forms the floor of the midbrain, whereas the tectum forms the ceiling.

Telencephalon. Largest division of the developing brain. Constitutes the anterior portion of the forebrain, including the cerebral hemispheres and related parts.

Temporal lobe. A region of the cerebral cortex that is located beneath the lateral fissure on both cerebral hemispheres of the mammalian brain. The temporal lobes are involved in the retention of auditory, rather than visual memories, processing sensory input, comprehending language, storing new memories, emotion, and deriving meaning.

Terminal bouton. A button-like swelling on an axon where it has a synapse with another neuron.

Thalamus. The middle and larger portion of the diencephalon that forms part of the lateral wall of the third ventricle and lies between the hypothalamus and the epithalamus. Considered important for relaying incoming sensory stimuli, with the exception of olfaction (smell), to the cortex.

Transcortical motor aphasia. An aphasia syndrome of nonfluent speech with markedly decreased word production. Speech repetition and comprehension are preserved despite the low speech output.

Transcortical sensory aphasia. Syndrome of fluent aphasia with preserved repetition of spoken language and poor comprehension.

Transcranial Doppler (TCD) ultrasonography. Noninvasive method of detecting the velocity of blood flow through the artery, using special Doppler probes placed at the front, sides, and base of the skull.

Transient ischemic attack (TIA). A transient episode of neurologic dysfunction caused by ischemia (loss of blood flow). The symptoms of a TIA are short-lived and usually last a few seconds to a few minutes and most symptoms disappear within 60 minutes. The most common cause is an embolus that blocks an artery to the brain.

Transmissible spongiform encephalopathy (TSE). See *Prion disease*.

Traumatic brain injury (TBI). A nondegenerative, noncongenital insult to the brain that can lead to permanent or temporary impairment of cognitive, physical, and psychosocial functions. The TBI may result in diminished or altered brain functioning due to an external mechanical force that may disrupt the individual's normal state of consciousness.

Treatment efficacy. Improvements in communication behavior that have resulted from the interventions of the speech-language pathologist.

Uncinate fasciculus. The uncinate fasciculus is a white matter tract in the human brain that connects parts of the limbic system such as the hippocampus and amygdala in the temporal lobe with frontal ones such as the orbitofrontal cortex. Its function is unknown, although it is affected in several psychiatric conditions. It is the last white matter tract to mature in the human brain.

Universal Precautions. Self-washing and other prophylactic procedures to protect health workers from infectious diseases while treating patients.

Vacuole. A small cavity in the cytoplasm of a cell, bound by a single membrane and containing water, food, or metabolic waste.

Vascular dementia (VaD). A decline in thinking skills caused by conditions that block or reduce blood flow to the brain, depriving brain cells of vital oxygen and nutrients (Alzheimer's Association).

Vigilance. An individual's ability to maintain attention in the presence of incoming stimuli that serve as distractors. Vigilance is one of the most complicated attention skills.

Visual agnosia. An impairment in the ability to recognize visual stimuli despite the absence of a visual deficit (i.e., acuity, visual field, and scanning).

Watershed stroke. An ischemia, or blood flow blockage, that is localized to the border zones between the territories of two major arteries in the brain.

Wernicke's aphasia. Described by Carl Wernicke in 1874 and named for him. This is a fluent aphasia characterized by poor auditory and reading comprehension, poor repetition ability, fluent speech with semantic and phonemic paraphasias, and, often, neologistic jargon.

Index

Note: Page numbers in **bold** reference non-text material.